How did doctors make a living? *Making a medical living* explores the neglected socio-economic history of medical practice, beginning with the first voluntary hospital in 1720 and ending with national health insurance in 1911. It looks at private practice and how this was supplemented by public appointments. In this innovative study, Anne Digby makes use of new archival sources of information to produce a compelling picture of ordinary rather than élite doctors, and of the dynamics of provincial rather than metropolitan practice.

From the middle of the eighteenth century doctors travelled to see ordinary patients, developed specialisms and expanded institutions. Despite limitations in treatment, doctors raised demand for their services, as illuminating case studies of women, children, the poor and the affluent show. But doctors did not limit their own numbers, and were largely unsuccessful in restricting competition from other practitioners, with the significant exception of women. Consequently, many GPs struggled to make a living by seeing numerous patients at low fees.

Doctors' entrepreneurial activity thus helped shape English medicine into a distinctive pattern of general and specialist practice, and of public and private health care.

Making a medical living

Cambridge Studies in Population, Economy and
Society in Past Time 24

Series Editors

PETER LASLETT, ROGER SCHOFIELD and E. A. WRIGLEY
ESRC Cambridge Group for the History of Population and Social Structure

and DANIEL SCOTT SMITH
University of Illinois at Chicago

Recent work in social, economic and demographic history has revealed much that was previously obscure about societal stability and change in the past. It has also suggested that crossing the conventional boundaries between these branches of history can be very rewarding.

This series exemplifies the value of interdisciplinary work of this kind, and includes books on topics such as family, kinship and neighbourhood; welfare provision and social control; work and leisure; migration; urban growth; and legal structures and procedures, as well as more familiar matters. It demonstrates that, for example, anthropology and economics have become as close intellectual neighbours to history as have political philosophy or biography.

For a full list of titles in the series, please see end of book

Making a medical living

Doctors and patients in the English market
for medicine, 1720–1911

ANNE DIGBY

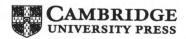

CAMBRIDGE
UNIVERSITY PRESS

PUBLISHED BY THE PRESS SYNDICATE OF THE UNIVERSITY OF CAMBRIDGE
The Pitt Building, Trumpington Street, Cambridge, United Kingdom

CAMBRIDGE UNIVERSITY PRESS
The Edinburgh Building, Cambridge CB2 2RU, UK
40 West 20th Street, New York NY 10011–4211, USA
477 Williamstown Road, Port Melbourne, VIC 3207, Australia
Ruiz de Alarcón 13, 28014 Madrid, Spain
Dock House, The Waterfront, Cape Town 8001, South Africa

http://www.cambridge.org

© Cambridge University Press 1994

First published 1994
First paperback edition 2002

A catalogue record for this book is available from the British Library

Library of Congress Cataloguing in Publication data
Digby, Anne.
Making a medical living: doctors and patients in the
English market for medicine, 1720–1911 / Anne Digby.
p.   cm. – (Cambridge studies in population, economy,
and society in past time: 24)
Includes index.
ISBN 0 521 34526 X (hardback)
1. Medicine – Great Britain – History.
I. Title.   II. Series.
R486.D54   1994
362.1′0941–dc20   93-34762   CIP

ISBN 0 521 34526 X hardback
ISBN 0 521 52451 2 paperback

For Charles

Contents

Illustrations

Maps

Tables

Acknowledgements

This book has taken a considerable time to research and write, and my sincere thanks go to a large number of people and institutions that have assisted its progress.

I am grateful to the Wellcome Trust and to Oxford Brookes University for generous financial assistance, and to the latter institution for a term's study leave. Efficient administrative support was provided for the research project first at the Institute for Research in the Social Sciences at the University of York, and then at the Institute of Economics and Statistics at the University of Oxford. Facilities generously placed at my disposal at Harvard and Stanford Universities facilitated my researches at an early stage during 1986–7, as did those later provided for me at the Australian National University during the summer of 1989, and more recently during 1992 at the University of Cape Town. I am most grateful to colleagues at each of these institutions for intellectual stimulation and friendly criticism.

Fundamental to the progress of my researches has been the assistance given by archivists and librarians at the Public Record Office, Scottish Record Office, British Library, Wellcome Institute for the History of Medicine, Royal College of Physicians (London), the Royal College of Surgeons (London), Royal Society of Medicine, the Royal College of Physicians (Edinburgh) and Friends Library (London). I should also like to recognise my intellectual debt to archivists at the county record offices of Buckinghamshire, Devon, Dorset, Durham, East Suffolk, Gloucestershire, Leicestershire, Lincolnshire, Norfolk, Somerset, South Yorkshire, Wiltshire and West Yorkshire; as well as to those at city, borough and hospital archives at Chester, Leeds, Manchester, Sheffield and York. Finally, I am appreciative of the access and support given to me at university, college, and medical libraries in Birmingham, Cambridge, Canberra, Cape Town, Harvard, Leeds,

xvi   *Acknowledgements*

Oxford, Stamford and York, as well as in public libraries in Bath, Birmingham, Bristol, Carlisle, Leeds and Manchester.

Helpful points were made following a number of conference and seminar presentations at Canberra, Cambridge (Mass.), Colchester, Durham, Exeter, Glasgow, London, Oxford and York. A number of people have assisted me with constructive comments, expertise and references including: Michael Bevan, Roy Campbell, Marguerite Dupree, David Fitzpatrick, Jim Gillespie, Alan Heeson, Jacqueline Jenkinson, Mark Lester, Colin Pedley, John Porter, Eric Richards, Nigel Sims, Roger Schofield, Paul Weindling, and Brenda White. Irvine Loudon and Barry Smith have each generously supplied me with much relevant information. Jessica Feinstein has kindly contributed her reader's expertise in improving the presentation of my draft and in compiling the index. I owe a particular debt of gratitude to Margaret Pelling who commented perceptively on the whole of the text, and to Derek Robinson for his helpful observations on part of Chapter 9. My thanks are also due to my editors, who have been very civilised whilst waiting an inordinate time for the text to be completed.

Practising authorship can seem at times almost as difficult as practising medicine and, in acknowledgement of invaluable intellectual stimulation, support and companionship, *Making a Medical Living* is dedicated to Charles Feinstein.

Copyright is acknowledged, and permission to reproduce the following, is gratefully acknowledged: the Wellcome Institute (Illustrations 1 to 9, 12 to 15); the Rev. D. V. Whale and the Norfolk Record Office (Illustration 10); Somerset County Council (Illustration 11); the Tate Gallery (Illustration 16). I am grateful to Sir John Clerk of Penicuick for permission to cite from the Penicuick papers held in the Scottish Record Office, and to Dr Jean Hugh-Jones for permission to reproduce the material in Table 3.1.

Abbreviations

BMJ	*British Medical Journal*
BHM	*Bulletin of the History of Medicine*
BMA	British Medical Association
JHM	*Journal of the History of Medicine*
MH	*Medical History*
PP	Parliamentary Papers
PRO	Public Record Office
RC	Royal Commission
RCPE	Royal College of Physicians, Edinburgh
RCPL	Royal College of Physicians, London
RCSL	Royal College of Surgeons, London
RO	Record Office
SC	Select Committee
SHM	*Social History of Medicine*
Wellcome	Wellcome Institute, London

Glossary

Alterative – a medicine changing the process of digestion

Analeptic – a restorative or strengthening medicine

Antimonial – a medicine containing antimony usually used as an emetic

Bolus – a large pill

Caries – bone or teeth decay

Chyle – a form of lymph occurring in the lacteals from the small intestine, and serving as the chief medium for the transfer of ingested fats to the blood

Consumption – an earlier term for TB

Electuary – a medicine in the form of a powder mixed with honey, jam or syrup

Elixir – a strong extract or tincture

Emetic – a medicine that causes vomiting

Empiric – one whose practice is based on experience rather than principle or scientific knowledge

Erysipelas – a highly infectious disease characterised by skin inflammation, often affecting the face

Febrifuge – an anti-febrile or cooling medicine

Fistula – a suppurating canal in the body

Gynaecology – a specialism concerned with the functions and diseases of women

Homeopathy – a practice founded by Hahnemann in which diseases are treated by very small doses which in the healthy would produce similar effects to the disease being treated.

Hydropathy – treatment by the external and internal applications of water

Hydrocele – a tumour with a collection of serous fluid

Julep – a liquid medicine sweetened with honey, syrup or sugar

King's Evil – scrofula (see below)

Laryngology – a specialism concerned with diseases of the larynx

Lithotomy – cutting for the stone: an operation that removed a stone or calculus that had formed in the bladder by making an incision in the lower abdominal wall

Lues – a generic term for a spreading disease of which syphilis was one manifestation

Medical galvanism – the therapeutic use of electricity

Nosology – the classification of diseases

Nostrum – a medicine prepared by the person recommending it – as in patent medicine

Ophthalmology – a specialism concerned with the structure and affections of the eye

Placebo – a medicine given to please rather than benefit the patient

Prognosis – art of forecasting the probable course of diseases

Scrofula – a condition which involved diseased neck glands and might lead to susceptibility to TB

Scald heads – narrowly defined as ringworm but more often applied to a range of infestations, usually in children

Stone – the formation of a calculus or concretion in the bladder

Strumous – affected with a scrofulous tumour or swelling

Sudorific – a medicine that promotes perspiration

Therapeutics – branch of medicine concerned with healing diseases

Introduction

The economic history of medicine is a strangely neglected field; relatively little is known as yet about the finances of institutions or the business side of medical practice. One reason for this may have been the emphasis given by an older tradition of medical historiography to the history of great men, clinical advances, and notable institutions. More recently, the expansion of the social history of medicine has directed attention to a much wider spectrum of concerns. Amongst these has been a desire to research more fully into the patient and the patient's experiences. Whether it is possible for the historian to gain direct knowledge of the patient independently of medicalisation is controversial.[1] One problem with this particular form of 'history from below', however, has been the difficulty of giving a coherent account that was more than a fascinating anthology of personal accounts of illness; a 'presentation and evaluation of ... attitudes and experiences.'[2] This volume is an attempt to advance the discussion by giving a more central place to the financial dimension of the patient's relationship with the practitioner, and thereby also to contribute to the economic history of medicine by looking at the doctor's income.

Doctors' incomes have a major influence on central issues in the social history of medicine. On the supply side, income affects the type of individual recruited to the medical profession; the status of the doctor in society; and the development of professional standards and professional attitudes. Remuneration has implications for the quality of medical care – most obviously in the time that the practitioner can afford to give to patients. On the demand side, the fees charged

---

[1] R. Porter, ed., *Patients and Practitioners. Lay Perceptions of Medicine in Pre-industrial Society* (Cambridge, 1985), p. 2.

[2] D. and R. Porter, *Patients Progress. Doctors and Doctoring in Eighteenth-Century England* (1989), prefatory explanation of rationale of volume.

1

clearly influence the numbers and types of patients who seek treatment. Ability to pay a qualified doctor affects the levels of health in society, and perceptions of what constitutes health. The fee levels also have an important bearing on the provision of related forms of medical care – as for example through private or public health insurance. Looking at the social history of medicine in the eighteenth and nineteenth centuries from a broad perspective, one of the major changes was the increasingly important role that professionals assumed in complementing lay care of the sick within the household. This change involved an extension of the market, so that ability to pay for the doctor became an important factor in standards of health care.[3] Patients' incomes were not the sole determinant of access to medical care, since normative considerations remained important, but capacity to meet the doctor's bill was a factor of growing significance. Ability to gauge the market in terms of demand for medical services at different fee levels was thus a crucial feature in successful medical practice. Whilst studies of professionalisation have drawn attention to ability to control the market,[4] there have been few studies of how this was attempted by members of the medical profession.[5] Two fine studies that give insight into this area from this point of view are those of Irvine Loudon and M. J. Peterson,[6] and this volume aims to complement them.

The concept of a market is sometimes used to refer to a particular institution (for example, Smithfield), or to a very specific exchange with a well-defined product and participant (for example, the housing market). It is used in this study in a less sharply defined sense to cover a looser relationship. On the one side are the suppliers of medical services – represented by a range of practitioners from the physician through the GP to the fringe practitioner. Their attempts to sell their own version of medical treatment, and thus to establish a practice by making a reputation which would attract and keep patients, are central to the analysis. The methods they used with different types of patients, and their concerns over fees and income from this medical custom are discussed. On the other side of the medical market were the patients, rich and poor, young and old, male and female; as

[3] P. Starr, 'Medicine, Economy and Society in Nineteenth Century America', *Journal of Social History*, 10 (1977).
[4] M. S. Larson, *The Rise of Professionalism. A Sociological Analysis* (Berkeley, 1977), p. xvi.
[5] For an interesting recent investigation see P. Weindling, 'Medical Practice in Imperial Berlin: the Casebook of Alfred Grotjahn', *BHM* , 61 (1987).
[6] I. S. L. Loudon, *Medical Care and the General Practitioner, 1750–1850* (1986); M. J. Peterson, *The Medical Profession in Mid-Victorian London* (1978).

consumers they had limited knowledge of what they were buying but needed to trust their practitioner. What they were purchasing, and what they thought they were buying, are also important in this investigation.

The time-span of *Making a Medical Living* is distinctive in looking at the longer-term dynamics of economic change for the practitioner and patient. This volume begins in the early eighteenth century, with the inception of the first voluntary hospital in 1720. The growth of these institutions gave social status to practitioners who held office in them, and an indirect means to expand private practice from the prominence that this élite position gave them. It also gave them direct access to clinical material. During the Georgian, Victorian and Edwardian eras discussed here, there was a significant increase in the number of offices – voluntary, charitable and public – and these, although frequently badly paid, formed an important element in attempts to construct medical practices that were financially viable. The end date of the volume is that of the National Insurance Act of 1911, which altered practice for many, by adding a large and publicly funded component to income from private practice. In looking at the financial relationships between practitioners and their patients, central attention is given to the GP (who treated most patients), but other types of doctor – notably the physician – are also discussed. In addition, an attempt has been made to direct attention much more onto the ordinary provincial practitioner rather than on the better-known London élite. In researching the book, much attention was given to archives in county record offices in order to try to recapture the realities of provincial practice, and thus to provide a more representative view.

The contemporary sources used in *Making a Medical Living* have been wide-ranging. The initial decision to attempt to provide greater insight into provincial practice resulted in many searches at county and borough record offices and local libraries, as well as at metropolitan libraries and archives. Whilst initial responses to enquiries indicated that relatively few repositories considered that they had much medical material, searches proved that the range and diversity of available material was very considerable. The time it has taken to research and write this book reflects their magnitude. Central to my understanding of medical relationships have been the diaries, letters, journals, autobiographical recollections, and accounts of patients, as well as those of practitioners. Institutional records in the form of hospital or dispensary casebooks, ledgers, reports, minutes, statutes and rule-books have been equally fundamental. To further illuminate practice with poor patients, poor-law overseers' accounts, contracts and bills, together with later medical officers' registers, have been consulted. For private practice, ledgers, casebooks, and correspondence kept by the individual practitioner have been eagerly perused. Supplementing these have been editorials, reports, letters and advertisements in contemporary medical journals, notably the *British Medical Journal* (*BMJ*) and the *Lancet*, together with material (especially fee schedules) published by professional medical organisations. Data in medical directories and medical registers, together with the enumerations in the *Census*, have been serviceable, as have the reports of some parliamentary inquiries. Finally, prescriptive material has given some helpful insights; notably, the records of formal homilies and lectures addressed to medical students; professional manuals addressed to entrants to the profession; and health manuals directed to sufferers.

There have been methodological problems both in addressing and selecting from these sources. Only a small proportion of practitioner–patient encounters is likely to have been recorded and, of these, only an uncertain amount have survived. A substantial number of these records have been consulted, and an illustrative selection of the records themselves are discussed. But the extent to which these are representative of past relationships remains a very difficult issue. Interpreting these sources is thus problematical, since there is no single answer to the question of how much this past experience was homogeneous or heterogeneous. In some respects the historical practice is likely to have been reasonably uniform and even a small sample would provide a reliable indication, whereas for other topics there was probably considerable variety and it would be unwise to generalise on the basis of small, and possibly unrepresentative samples. Inferences as to what is typical or unusual are – at this stage of scholarship in the social history of medicine – a matter of judgement, informed by a partial insight which, as further detailed biographical or local studies are made, is likely to be modified. In part this is a familiar chicken and egg historiographical dilemma of whether it is best to direct research to general contextual studies or detailed individual subjects. Since each informs, and is mutually dependent on the other, there is no obvious intellectual priority to be given to one or the other approach.

The economic perspective of *Making a Medical Living* was an intrinsically interesting and significant one to investigate. However, a central focus on financial aspects of doctor–patient encounters – where objective quantitative material is plentiful – also facilitated generalisation. In discussing both quantitative and qualitative data a range of confidence in its credibility is involved: at one extreme an upper limit involves hard information on incomes and fees which is unlikely to be disputed, whilst at the other end of the spectrum, a lower limit is concerned with subjects such as inferences on motivation, where subjective judgements may be more controversial. Predictably, there was no uniformity in the richness of sources of information; this has influenced the treatment of class, gender and age in Part III. It was found that the propertied groups were well-served by correspondence with physicians; the poor and children by institutional records, and women by abundant and varied sources. The chronological coverage is variable since sources for the later period are generally better; this is especially true for quantitative data. However for some subjects, notably the correspondence between affluent patients and physicians, this situation is reversed.

The two centuries that have been investigated have not only an economic, but also a therapeutic, coherence in that this was a period of what has been termed 'traditional medicine.'[7] Despite Foucauldian interpretation of this period as including the birth of modern medicine with the inception of the clinic, and the 'medical gaze' on 'what for centuries had remained below the threshold of the visible',[8] this volume emphasises that the forces for continuity in general (as distinct from surgical), practice were still resilient. So too was the continued importance of domiciliary as against institutional care of the sick. The overlap between older and newer practices and beliefs was thus considerable; the interplay between traditional and scientific, or between popular and élite conceptions of health and sickness was significant.[9] This suggests that Illich's allegations of the 'disabling impact of professional control over medicine',[10] need to be applied circumspectly, if at all, to the period in this book. Practitioners' potential influence was limited both by many sufferers' inability to pay for their services, even if they were desired, and by cultural assumptions which made other responses to illness more appropriate.[11]

---

[7] E. Shorter, *Bedside Medicine* (New York, 1985), p. 26. Shorter uses the term for the period up to 1850, but for reasons advanced in Chapter 3 I have extended this to 1911.

[8] M. Foucault, *The Birth of the Clinic. An Archaeology of Medical Perception* (New York, 1973), pp. ix–xii.

[9] M. Macdonald, 'Anthropological Perspectives in the History of Science and Medicine', in P. Corsi and P. Weindling, eds., *Information Sources in the History of Science and Medicine* (1983).

[10] I. Illich, *Limits to Medicine* (1977), p. 11.

[11] See, for example, M. Fissell, *Patients, Power, and the Poor in Eighteenth-Century Bristol* (Cambridge, 1991), Chapter 2.

In this volume, the longer-term perspective adopted makes it possible to suggest some of the shortcomings of the conventional, and somewhat simplistic, view of the changes to the modern from the traditional,[12] not just in clinical practice but in professionalisation as well.[13] A closer look at the importance of the financial relationship between practitioner and patient soon suggests some of the deficiencies of seeing the process of medical professionalisation as a simple power relationship in which doctors increasingly dominated their clients. Instead, a complicated picture emerges in which there is a more even balance between the financial standing of the patient and the clinical expertise of the doctor. To see this as an uncomplicated act of patronage would be misleading, however, since an economic transaction between doctor and patient was infused with cultural assumptions and expectations. These attitudes were themselves highly differentiated, as chapters on selected groups of patients indicate. Medicine, even for the regular members of the medical profession or Faculty, was an occupation which still retained strong elements of trade. To counteract this, both medical education and medical etiquette emphasised the importance of social aspects of practice, with appropriate demeanour, appearance and behaviour befitting not just professional but, crucially, genteel status.

In his famous preface to *The Doctor's Dilemma*, George Bernard Shaw wrote a savage indictment of the predominantly private medicine that is the subject of *Making A Medical Living*. 'Nothing is more dangerous than a poor doctor ... Of all the anti-social vested interests the worst is the vested interest in ill-health.'[14] Does the historical record indicate that doctors were in reality poor and their conduct anti-social? Part II of this volume (Chapters 4–6), on the finances of medical practice, indicate that there was very considerable variation in medical income. When Shaw was writing, in the early twentieth century, the struggle to make a living from medicine was certainly becoming much more difficult. The financial imperative was therefore even stronger than had usually been the case earlier. During the two centuries discussed in this volume, doctors' struggles to first create and then maintain an economically viable practice – either through fees from private practice or through remuneration from public or charitable appointments

---

[12] For example, 'the professions as we know them are very much a Victorian creation' in W. J. Reader, *Professional Men. The Rise of the Professional Classes in Nineteenth Century England* (1966), p. 2.

[13] L. J. Jordanova, 'The Social Sciences and the History of Science and Medicine', in Corsi and Weindling, eds., *Information Sources*, pp. 90–2.

[14] G. B. Shaw, *Prefaces*, (1934), p. 280.

– were unremitting. Success in the form of wealth went to a very small minority of doctors. Rather more made a comfortable income, many scraped by on an income that scarcely bought gentility, and a surprising number failed to make a living at all. That there were so many less-than-affluent doctors exposes the hidden contradiction in the quotation from Shaw, since if they had been sufficiently mercenary, more should have been able to make a decent living. However, this also assumes that there were sufficient affluent patients for the number of practitioners, and that these were distributed equitably between them – assumptions that were belied by historical reality.

Part I of the book (Chapters 1–3) provides the context for understanding the practitioners' predicaments. These chapters attempt to synthesise a large amount of primary and secondary sources in order to provide the essential historical building blocks on which the more original interpretation can be erected elsewhere in the book. It is suggested that the presence of fringe practitioners (variously termed irregulars, empirics or quacks), continued to give strong competition to the regular practitioner, not least because of the considerable overlap in the kind of therapeutic help they offered to sufferers. However, the availability of regular practitioners varied, as did that of unorthodox practitioners, so that sufferers' choice of the kind of practitioner they consulted showed marked regional variation. Nineteenth-century legislation failed to give a medical monopoly to regular practitioners despite their attempts at professionalisation which were driven by a desire to restrict competition. Competition for patients thus remained severe, and from the mid-eighteenth century doctors showed marked commercial flair and versatility in their attempts to expand the medical market by keeping business records, by actively pursuing patients through increased travel, and by flexibility in the exploitation of changing market opportunities.

The incidence of morbidity (sickness) was only slowly reduced by preventive measures in public health, by improvements in living standards, and by the relatively few scientific advances in the prevention and cure of diseases. In winning the patient's confidence the social attributes and personal manners of the doctor were thus imbued with considerable importance. Increasingly this was reinforced by some enhancement in medical authority which derived substantially from the considerable achievements of surgeons, yet in popular perception was also attributed to the physician and GP. Routes to the achievement of a viable medical practice in a rapidly increasing Victorian population were differentiated into a three-tier medical market. Part III (Chapters 7–9) of *Making a Medical Living* looks at selected groups of patients within this market in analysing the extent to which relationships between practitioner and client were shaped by economic rather than other factors. Chapter 7 discusses the interaction between physicians and affluent Georgian and Victorian patients which, on *a priori* grounds, might be thought to exemplify most clearly a patient-dominated patronage relationship.[15] Instead, it suggests that the physician offset patient power by claims to medical expertise in health as well as sickness. Similarly, Chapter 8 examines a marked growth of remunerated medical practice amongst the poor from the mid-eighteenth century, through voluntary, charitable and publicly-funded initiatives which benefited the surgeon, surgeon-apothecary and the GP. Whilst these offered a variety of financial rewards it is also suggested that there was a substantial amount of professional altruism provided by practitioners to poor patients in the form of free treatment. Chapter 9 analyses practice in two linked areas in which expansion in medical practice was also found during the late eighteenth and nineteenth centurries – that of women and children, and suggests that remunerative practice resulted. This is linked to inter-professional rivalry with midwives, and with hostility to women entering the medical profession, since each would offer strong competition.

In Part IV, a final chapter, 'Reflections', attempts to draw out some more general implications of the nature of the relationship between practitioners and patients within the medical market. It examines the extent to which the patient prospered, in the sense of achieving well-being, and thus an absence of dis-ease. And it underlines the point that it is not just the financial prosperity of doctors that is the focus of attention in this volume, but the extent to which they were respected, and their views accorded authority. In doing so it returns to what was the underlying issue in the best-known discussion of this issue – Shaw's *The Doctor's Dilemma* – in which there is an idealisation of motives and self-justificatory processes by the practitioner.[16] The volume ends by asking whether doctors prospered in this wider meaning of self-worth, of making sense of what s/he did, rather than in the narrower sense of wealth.

[15] N. D. Jewson, 'Medical Knowledge and the Patronage System in 18th Century England', *Sociology*, 8 (1974), pp. 369–85.
[16] M. Holroyd, *Bernard Shaw. Vol. II, 1898–1918. The Pursuit of Power* (1989), p. 159.

PART I

The professional structure of practice

1

Medical practitioners

This chapter begins with a discussion of the number, diversity, distribution and availability of medical practitioners, and goes on to analyse the nature and structure of the occupation and the relevance to it of discussions on professionalisation. It ends with a brief look at the ambivalent status of medicine as an occupation and its connection to economic rewards. Interesting issues are raised about the regionalisation of the market, and of the importance of economic factors – in the conceptualisation of medicine as an occupation or profession – in attempts to control it.

Numbers, composition and distribution

There are a variety of sources from which to compile estimates of regular medical practitioners who practised: numbers of medical students graduating, medical directories, the *Census*, and numbers of qualified doctors under the provisions of the Medical Act of 1858 who were on the *Medical Register*.[1] These give approximate figures but also pose problems; numbers of graduating students will include some who did not subsequently make a successful career in medical practice; medical directories may also include the recently deceased; whilst medical directories and *Census* figures do not always distinguish clearly between those active in the profession and those who are retired.[2]

[1] The basis of these three sources was different in that an enumerator provided the wording of the occupational return in the *Census* on the basis of information supplied by the individual, whilst for the directory, individual practitioners submitted an entry, and in the case of the *Register* the entry followed a voluntary process of legal registration as a member of the profession that resulted from the 1858 act.
[2] See *Lancet*, 26 May 1877, p. 775; also, W. Rivington's comparison of the *Medical Register* and Churchill's *Medical Directory* in 1878 where the latter had 900 more practitioners listed (*The Medical Profession* (Dublin, 1879), p. 1).

Estimating numbers in the profession by calculating numbers of entrants poses problems. Until the mid-eighteenth century the Universities of Oxford and Cambridge were important – if declining sources – of medical graduates; smaller numbers qualified at continental schools, especially Leiden; and a few at Trinity College, Dublin.[3] By the early nineteenth century the rise of medical education in the four Scottish Universities of Aberdeen, Edinburgh, Glasgow, and St Andrews had transformed this situation. Edinburgh, in particular, attracted many English students. Rosner's study of medical education in Edinburgh after 1760 indicates that the distinction between those who followed a formal medical education and those who pursued a practical apprenticeship was breaking down, since substantial numbers of apprentices attended university lectures. The fluidity of the student body was remarkable. A group previously discounted by historians, but at Edinburgh the largest group, were the occasional auditors who attended lectures but left without certification.[4] Similarly, at Glasgow, while the numbers of those graduating by the late 1820s had only reached an average of 30, the numbers enrolling in classes may have been as great as 1000 annually.[5] This indicates the fragmentary process of medical education pursued by many, and therefore underlines the inadequacy of estimating the extent of medical education and numbers of entrants into the profession by looking at graduation figures alone. Another important group were those studying in London hospitals. In 1815 numbers of pupils at the more important hospital schools had reached 350; a large increase from the 100 to 150 in the 1780s and 1790s.[6] By 1850 London medical schools had been established at Guy's, the London, the Middlesex, the Royal Free, St Bartholomew's, St George's, St Thomas', University College and the Westminster Hospitals.[7] Prospective doctors were also trained during the late eighteenth and early

[3] F. N. L. Poynter, ed., *The Evolution of Medical Education in Britain* (1966); C. Webster, 'The Medical Faculty and the Physic Garden' in L. S. Sutherland, *The History of the University of Oxford: the Eighteenth Century* (Oxford, 1986), p. 685; R. B. Mcdowell and D. A. Webb, *Trinity College, Dublin 1592–1952* (Cambridge, 1982), pp. 88, 524. Whilst 40 matriculated each year, only 2 graduated.
[4] L. Rosner, *Medical Education in the Age of Improvement. Edinburgh Students and Apprentices, 1760–1826* (Edinburgh, 1990), pp. 95–7, 104.
[5] D. Dow and M. Moss, 'The Medical Curriculum at Glasgow in the Early Nineteenth Century', *History of Universities* (1988), p. 239.
[6] S. C. Lawrence, 'Science and Medicine at the London Hospitals: The Development of teaching and Research, 1750–1815' (unpublished PhD thesis, University of Toronto, 1985), p. 646.
[7] A. H. T. Robb-Smith, 'Medical Education at Oxford and Cambridge Prior to 1850' in Poynter, *Medical Education*, p. 49.

nineteenth century both by anatomy schools run by notable surgeons,[8] and by dispensaries in London and the provinces.[9] Unfortunately, there are no estimates of the numbers involved. Beginning in
1824 a number of provincial medical schools were set up, and by 1858
there were facilities in Bristol, Birmingham, Exeter, Hull, Leeds,
Liverpool, Manchester, Nottingham, Newcastle, Sheffield and York.[10]
In 1841 London medical schools had 951 medical students, with the
largest school – that at University College Hospital – having nearly 200
students. This contrasted with provincial medical schools where even
the largest – Manchester – had only 50 students at this date.[11]

Statistical information became more plentiful after the Medical Act
of 1858. From Figure 1.1 we can see the numbers of medical students
registered in England, and also in Scotland, Ireland, and in the United
Kingdom as a whole. Whilst the figures for England are the most
directly relevant to our discussion they cannot be taken in isolation
since it is important to recognise that many Scottish and some Irish
trained doctors came to practise in England. (There was also a very
small number trained in Wales.)[12] There was a very considerable
growth in student numbers from the 1860s to the 1890s, and a slow
decline thereafter. The *BMJ* estimated that about 1800 students registered annually at the close of the nineteenth century, and about 1400
in the years before the First World War.[13]

Turning now from potential entrants to practising doctors, an
analysis of the earliest, reasonably reliable medical directory of 1783,
Simmons *Medical Register*, indicated 3166 provincial practitioners, of
whom one in ten were physicians, more than four-fifths were
surgeon-apothecaries, and the rest divided between those returning
themselves solely as surgeons, or solely as apothecaries.[14] In London

[8] Z. Cope, 'The Private Medical Schools of London (1746–1914)', in F. N. L. Poynter, ed., *The Evolution of Medical Education in Britain* (1966).
[9] Z. Cope, 'The Influence of the Free Dispensaries upon Medical Education in Britain', *MH*, xii (1969), pp. 29–36.
[10] S. T. Anning, 'Provincial Medical Schools in the Nineteenth Century' in F. N. L. Poynter, ed., *The Evolution of Medical Education in Britain* (1966), pp. 121–2.
[11] S. T. Anning and W. K. J. Wallis, *A History of Leeds School of Medicine* (Leeds, 1982), p. 34.
[12] Seventeen degrees in medicine and dentistry were gained in Wales in 1919–20 compared with 405 in England, 381 in Scotland and 205 in Ireland (*Returns from Universities in Receipt of Treasury Grant*, PP 1921, Cmd 1263, viii, p. 619).
[13] *BMJ*, 4 September 1937, p. 444.
[14] Simmons acknowledged that some towns had incomplete entries. See also J. Lane, 'The medical practitioners of provincial England in 1783', *MH*, 28 (1984), pp. 354, 356, which analyses Simmons *Medical Register*.

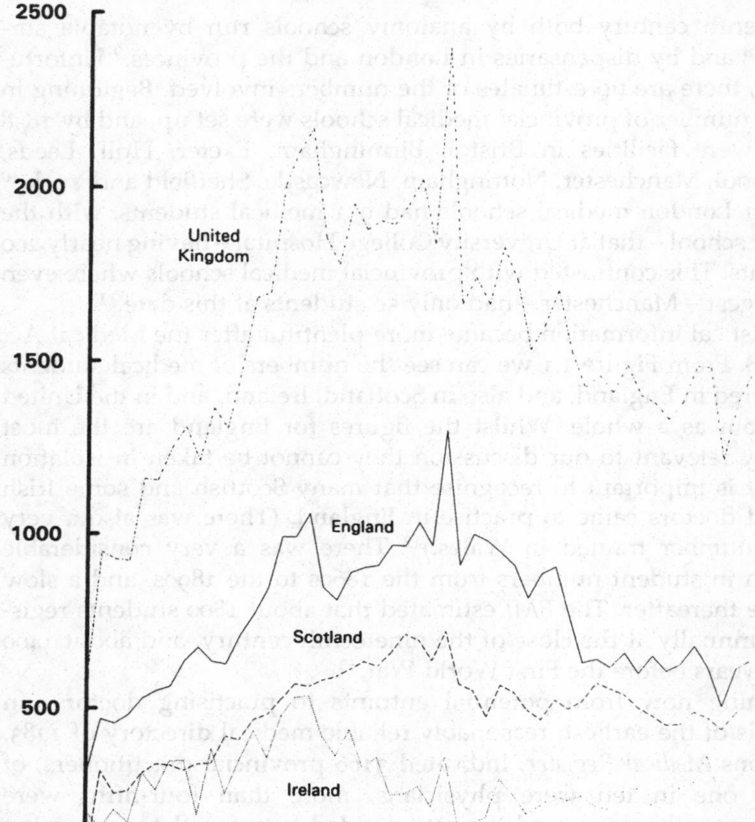

Making a medical living

Figure 1.1   Medical students registered, 1865–1913

there were another 968 physicians, surgeons and apothecaries.[15]
Accurate returns of medical practitioners were enumerated for the
first time in the *Census* for 1841. Comparisons over time are problematic, however, because the *Census* headings for returns varied.[16] Also,

[15] W. F. Bynum, 'Physicians, hospitals and career structures in eighteenth-century
London' in W. F. Bynum and R. Porter, eds., *William Hunter and the Eighteenth-Century
Medical World* (Cambridge, 1985), p. 107.

[16] It was not until 1931 that the retired were excluded from the figures. Medical
assistants and students were listed with other practitioners until 1881. Physicians and
surgeons were listed separately until 1881.

Table 1.1. *Ratios of regular practitioners to population in England and Wales, 1851–1911*

Date	Doctors (i)	Doctors (inc.assistants and students) (ii)	Population (iii)	Population per doctor 1[a] (iv)	Population per doctor 2[a] (v)
1851	17,491	21,146	17,983,000	1028	850
1861	14,415	17,981	20,119,000	1396	1119
1871	14,684	19,198	22,789,000	1552	1187
1881	15,116	20,772	26,046,000	1723	1254
1891	19,037	–	29,086,000	1527	–
1901	22,653	–	32,612,000	1439	–
1911	23,469	–	36,136,000	1539	–

Note: [a]Ratio 1 is of medical practitioners and includes physicians, surgeons and apothecaries only, whilst ratio 2 also includes medical assistants and medical students.
Source: Census

professional regulation in 1858 meant that individuals could no longer style themselves as a surgeon or physician as had been possible earlier, and this was largely responsible for a fall in the *Census* returns between 1851 and 1861.

In the longer term cumulated numbers of registered practitioners continued to grow, as Figure 1.2 indicates. One important reason for this was the growing numbers of graduate entrants in the *Medical Register*.[17] Precise numbers of practising practitioners are probably unattainable but discrepancies between the figures in the *Medical Register* and the *Medical Directory* were not vast.

The *Census* gave information on the age structure of the profession and from this it is apparent that some doctors worked well beyond 65, the modern age of retirement. The concept of retirement (ideally, aided by an occupational pension) was one that had hardly been taken up by 1900.[18] From the age breakdown of the *Census* it appears that between six and ten per cent of medical practitioners were aged 65 or over. Doctors were as actively employed as circumstances allowed but 'death vacancies' in practice advertisements suggested that the average doctor could not afford to retire even when in poor

---

[17] *BMJ*, 4 September 1937, p. 446.
[18] In 1900 only 100,000 million occupational pensions were paid (L. Hannah, *Inventing Retirement. The Development of Occupational Pensions in Britain* (Cambridge, 1986), pp. 45, 51, 115, 125).

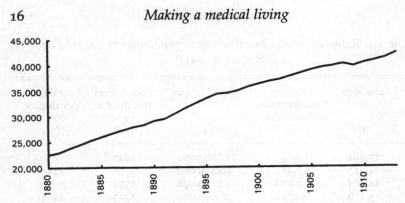

Figure 1.2   U.K. total numbers of practitioners on *Medical Register*, 1880–1913

health. For the affluent minority for whom the issue of when to retire was a matter of professional judgement, important ethical issues were posed. Dr Heberden commented in 1794 that 'When I retired a few years ago from the practice of physic, I trust it was not with a wish to be idle ... but because I was willing to give over before my presence of thought, judgement and recollection were so impaired that I could not do justice to my patients.'[19]

Whilst there was a fair spread in age distribution, the gender composition of medical practitioners was skewed. Before the Georgian period women had practised as apothecaries and surgeons.[20] Georgian gentry households had used women practitioners,[21] and the Blundell household in Lancashire was probably not untypical in its reliance on five of them. The extent to which they were all full-time professionals is doubtful, since one ran a boarding school, and another was described as being a housekeeper. However, two – Mrs Morrice and Mrs Bolton – were termed chirurgeonesses (i.e. surgeonesses), which implied a greater expertise than might be possessed by a skilled domestic healer. Certainly, Bolton appears to have had a local reputation since she was described as treating others in the neighbourhood. More ambiguously, however, early in his acquaintance with Morris, Nicholas Blundell recorded that 'I gave Betty Morrice a good

[19] T. Percival, *Works* (1807), vol. I, p. clxxxiii, letter from Heberden to Dr Percival 28 August 1794. See also *An Autobiogrpahy of the late Sir Benjamin Brodie* (1865) for similar sentiments.

[20] M. Pelling, 'Medical Practice', p. 101; M. Pelling and C. Webster, 'Medical Practitioners' in C. Webster, ed., *Health, Medicine and Mortality in the Sixteenth Century* (Cambridge, 1979), p. 186; A. L. Wiseman, 'The Surgeoness: the Female Practitioners of Surgery, 1400–1800', *MH*, 28 (1984), p. 37.

[21] For example, *Margaret Maria, Lady Verney, Verney Letters of the Eighteenth Century from the MSS at Claydon House* (1930), vol. II, p. 93.

book of physic and chirurgery'. Nevertheless, she earned a professional level of payment; receiving one pound for physic and treatment. Female practitioners repeatedly treated Mrs Blundell, in addition they treated the children for 'mouth canker' or worms, and on a couple of occasions bled, and prescribed for, the male head of the household. The success of their treatment was as variable as that of male doctors but the fact that they were each called in several times suggests their patients' confidence in their ministrations. So too does the fact that they alternated with male practitioners; sometimes a female failure to effect a cure led to a male counterpart being called in, and sometimes these roles were reversed.[22]

Eighteenth-century overseers' accounts for the poor also reveal that women were employed in a variety of ways: dressing wounds; effecting diverse cures; or, more rarely, acting as the parish surgeon. Particularly in remote country areas their use continued into the late eighteenth century, and they were paid to change dressings, treat simple wounds, or cure ringworm and similar infestations. Women were also present in the so-called medical fringe at this time, exemplified by well-known figures such as Mrs Joanna Stephens, with her stone-dissolving medicine, but also involving more obscure practitioners. One such was Mrs Anne Stanley, reputedly the deaf and dumb daughter of a Hampshire doctor, who advertised with an admixture of cautious and bold claims which suggested a shrewd eye for the state of the medical market:

By her close application, constant practice, [and] thro' divine assistance she can cure complaints with speed and safety, if not too far gone viz dropsey, [sic] rheumatism, convulsion, hysteric fits ... She has a speedy and effectual cure for worms in old and young; and has a peculiar method in curing most calamities incident to women and children for which she is famous, with many other distempers too tedious to enumerate here ... She is honest and prosperous, and knows people's diseases at first sight, and takes none in hand, but those she does good to.[23]

The reference to a conditional contract at the end of the advertisement is interesting in indicating a survival in the fringe of what had formerly been a mainstream practice. That this custom was declining in importance suggests a weakening in the bargaining power of the patient in the medical market. Equally, Mrs Stanley's claim to prosperity is significant in asserting the financial success of her practice, and hence – by implication – the popularity of her remedies.

[22] *The Great Diurnall of Nicholas Blundell* (Record Society of Lancashire and Cheshire, 1968), iii, August 1725: ii, 14 March 1714.
[23] Glos. RO, Pc 1159.

Professionalisation marginalised female practitioners and one of the intra-professional disputes was that between females and males in midwifery during the late eighteenth and early to mid-nineteenth centuries. (This is discussed in Chapter 9.) Later attempts by women to achieve formal medical qualifications were bitterly opposed by the male faculty. Two professional handbooks from the 1870s illustrated this well. W. Dale in *The State of the Medical Profession in Great Britain and Ireland* commented that women doctors had 'opened the door to further trouble and given grave offence to the profession',[24] whilst W. Rivington in his analysis of the same issue in *The Medical Profession* thought that it had led 'to the display of an antipathetic feeling unsurpassed by any other professional topic.'[25] However, a rival publication by Keetley, *The Student's Guide to the Medical Profession*, stole a march on its competitors by requesting Dr Elizabeth Garrett Anderson, the first woman to qualify in England, to write a special chapter, 'For Ladies who Propose to Study Medicine.' She stated:

It is necessary, however, to recognise that the standard of professional attainment expected to be reached by women, will for some years be higher than expected by the ordinary male practitioner. Women can less easily afford to be second-rate; their professional work will be more closely scrutinised; mistakes will ruin them more quickly than they will men ... In conclusion, I would beg female students of medicine not to be discouraged either by the magnitude of the work to which they have put their hands, or by the disapproval of many of their friends and acquaintance.[26]

Changing social attitudes to medical women are evident in the *Census* returns. Although the 1851 Census noted that there were 13 females who were termed 'doctors' by local Census enumerators, these were not given the status of regular practitioners. In the next Census women practitioners were listed as: 'chiefly of druggists 388 and midwives 1,913.' The 1881 Census was the first to note female practitioners using the same definition as men, when 25 were returned as physicians, surgeon-apothecaries and GPs. Numbers then increased to 101 in 1891, 232 by 1901 and 477 in 1911.

How adequate were numbers of practitioners for the population? Today, a ratio of one doctor to 950 patients is seen as appropriate for good primary care in Britain.[27] By 1800 London had apparently achieved that provision in the ratio of *regular* practitioners to popu-

---

24 W. Dale, *The State of the Medical Profession in Great Britain and Ireland* (Dublin, 1875), p. v.
25 Rivington, *Medical Profession*, p. 135.
26 C. B. Keetley, *The Student's Guide to the Medical Profession* (1878), pp. 43–4.
27 Ratio quoted in Bynum, 'Physicians, hospitals', p. 106.

lation, and in 1841 the nation as a whole was not far from this.[28] Thereafter, as Table 1.1 indicated, ratios worsened between 1851 and 1881 as population growth outstripped even the increasing numbers in the medical profession. After 1881 the ratio of doctors to population improved since numbers of entrants to medical practice expanded more rapidly. Until 1881 the Census also returned numbers of medical students and medical assistants and doctor-patient ratios for the mid-Victorian period are naturally rather better if they were included (see Table 1.1, cols. (iv) and (v)). Given the use made by practitioners of medical assistants to treat their poorer patients, this second, and slightly better, ratio is more realistic, and may be taken as an upper bound to the ratios.

Evaluating whether past provision was adequate in terms of a modern ratio does, however, raise complex issues. The modern ratio is presumably predicated on assumptions about clinical care in relation to contemporary expectations of health, the financing of health provision, current therapeutics and state-of-the-art medical technology. It is important to appreciate that the issue that exercised many commentators in the past – particularly medical observers – was based less on medical, than on *economic*, criteria. Since medicine was a business as well as a vocation, professional discussion focused on the supply of practitioners in relation to patients' ability to pay for their treatment. Practitioners recognised that they were not able to charge the majority of the population for medical services; the 'poor' obtained their medical assistance from collective forms of medical assistance – whether this was from the poor law, voluntary hospitals or private 'clubs' – as well as from large numbers of alternative practitioners who offered medical care at a cheaper rate.

The greater the numbers of regular medical practitioners in relation to population the louder the anxiety medical commentators expressed about their 'unqualified' rivals and competitors. The *Lancet* fulminated about this allegedly serious situation in 1843, 'That "the profession is overstocked" we daily hear exclaimed, and the assertion is true. The "profession" *is* overstocked, and with a superabundance of unqualified men, mere speculators in drugs and chemicals.'[29] The failure of the Medical Act of 1858 to legislate against 'quackery' disappointed many practitioners, since they suspected that their competition impeded regular doctors in making an adequate living. Others were anxious for more altruistic reasons. William Farr, the Registrar

---

[28] In London in the late sixteenth century the ratio was estimated to be as high as 1:400 (Pelling, 'Medical Practice', p. 100).

[29] *Lancet*, (i) 1842–3, p. 795.

General, commented in 1877 that 'a considerable number of people die without the attendance of qualified medical men ... and hundreds of thousands are treated by quacks, ignorant midwives, unqualified assistants, and chemists and druggists.'[30] Potential patients therefore had a wide range of choice in deciding whom to consult, although only two-fifths of those classified as having a medical occupation in the *Census* of 1861 were registered, qualified practitioners in terms of the Medical Act of 1858.

The availability of doctors varied according to region and locality.[31] In 1783 the provinces had a ratio of one practitioner to 2224 people, whereas the capital had a ratio nearly three times better.[32] This situation continued; in 1841, for example, London had four times as many practitioners, relative to population, as had the worst provided county.[33] Fashionable seaside and watering places were well-endowed with physicians (see Table 6.1). Hospital towns and prosperous market towns were equally well serviced. Less-populated country areas, particularly if geographically remote, were at a disadvantage in relation to more accessible ones: Simmons' *Medical Register* of 1783 returned far more practitioners for Kent than for the much larger county of Devon. During the early nineteenth century a greater supply of medical practitioners meant more even coverage in the provinces. The disparity between urban and rural provision remained, however, so that in 1901, whilst one in four of the population lived in rural areas, only one in seven medical practitioners resided there.[34]

Three historical snapshots of the changing distribution of the regular faculty in relation to population in English provincial counties (excluding London) have been drawn up in maps for 1783, 1861 and 1911. These years were selected because 1783 was the date of the first reasonably inclusive medical directory, 1861 was the first *Census* after the Medical Act of 1858 and therefore represented fairly accurately the numbers of regular practitioners, whilst 1911 was the endpoint of our analysis. No great precision is claimed for these maps except in indicating broad regional disparities over time.

Map 1 suggests that there were some marked changes in the distri-

---

30 *Lancet*, 26 May 1877, p. 775.
31 The Registrar General in his analysis of the *Census* of 1861 considered medical attendance defective from the 1850s onwards, with the fear that it was becoming inaccessible for large numbers (quoted in Rivington, *Medical Profession*, p. 2).
32 Lane, 'Medical practitioners', p. 354; E. A. Wrigley and R. S. Schofield, *The Population History of England 1541–1871* (1981), p. 577; Bynum, 'Physicians, hospitals', p. 106.
33 I. Loudon, *Medical Care and the General Practitioner, 1750–1850* (1986), p. 306.
34 The 1901 census had 22,486 doctors in urban areas, compared with 3786 in rural ones in England and Wales. See also the comments of Rivington, *Medical Profession*, p. 4.

bution of regular practitioners in relation to population. The map for 1783 is based on figures in Simmons' *Medical Register*, and thus was much less reliable in its coverage than the maps of 1861 and 1911, based on *Census* returns. The first map may therefore be taken as impressionistic rather than accurate, particularly for the counties around London such as Surrey. In 1783 there were counties with ratios of practitioners to population as low as 1:2500 or above: four (Surrey, Bedfordshire, Lancashire and Cheshire) had ratios of between 1:2500 and 1:2999; whilst a further four (Cambridgeshire, Buckinghamshire, Gloucestershire and Staffordshire) had ratios even lower than this. Of these eight, only two (Lancashire and Staffordshire) again scored particularly badly in 1861, although by then their ratios had improved to the range of from 1:2000 to 1:2499. In this band of the worst-doctored counties they were joined by Huntingdonshire. By 1911 there were more counties in this band than had been the case earlier: there were six Midlands counties (Huntingdonshire, Northamptonshire, Leicestershire, Nottinghamshire, Derbyshire, and Staffordshire) and one northern one (Durham). Well-doctored counties, with fewer than 1499 patients per regular practitioner, were to be found mainly in the south in counties such as Sussex, Kent, Hampshire, or Somerset, together with a few outliers in the border counties.

Map 2 explores this point further and shows the counties with an above-average proportion of regular practitioners to population, taking the mean for each date. From this an important point emerges. It can be seen that there was a growing regional split; southern England became increasingly well-doctored by comparison with the northern counties. Whereas in 1783 the dividing line ran from the Severn to the Humber, by 1861 this had moved south from the Severn to the Wash. Outlying areas of well-doctored counties remained in the extreme north, probably influenced by the large production of medical graduates by Scottish universities. The regionalisation of medical practice is brought out further in later chapters since sufferers in the north of England were more prone to consult a member of the medical fringe, and were also less inclined to consult a poor-law medical practitioner. The orthodox medical practitioner had thus been much more successful in penetrating the medical market of the south than the north of England.

Affluent areas attracted a good supply of practitioners, but even at the inception of the National Insurance Scheme in 1911 the poorest urban areas were still thinly doctored. One London doctor, with 30 years experience, commented that, 'well trained, fine young doctors

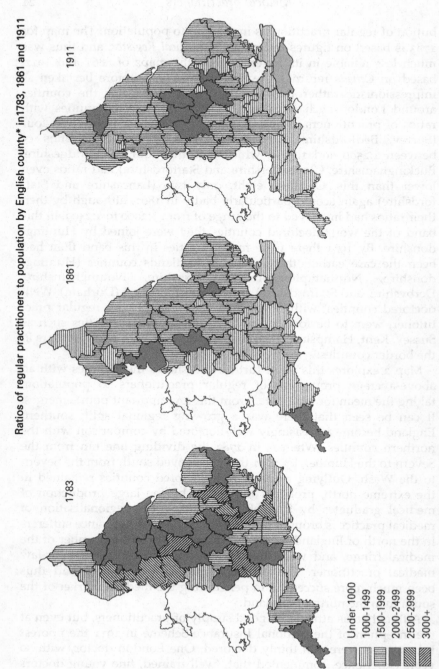

Map 1 Ratios of regular practitioners to population by English county* in 1783, 1861 and 1911. *Source:* Simmons's *Medical Register* 1783. *Note:* *excludes London

1783

1861

1911

Under 1000
1000-1499
1500-1999
2000-2499
2500-2999
3000+

English counties with an above average ratio of regular practitioners to population

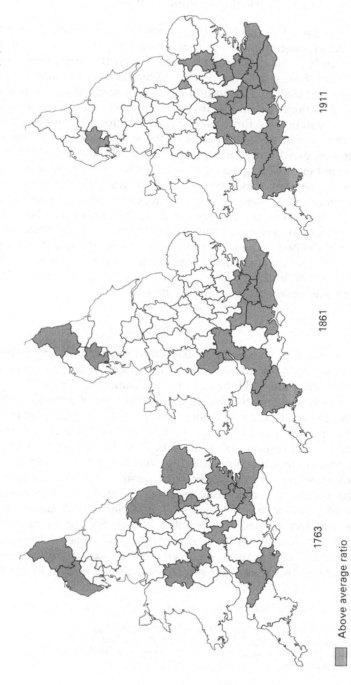

1763   1861   1911

Above average ratio

Map 2   *Sources: Simmons's Medical Register 1783; Census 1861 and 1911.*

could not stomach practice in these areas'.[35] Experience during the
First World War threw some light on the vexed question of the supply
or over-supply of medical practitioners. Given the large numbers of
doctors in the forces, and the continued availability of colleagues for
the civilian population a Dean of a university medical school told the
Ministry of National Service in 1917 that, 'the present conditions show
that there are in normal times far too many doctors.'[36] Revealingly, he
was concerned not with the needs of the entire population for adequate medical care but with the market conditions that would support
a given number of GPs, given the finite numbers of those able to pay
the doctor's fees. Insurance payments from the panel system meant
that later more GPs were enabled to make an adequate living, but
despite these interwar improvements disparities remained. The extent
of these can be gauged by the continued presence of inequalities at the
inception of the NHS when 'the number of residents per GP was twice
as great in Kensington as Hampstead: thrice as great in Harrow; four
times as great in Bradford; five times in Wakefield; six times in West
Bromwich and seven times in South Shields.'[37]

Occupational character

'The professions ... live by persuasion and propaganda, by claiming
that their service is indispensable to the client or employer and to
society and the state.'[38] Until recently the claims of the medical profession in defining and constructing an ideal type of profession have
been accepted uncritically by historians as representing a past reality.
Some of the key elements in a profession included: a possession and
extension of, and responsibility for, a body of knowledge; a standard
of professional qualification; a self-governing organisation for the
group directed at service rather than profit, and the existence of
sanctions to enforce responsibilities; finally, a recognition by the state
of monopoly status and of privilege.[39] Associated with these were a
sense of mystery related to specialist knowledge; of exclusiveness
related to the formal entry qualifications and thus of instruction
undergone and certification achieved; and of autonomy related to
self-regulation. There was also seen to be a strong ethical component

[35] B. N. Armstrong, *The Health Insurance Doctor. His Role in Britain, Denmark and France* (Princeton, 1939).
[36] J. M. Winter, *The Great War and the British People* (1985), p. 186.
[37] J. and S. Jewkes, *The Genesis of the British NHS* (Oxford, 1962), p. 13.
[38] H. Perkins, *The Rise of Professional Society. England Since 1880* (1989), p. 6.
[39] R. Lewis and A. Maude, *Professional People* (1952), pp. 55–6.

of disinterestedness and moral responsibility in the discharge of one's specialism, and of propriety in competition with colleagues. Whether this corporate image reflected historical reality at any one time, or was to a greater or lesser extent a useful political ideology in justifying privilege is an important issue.[40] It is particularly germane to any study of the medical market since the pretensions of the orthodox practitioner for a privileged status within it were dependent on superior claims as a professional to give a better service to the consumer or patient.

Recent work by early modernists has challenged previous studies of professions which assumed a discontinuity around 1800, and foreshortened the past by neglecting the pre-1800 period, since interest then was focused on the formative influence of industrialisation in shaping the Victorian professions.[41] Instead it has been persuasively argued that there is no clear or simple linear progress to be discerned in the 'rise' of the professions. Professions, it is suggested, existed in pre-industrial England despite their lack of conformity to what are usually seen as key elements in a modern profession. Thus, there was occupational differentiation within a single profession; part-time as well as full-time followers of an avocation; a lack of monopoly powers in relation to practice; frequently a lack of, or an imperfect, institutional structure within the profession; and finally, a more active role by clients in their relationships with practitioners.[42] Margaret Pelling's thought-provoking analysis of the medical profession in the early modern period challenges many of the stereotypes about medicine as a profession. She makes a case for seeing both similarities and differences, continuities and discontinuities before and after 1800, and thus for the profession having a non-linear development. She emphasises that the medical profession in this earlier period needs to be seen on its own terms; with a variety of practitioners, both full- and part-time; practice that was 'neither well organised nor firmly controlled'; and with a complex interrelationship with other economic and social

[40] A. K. Daniels, 'How Free Should Professions Be', in E. Friedson, ed., *The Professions and their Prospects* (1971), p. 56.
[41] W. R. Prest, 'Why the History of the Professions is not Written', in G. R. Rubin and D. Sugarman, eds., *Law, Economy and Society. Essays in the History of English Law, 1750–1914* (1984); A. M. Carr Saunders and P. A.Wilson, *The Professions* (1933); I. Waddington, *The Medical Profession in the Industrial Revolution* (1984), p. 176; W. J. Reader, *Professional Men. The Rise of the Professional Classes in Nineteenth-Century England* (1966), p. 2; E. Friedson, 'The Theory of the Professions: State of the Art', in R. Dingwall, and P. Lewis, eds., *The Sociology of the Professions* (1983), p. 22.
[42] W. Prest, ed., *The Professions in Early Modern England* (1987), pp. 14–18.

groups.[43] By implication, medical practice thus partook both of trade and profession; each being an honourable avocation. This interpretation – that those engaged in medicine were members of an *occupation* – has much to commend it, not only for the period before 1800 but to a more limited extent thereafter. It contrasts with that of Holmes, in his study of the Augustan period, who has argued that there occurred, 'between the 1660s and the 1740s the rise of a true medical profession, and one that already had a measure of homogeneity.'[44]

Professionalisation was a drive towards an ideal rather than a static attainment of a set of essential criteria. Georgian and Victorian patients regularly consulted a variety of regulars and irregulars and thus accepted that medicine was a very differentiated occupation. The defining conceptual and historical boundaries between regular and irregular were in any case arbitrary and (particularly in the earlier part of the period) permeable. Two of the foremost practitioners of the Georgian age exemplified this. The physician Dr Fothergill, admitted that 'I own I think the Faculty too much indebted to empiricism to frame a wish to suppress it',[45] whilst the surgeon William Cheselden, had a healthy respect for bonesetters and acknowledged that he had learned from their techniques.[46] This situation continued, albeit to a lesser extent, into the nineteenth century, when eminent physicians or surgeons could practise in so-called irregular fields such as acupuncture, phrenology or mesmerism. Mesmerism, together with hydropathy, homeopathy and herbalism were the big battalions by the Victorian period but there were a host of smaller regiments and platoons, some lasting (like osteopathy), and others more transient (such as medical galvanism).[47] Irregular activity – in the eighteenth century especially – was encouraged by the low therapeutic efficacy of regular practitioners, which in turn facilitated eclecticism amongst patients in whom they consulted.

The growth of a secular and consumer society, in which health was increasingly seen as a commodity to be purchased like any other, underpinned this. This provided a dynamic to sustain and encourage a vigorous commercialism in a medical market in which many different kinds of practitioners were able to compete. In eighteenth-century England, unlike the situation in France or Germany, supervision by

43 M. Pelling, 'Medical Practice in Early Modern England: Trade or Profession', in Prest, *Professions*, pp. 90–128.
44 G. Holmes, *Augustan England, Professions, State and Society, 1680–1730* (1982), p. 206.
45 Wellcome MSS 3246–8, Letter from Fothergill to Lettsom in J. C. Lettsom, 'Fugitive Pieces'.
46 Z. Cope, *William Cheselden, 1688–1752* (1953), p. 85.
47 R. Cooter, ed., *Studies in the History of Alternative Medicine* (1988), p. xiv.

the regulatory bodies, notably the College of Physicians was inadequate. By the nineteenth century growing pressure from regular practitioners to create an exclusive medical profession was insufficiently powerful, within what was by then a prevalent free-trade and *laisser-faire* ethos, to create a monopoly for the Faculty.[48]

This contest between the forces of orthodoxy (represented by the regulars) against heterodoxy, (the irregulars), may look sufficiently complicated, but there was a further seemingly ubiquitous group, the 'quacks'. Like the mad, these were always other people, and the term appears to have been frequently used as a non-specific kind of abuse. However, variety in medical practice, particularly in the earlier part of our period, meant that methods developed by quacks might enter the realms of the orthodox, or *vice versa*.[49] Quack was used variously during the eighteenth century to mean a pretender, an ignoramus, an advertiser, an empiricist, or an untrained practitioner.[50] Roy Porter has argued that 'most of the litmus tests that might be proposed to divide quacks from pukka doctors, in the event confuse rather than clarify the issues.'[51] Amongst these are the tests of ignorance, deceit, empiricism, therapeutic competence, and entrepreneurialism. Given the extent of the overlap in the actual roles of regular and irregular, or quack and orthodox, practitioners, much contemporary rhetoric on empiricism, competition and entrepreneurialism should be discounted. Concern about quackery waxed and waned according to the state of the medical market; it was particularly prevalent in the period between 1815 and mid-century when large numbers of practitioners meant that further competition was unwelcome.[52] The *Lancet* was extremely concerned about 'the infatuated ignorance which prompts men to prefer the charlatan to the educated practitioner.'[53] Economic self-interest was camouflaged by assertions about the public interest in attempts to promote a greater regulation of medical practice by the Faculty. Thus, William Heberden the Younger spoke of the need to secure 'the public from the bold intrusion of empirics or the unlicensed practice of the ignorant.'[54]

[48] R. Porter, *Health for Sale. Quackery in England, 1660–1850* (1989), Chapter 2 and Conclusion, *passim*.
[49] L. R. C. Agnew, 'Quackery' in A. G. Debus, ed., *Medicine in Seventeenth-Century England* (Berkeley, 1974), p. 322.
[50] L. S. King, *The Medical World of the Eighteenth Century* (Chicago, 1958), Chapter 2, *passim*.
[51] Porter, *Health for Sale*, p. 6.
[52] M. Neve, 'Orthodoxy and Fringe: Medicine in Late Georgian Bristol' in W. F. Bynum and R. Porter, eds., *Medical Fringe and Medical Orthodoxy, 1750–1850* (1987), p. 45.
[53] *Lancet*, i (1837–8), p. 523.
[54] RCPL, Letter of William Heberden the Younger to Dr Mason, 20 August 1820.

Between the Apothecaries Act of 1815 and the Medical Act of 1858 was a period of transition, when the training and qualification of regular practitioners was increasingly specified and tightened up. The legislation of 1815 laid down that apothecaries, having undergone a five year apprenticeship and attended some courses, had to pass an examination of the Society of Apothecaries, and thus be licensed, before they could practise.[55] The act of 1858 made a clear demarcation between the orthodox practitioner who qualified under the provisions of the act, and thus went on the *Medical Register*, and the fringe practitioner who did not.[56] Nevertheless, it did not in any sense outlaw fringe practice, and so it was alleged by a disgruntled Faculty that England retained the reputation of being a 'Paradise of Quacks.'[57] In this context it is interesting to find that certain local medical associations were prepared to attempt the job that they saw the 1858 act as having failed to do. In 1863 Herefordshire Medical Association confronted a Dr Evans of Gloucester for his association with an unqualified druggist, but were rebuffed by Evans who stated that, 'it would be better for them to avoid interference in a matter over which they have no authority.'[58] Even an official report concluded in 1910 that medical legislation had failed to enable the public, 'to distinguish qualified from unqualified practitioners.'[59] English medicine thus only very slowly moved towards important professional elements: an increasing homogeneity and a minimum level of standards of practice, acquired through education and training, together with a greater control over entry in order to try to achieve a monopoly in practice.

Occupational structure

Traditionally, the historiographical view of eighteenth-century English medical practitioners has been influenced by that of the medical professsion in seeing this as a tripartite structure composed of physicians, surgeons and apothecaries.[60] This is interesting in drawing attention both to differences in the relative social status of medical practitioners and to a division of labour, but misleading since it related

[55] See S. W. F. Holloway, 'The Apothecaries Act', *MH*, 10 (1966) for a fuller analysis of the extent to which the act merely rationalised existing practice rather than initiating new.
[56] 'Introduction' to Bynum and Porter, *Medical Fringe*, p. 2.
[57] Dale, *Medical Profession* (1875), pp. 24–5.
[58] Glos. RO, D637 II/3/c6, correspondence dated December 1863 to January 1864.
[59] *Report as to the Practice of Medicine and Surgery by Unqualified Persons in the UK*, PP, 1910, XXXVII, p. 10.
[60] Carr Saunders and Wilson, *Professions*, p. 75.

personnel too stringently to different kinds of medicine. This stereotypical division of labour supposedly meant that: physicians dealt with
diseases amenable to physic or medicine under intellectual direction or
management; surgeons treated conditions for which manual or operative interventions of a mainly local and external character were
involved; and the apothecaries prepared or compounded drugs and
medicines. However, a more nuanced and complex interpretation is
needed since these distinctions were less than clear-cut. Studies of
sixteenth- and seventeenth-century medicine have emphasised the
dominance of general practice rather than a tripartite division of
medical labour.[61] Even in London, where specialism was facilitated by
the numbers of practitioners, the apothecaries and surgeons who
treated most of the population, increasingly resembled one another.[62]
Burnby saw the Georgian apothecary turning 'more and more to the
practice of medicine' rather than dispensing in the shop, while in a
study of provincial practice Kett argued that the apothecary had
largely abandoned trade for full-time medical practice by 1800.[63]
Indeed, a contemporary study of the apothecary in 1795 commented
that 'there are few apothecaries in the country who do not engage in
the practice of surgery, and by far the greatest number in London do
the same.'[64] Also influential were the growing numbers of chemists
and druggists, particularly after 1780, who challenged the apothecary's
shop trade and successfully met demand for cheap medicines. Overlapping in the forms of practice was also found amongst physicians
and surgeons where older demarcations – between 'the internal and
the external, what one knows and what one sees'[65] – were undercut by
scientific advances associated with the 'birth of the clinic', discussed in
Chapter 3. The necessity for the physician to be aware of anatomy and
the surgeon to be knowledgeable in prescription were repeatedly
stressed in the late eighteenth and early nineteenth centuries. With
this came a recognition that each needed to assist the other.[66] Indeed,

---

61 Pelling and Webster, 'Medical Practitioners' in Webster, *Health, Medicine and Mortality*,
    pp. 234–5; R. S. Roberts, 'The Personnel and Practice of Medicine in Tudor and Stuart
    England. Part 1. The Provinces', *MH*, VI (1962), p. 376.
62 R. S. Roberts, 'The Personnel and Practice of Medicine in Tudor and Stuart England.
    Part 2. London', *MH*, VIII (1964), p. 229.
63 J. G. L. Burnby, *A Study of the English Apothecary from 1660 to 1760* (Medical History
    Supplement Number 3, Wellcome Institute, London, 1983), p. 114; J. F. Kett, 'Provin-
    cial Medical Practice in England, 1730–1815', *JHM*, XIX, 1964, p. 18.
64 John Mason Good, *The History of Medicine, so far as it relates to the Profession of the
    Apothecary* (1795), pp. 146–7.
65 Foucault, *Clinic*, p. 81.
66 R. C. Brock, *The Life and Work of Astley Cooper* (1952), p. 111. In his thinking Astley
    Cooper was following the dictums of his esteemed predecessor, John Hunter. See

Sir Anthony Carlisle, Surgeon to the Westminster Hospital, went further in 1834 in asking, 'can any definite line be drawn in practice between medical and surgical diseases?' and answering, 'I think not.'[67] Although Acts of Parliament and decisions in the courts had pre-scribed a division of labour there were many intermediate areas between the task of surgeons and that of physicians as, for example, in the treatment of skin diseases or venereal diseases. Medical practice was therefore fluid, with much overlapping of professional roles, not least because practitioners were quick to seize changing market opportunities as R. Campbell had emphasised in 1747. 'The physician should know something of the surgeon's business, and he of the doctor's [i.e. physician's], and the apothecary of both.'[68] The social status of the practitioner, in which the physician alone had tradi-tionally possessed genteel status, informed the kind of patients seen.[69] However, in a competitive medical market the relative levels of fees helped demarcate different kinds of practitioner, as well as stratifying practices. Parts II and III suggest the ways in which both poverty and property expanded openings in the medical market (albeit in different ways), and how a disregard of the stereotypical role, function and status of different types of practitioner shaped a remarkably fluid occupation.

By the early nineteenth century the obselete nature of a tripartite division in medicine was acknowledged.[70] No consensus as to what should replace it emerged, although there were hopes of radical reform that would have brought about more integration. This differ-entiated culture contrasted with that of France, where medicine and surgery had become united after 1794.[71] In England there was much criticism by surgeons and general practitioners of what were per-ceived as artificial divisions.[72] However, physicians were prominent in defending the *status quo*, since they had the most to lose from a

also evidence by Astley Cooper and Benjamin Brodie to the *SC on Medical Education*, PP 1834, XIII, QQ 5447–8, 5755–6.

[67] *SC on Medical Education*, Q 5983.
[68] R. Campbell, *The London Tradesman* (1747, reprinted Newton Abbot, 1969), p. 52.
[69] B. Hamilton, 'The Medical Professions in the the Eighteenth Century', *Economic History Review*, IV, second series, (1951), p. 141. The College of Physicians in London admitted only graduates of the universities of Oxford and Cambridge and of Trinity College, Dublin.
[70] *SC on Medical Education*, QQ 2121–31, 2467.
[71] M. Ramsey, *Professional and Popular Medicine in France, 1770–1830. The Social World of Medical Practice* (Cambridge, 1988) p. 123.
[72] R. C. Maulitz, *Morbid Appearances* (Cambridge, 1987), pp. 226–7; T. Alcock, *Essay on the Education and Duties of the General Practitioner in Medicine and Surgery* (1823) p. 128; T. Hodgkin, *Medical Reform. An Address read to the Harveian Society* (1847), p. 13.

blurring of professional roles.[73] In any case, radical arguments ran up against powerful and conservative interest groups in the Royal Colleges of Physicians and Surgeons, and these bodies were successful in limiting the changes that were eventually to emerge in the legislation of 1858.[74]

The Medical Act of 1858 failed to integrate medicine and to specify a single means of entry to it. It was not until the Medical Amendment Act of 1886 that all medical students had to have a qualification in surgery, midwifery and medicine. What was worse from the practitioners' viewpoint, was that the 1858 legislation failed to give the profession a medical monopoly: quackery was not outlawed nor were chemists and druggists regulated. GPs had to practice in an open medical market, where – as Figure 1.3 indicates – numbers of chemists and druggists increased even more rapidly than did surgeons, physicians and GPs.[75] The 1858 Act did have the virtue of establishing a new category of doctor 'the registered medical practitioner', who gained entry to a *Medical Register* through either a single or a double qualification in medicine and/or surgery. A control of standards in the profession was initiated by the creation of the General Medical Council, since this could not only register names but also strike them off the list. There was therefore a central coordinating body responsible for standards in medical practice and for professional self-regulation. Earlier, the 1858 act had been seen as a landmark in that it went 'a long way towards establishing the approved pattern of a Victorian profession.'[76] But more recent historiography has emphasised its limitations;[77] in key respects of professionalisation the act established neither complete control over standards, nor monopoly – and thus control over entry and selling power.[78]

One of the chief competitors of the medical practitioner was the druggist or chemist and this became a distinct occupation during the eighteenth century, first in London and then in the provinces. With the advent of new patterns of consumerism and new patterns of retailing, their numbers increased rapidly. The occupation was diffuse – ranging from the skilled, high-class specialist establishment to the poor corner-shop that sold medicaments alongside other goods. Holloway has made an interesting, but not wholly convincing case,

---

[73] Loudon, *Medical Care*, pp. 193–4.   [74] Waddington, *Medical Profession*, p. 132.
[75] See H. Marland, 'The Medical Activities of Chemists and Druggists with Special Reference to Wakefield and Huddersfield', *MH*, 31 (1987), pp. 420–6 for the way in which doctors felt threatened by this increase.
[76] Reader, *Professional Men*, p. 66.   [77] Loudon, *Medical Care*, pp. 297–301.
[78] E. Friedson, *Professional Powers. A Study of the Institutionalisation of Formal Knowledge* (Chicago, 1986), pp. 63–4, 186–7.

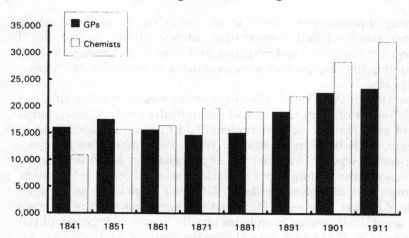

Figure 1.3   Chemists and general practitioners, 1841–1911
Note: Between 1841 and 1881 practitioner numbers included medical assistants
and medical students.

that contrary to the statements of rival GPs and apothecaries there
was nothing unorthodox, irregular, or fringe about chemists: their
pharmacy was based on the London, Edinburgh and Dublin *Pharmacopoeias*, as was the prescription of physicians, surgeons and apothecaries; and the apprenticeship served by chemists conferred expertise.
Chemists had standing in their local community, shown by their
public offices, and thus were in no sense marginal.[79] They depended
on their reputation and the trust of their customers for their business
and their constantly supervised chemist's shop offered clients a more
regular skilled service than many mobile regular practitioners.

The fluidity of medical roles during the nineteenth century also
involved a distinction between consultants and ordinary practitioners;
those who practised purely as surgeons or physicians were perceived
increasingly as consultants.[80] This was an élite in social and financial
as well as medical terms, consisting of Fellows of the Royal College of
Surgeons, or of the Royal College of Physicians. Central to their
evolving role was the growth in hospitals which had begun in the
eighteenth century; the importance of the general hospital as a route
to a career as a consultant, grew in importance.[81] Beginning in 1720,
with the foundation of the Westminster Infirmary, by 1861 there were

[79] S. W. F. Holloway, *Royal Pharmaceutical Society of Great Britain, 1841–1991. A Social and
Political History* (1991), pp. 36–7, 42, 45, 46, 50–1.
[80] Loudon, *Medical Care*, p. 187.
[81] M. J. Peterson, *The Medical Profession in Mid-Victorian London* (Berkeley, 1978), p. 138.

more than 150 general hospitals in England and Wales.[82] Honorary hospital appointments were of even greater importance to the career of a surgeon than to a physician, as can be seen from an analysis of membership of the respective Royal Colleges.[83] (A considerable growth in the numbers of rural cottage hospitals from the 1860s was also helpful to the status and career of the provincial GP.)[84] During the Victorian period the position of the general hospital consultant was challenged by an increasing number of specialists. General consultants saw the specialist within the specialist hospital as a threat to the viability of the general hospital, the pattern of medical education linked to it, and hence of their own positions in the voluntary institution. The growth in private *specialist* hospitals during the nineteenth century which, by 1900, numbered 128 in England and Wales,[85] was strategically important. Granshaw has argued that this institution converted the medical specialist from possessing a status not much different from that of the 'quack' in the early nineteenth century to a position at the pinnacle of the profession a century later. This is too optimistic since ambivalence towards the idea of specialism continued, and the concept of the consultant surgeon as generalist retained its hold. As a result, some surgeons who had held positions at specialist hospitals early in their career went on to prestigious consultancy posts as generalists at ordinary hospitals.[86] Others appear to have retained a dual appointment.[87] Significantly, however, there had to be some concessions to the manifest appeal for patients of specialisms, so that even in general hospitals special wards were set up, and junior posts were created in specialities such as ophthalmology or laryngology.[88] Within the hierarchy of the voluntary general hospital, specialists were therefore subordinate to generalists who retained their supremacy. Typical English consultants were not – as in other countries – scientific researchers; instead, the emphasis of their work was on *general* clinical observation.[89] Consultants, as generalists, considered that specialists – in concentrating on local manifestations of

---

[82] J. Woodward, *To Do The Sick No Harm. A Study of the British Voluntary Hospital System to 1875* (1974) p. 36.

[83] Peterson, *Medical Profession*, p. 151.

[84] B. Abel Smith, *The Hospitals* (1964), p. 102. There were 18 cottage hospitals in 1865, 180 by 1880, and 600 by 1934.

[85] R. Stevens, *Medical Practice in Modern England. The Impact of Specialization and State Medicine* (New Haven, 1966), p. 27.

[86] L. Granshaw, ']Fame and Fortune by Means of Bricks and Mortar: the Medical Profession and Specialist Hospitals in Britain', in L. Granshaw and R. Porter, eds., *The Hospital in History* (1989), pp. 199, 214.

[87] Stevens, *Medical Practice*, p. 28.   [88] Peterson, *Medical Profession*, p. 277.

[89] Stevens, *Medical Practice*, p. 33.

disease – were giving insufficient attention to the state of the rest of the body. From a historical perspective, however, it is clear that specialists showed a greater appreciation of the new scientific insights of the 1870s and 1880s, whereas consultants retained a greater faith in traditional medical conceptions. Reflecting on specialism from the standpoint of the 1930s one eminent doctor concluded that, 'one of the most important events has been the complete recognition of legitimate specialism.'[90]

By the late Victorian and Edwardian period these divisions in medicine, and a related competition for patients, produced professional bitterness. Tensions arose between the specialist and the GP over their division of labour; under a referral system specialists saw cases of particular interest or difficulty for their colleagues – the ordinary medical practitioners – whilst the latter customarily retained overall continued care of the patient. Patients' growing recourse to specialists was said in 1885 to make GPs view 'the specialist as a receiver of stolen goods, if not as the actual thief' of patients whom the GP had been able earlier to view 'as his private property.'[91] GPs also criticised specialists for their lack of holistic knowledge and – from their perspective as family doctors – for their ignorance of the hereditary predispositions of the patient. Relationships between GPs and consultants were also less than happy. From the 1830s GPs articulated their bitterness at what they saw as socially indiscriminate treatment at hospital out-patients' clinics where the not-so-poor, who could afford private treatment by a GP, were allegedly given gratuitous attention. This 'monster evil of the day' led in 1876 to the creation of a Hospital Outpatients Reform Committee by the British Medical Association.[92] In addition, GPs considered that consultants were becoming rivals in private practice and, as competition in the medical market intensified in the 1880s, this was seen as aggravating an already very difficult economic situation. In 1866 an association of GPs was formed to defend their interests against the perceived depredations of the consultant.[93] In turn, consultants accused general practitioners of greed; a physician complained in 1910 that 'Just as the dishonest consultant steals a patient, so a dishonest general practitioner keeps a patient to himself long after he has discovered that he cannot without further

[90] H. Rolleston, 'The Changes in the Medical Profession and Advances in Medicine during the Last Fifty Years', _BMJ_, 23 July 1932.
[91] M. Mackenzie, 'Specialisms in Medicine', _Fortnightly Review_, 37 (1885), p. 777.
[92] For example, _BMJ_ i (1853), pp. 201, 315, 429; 10 January 1866, p. 66; 10 March 1876, pp. 870–1, and 14 July 1883, p. 64 (quoting resolution of Fifth BMA Meeting in 1836).
[93] _BMJ_, 18 December 1886, p. 1190.

advice on diagnosis or treatment do the best for such a patient.'[94] In large cities domiciliary care came to be provided by the GP and hospital care by the consultant or specialist,[95] whereas in smaller towns, GPs managed to retain a foothold in hospital practice, with an honorary post at a local infirmary or cottage hospital. Accurately encapsulating the nub of the dispute, one aggrieved GP stated that 'The whole struggle between the general practitioner and the consultant is one of bread.'[96]

Status and reward

In discussion of professionalisation attention has only recently switched to finance from structure. Schumpeter has seen the professions in terms of their monopoly over certain resources, whilst Illich has perceived modern professions' recent activity as 'a new kind of cartel', with disabling consequences for society.[97] Since professional practice was undoubtedly a business, there was a tension between the service function of professions and their need to make money. Larson, particularly, has developed the implications of this in defining 'professionalisation as the process by which producers of special services sought to constitute and control a market for their expertise.' There was thus 'an attempt to translate one order of scarce resources – special knowledge and skills – into another – social and economic rewards.'[98] Contemporary practitioners were only too well aware of this: Thomas Beddoes remarked that 'Our dignity is unfortunately placed in the quantity of our gains, not of the good we do.'[99] And, as members of the medical profession became more homogeneous, the gulf that separated them from those who were not professional widened, and typically this then led to a move to exclude or restrict fringe practice. Increased control over the privileged area could then accommodate growing numbers of professional practitioners.

Between 1660 and 1730 Holmes has concluded that 'a prime attraction of the profession of medicine lay in the growing professional

94 *BMJ Supplement*, 1910, p. 304. Statement by Dr Lauriston Shaw, Dean of Guy's Hospital and the Chair of the BMA's Central Ethical Committee.
95 F. Honigsbaum, *The Division in British Medicine. A History of the Separation of General Practice from Hospital Care, 1911–1968* (1979), pp. 1–4.
96 *BMJ*, 10 July 1886, p. 89.
97 J. A. Schumpeter, *Imperialism and Social Classes* (Oxford, 1951), pp. 133–221; I. Illich, *Disabling Professions* (1977), p. 15.
98 M. S. Larson, *The Rise of Professionalism. A Sociological Analysis* (Berkeley, 1978), pp. xvi, xvii. See also H. Perkin, *Rise of Professional Society. England since 1880,* (1989), p. 7.
99 Quoted in R. Porter, *Doctor of Society. Thomas Beddoes and the Sick Trade in Late-Enlightenment England* (1992), pp. 142–3.

rewards which the successful practitioner at all levels came to antici-
pate.'[100] And, by the late eighteenth century there was, as Irvine
Loudon has aptly commented, a golden age for doctors. But an
increased supply of practitioners after the end of the Napoleonic Wars
meant that the medical profession became 'grossly overcrowded'
during the early nineteeth century.[101] An analysis of 1845 estimated
that more than one thousand entrants annually were licensed to enter
the medical profession whereas there were viable economic openings
for only half that number.[102] But the state of the medical market is
much less clear for the period between 1850 and 1911. Waddington has
asserted that 'within two decades of the passing of the [1858] Act . . .
there was a serious shortage of qualified practitioners.'[103] If this were
the case then medical incomes would have been buoyant, but Peterson
takes a more sober view in concluding that medical incomes were
broadly static from the 1870s to 1911.[104] Chapter 5 therefore examines
in considerable detail the state of medical incomes in the late nineteenth and early twentieth centuries in order to resolve this issue.

The economic relationship between practitioner and patient
involved a tension between the service function of personal commitment to the individual patient as against a market orientation needed
for financial survival. Equally, there were discrepancies between the
higher conduct to be expected of a member of an ancient profession
and the tradesmanlike pursuit of profit. There were a number of
similarities between medical practice and a trade. It is indicative that
in the eighteenth century the surgeon-apothecary ran his practice
from a 'shop' rather than the later designation of the 'surgery'. And on
the fringes of respectable practice was a continuation of the earlier
habit of conditional contract – or bargaining for an agreed improvement as one would purchase a commodity – and thus not paying in
full until the 'cure' had been effected. Another aspect of a continuing
trade element in medicine was a short-lived use of tendering in
medical appointments during the first years of the New Poor Law.

The ambiguity of the mid-Victorian practitioners' status was
described by Thackeray, in that they 'would condescend to sell a
brown-paper plaster to a farmer's wife across the counter or to vend
toothbrushes, hair-powder and ladies perfumery.'[105] The crucial

---

[100] Holmes, *Augustan England*, p. 218.
[101] I. Loudon, 'Two Thousand Medical Men in 1847', *Bulletin of the Society for the Social History of Medicine*, 33 (1983) pp. 4–8.
[102] A. S. Taylor, 'On the Numerical Relation of the Medical Profession to the Population of Great Britain', *London Medical Gazette*, New Series (1844–5), pp. 497–504.
[103] Waddington, *Medical Profession*, p. 149.   [104] Peterson, *Medical Profession*, p. 129.
[105] W. Thackeray, *The History of Pendennis* (1848–50), p. 5.

distinction being made here was the sale of commodities, rather than services; it was this which signalled to a Victorian as it had not to a Georgian, that this was trade not profession. In this context it is significant to find doctors themselves urging that their charges should be made for advice and not for medicines. One argued feelingly in 1842 that:

The galling evil ... like an incubus, weighs down the independence and honourable feeling of so large a body of intelligent and respectable men is to be found in the practice of the profession ... I allude to our dependence on the sale of medicines as a remuneration for our professional services ... Give us but emancipation from this, and we become a new order of men: no longer to be regarded as petty traders, whose profits are elevenpence in the shilling, but men of science, whose proper business consists in supplying the art of medicine at its proper value.[106]

This change came about slowly in the mid-nineteenth century and contributed to the rising social status of doctors in Victorian society. However, once doctors began to charge for services rather than medicaments attention then focused on how such services were remunerated. The doctor who had a cash practice held a more lowly status than a colleague who sent out an annual bill. Of course, this was also inextricably mixed up with the fact that cash patients were almost invariably the poorer ones. Equally, autonomy in professional practice was also seen as a mark of professional status. Doctors who accepted club practice with friendly societies were looked down upon by those who could afford not to do so, since the direct power of the lay person over the doctor was implicitly seen as diminishing professional authority.

Throughout the period, an individual doctor's acceptance in polite society (and thus his access to more affluent patients) depended crucially on birth, independent wealth and cultural attainments. Those who failed to score positively here were regarded as 'also rans' along with others of ambiguous status in polite society. R. S. Surtees described in 1874 how 'The first to arrive were the gentlemen of the second class ... [including] Mr Pillerton, the doctor ... who were all very polite and obsequious [enunciating], "your lordship" ... the Earl at every opportunity.'[107] For the very best circles even finer distinctions had to be made, as Lady Warwick pointed out in 1890. 'Doctors and solicitors might be invited to garden parties, though never, of

---

[106] Letter by 'A Member of the Provincial Medical and Surgical Association', *Provincial Medical and Surgical Journal*, (1842), p. 167.
[107] R. S. Surtees, *Ask Mamma. The Richest Commoner in England* (1874), Chapter xix. I am grateful to Alan Heeson for this reference.

course, to lunch or dinner.'[108] She was presumably discussing the country GP, yet for all doctors the range was immense – from the unfortunate individual struggling to keep a hold on respectability to the comfortably-off member of the bourgeoisie.

A valuable insight into the extent to which the ordinary practitioner had achieved status and a comfortable life style is revealed by late-Victorian and Edwardian advertisements of practices for sale. The life of the Edwardian GP appears to have become increasingly pressurised since less was made of the sporting and recreational opportunities of a practice. Instead there was emphasis on its economic potential; information on fees became routine rather than exceptional. Being a doctor was apparently perceived much more as a matter of running a business than of possessing a genteel lifestyle. There were fewer lofty references to 'guinea midwifery refused', 'no club appointments held', or to 'no night work undertaken.' Rather, the physical attributes necessary to sustain a successful practice were emphasised: the possession of a corner or double-fronted house together with a separate surgery entrance. Preferably, this would be situated in a growing residential area if a town practice, or be unopposed by rival colleagues if a country one. There were more frequent, and precise, references to the class or classes of patient attended by the doctor. Fortunate country practitioners might advertise that they had the patronage of 'hunting and titled patients' or that 'patients include all classes from nobility downwards.'[109] The advertisement for the seaside practice might boast that it included 'all the best residents in the place', whilst the urban one might indicate that 'substantial tradespeople' or 'the respectable artisan class' were its patients.[110] A few GPs aspired to run a family practice where 'patients are good residents and families attended for half a life-time.'[111]

The English profession was thus a bifurcated one, with a small élite and a much larger group of ordinary practitioners, as was the case in France and the United States.[112] In England practitioners encompassed a wide range of status, income and life-style, and more of the formative influences upon them will be further explored in the next chapter.

[108] A. Glynn, *Elinor Glynn – A Biography* (1955), p. 64,
[109] *BMJ Advertiser*, 26 June and 25 December 1909.
[110] *BMJ Advertiser*, 26 June, 21 August, and 31 July, 1909.
[111] *BMJ Advertiser*, 9 October 1909. See also I. Loudon, 'The Concept of the Family Doctor', *BHM*, 58 (1984), p. 353.
[112] Rosenberg, 'The Practice of Medicine', p. 56; Ramsey, *Professional and Popular Medicine*, p. 110.

2

The context of practice

Doctors operated within an external set of constraints and a framework constructed by practitioners themselves. We begin by looking at the economic context of practice. This is followed by a discussion of the immediate forces helping to mould the context of practice: the role played by medical education in shaping practitioners' expertise and expectations; the insight given by medical ethics and etiquette into practitioners' preoccupations; and the appeal of 'quackery' to the patient, and hence the competition offered by the 'fringe' to the regular practitioner.

The economic context

The aim of this section is to signal some key points of interest that are discussed in more detail elsewhere in this volume. In considering the general development of the market academic discussion has focused on eighteenth-century consumption. Unfortunately, much of this is not directly relevant since debate has been: on its timing in relation to the industrial revolution; on the relative importance of home as opposed to export-led demand; and on goods rather than services. The discussion has been criticised as being reductionist and circular in its reasoning, with a consequent need to refocus attention on the change in sensibility that 'modern' consumerism involved.[1] However, there are dangers in inferring attitudes from behaviour, and of confusing imitation with emulation in studying consumption, which is as yet an underdeveloped field of historical study.[2] Bearing these admonitions in mind, the cult of sensibility and of idealised self-image which

[1] C. Campbell, *The Romantic Ethic and the Spirit of Modern Consumerism* (Oxford, 1987), Chapter 2 *passim*.
[2] J. Brewer and R. Porter, eds., *Consumption and the World of Goods* (1993), pp. 40–1.

peaked in the period from the 1750s to the 1770s[3] appears to have been important in changing beliefs and values as to the desirability of consumption, not least in terms of health. This sentimental revolution has also been linked to a more relaxed society with a less élitist culture,[4] which benefited the middle classes and gave them more self-confidence in their 'emulation', as in their patronage of élite doctors. The growth of a middle-class take-up of commercialised leisure contributed to increased expenditure in the development of leisure towns and spas,[5] which assisted the medical profession. Also important for the growth of a medical market were the growth in the 'numbers, wealth and self-confidence' of this middle class in London, together with a competition for status between a provincial urban middle class and the rural gentry within an urban cultural and social renaissance of the late seventeenth and early eighteenth centuries. Here an expanding medical profession included those who built conspicuously handsome town houses to display their affluence.[6]

What of a Georgian mass market? Population increased dramatically during the eighteenth century so that practitioners were operating in a potentially expanding market. Between 1700 and 1800 the number of towns with more than 2500 inhabitants increased from 104 to 188,[7] thus making retailing of goods and services easier. There was cash to spare in 1700 that had no place in 1550. Whereas most of this consumption was in material goods such as clothing and household items, certain services also benefited, amongst them medicine.[8] And by 1780 an earlier guesstimate had suggested that up to a quarter of the population had incomes that allowed an expenditure of around £30 per annum on services or manufactured goods.[9] The third quarter of the eighteenth century is said to have witnessed a 'convulsion of getting and spending', of a 'feverish' consumerism such that the

---

3 Campbell, *Romantic Ethic*, pp. 28–30, 173.

4 P. Langford, *A Polite and Commercial People: England, 1727–1783* (Oxford, 1992), p. 464.

5 J. H. Plumb, 'The Commercialisation of Leisure' in, N. McKendrick, J. Brewer and J. H. Plumb, eds., *The Birth of Consumer Society. The Commercialization of Eighteenth Century Society* (1983), pp. 283–5.

6 P. Earle, *The Making of the Middle Class. Business, Society and Family Life in London, 1660–1730* (1989); P. Borsay, *The English Urban Renaissance. Culture and Society in the Provincial Town* (Oxford, 1991), pp. 231, 207; G. Holmes, *Augustan England. Professions, State and Society, 1680–1730* (1982), p. 206.

7 P. Corfield, *The Impact of English Towns, 1700–1800* (Oxford, 1982).

8 J. Thirsk, *Economic Policy and Projects. The Development of a Consumer Society in Early Modern England* (Oxford, 1988), pp. 174–5. See also L. Weatherill, *Consumer Behaviour and Material Culture* (1988).

9 D. E. C. Eversley, 'The Market and Economic Growth in England, 1750–1780' in E. L. Jones and G. Mingay, eds., *Land, Labour and Population in the Industrial Revolution* (1967), p. 257.

'boom reached revolutionary proportions', and 'market opportunities were protean, the possibility of profit high.'[10] A growing market encouraged innovations in commerce, and the Georgian period witnessed a revolution in retailing, with an expansion in the number and variety of shops and in methods of selling goods. The development of a provincial press facilitated advertisements, whilst trade cards, billheads and handbills further promoted goods and services, so that by the 1770s advertisements and price competition had become keen. The apothecary, the chemist, and the vendors of patent medicines, were all beneficiaries of these developments.[11] Apothecaries' shops were a good business prospect since there were low start-up costs, a relatively low debt burden, and high returns.[12]

In terms of this developing market it is interesting to see that the distribution of mid-eighteenth century shops of all types – where there was a marked preponderance of retail outlets in the Lowland Zone of the English midlands and south – showed similarities with the distribution of counties having an above average number of late-eighteenth century practitioners shown in Map 2.[13] During the turnpike mania of the 1750s and 1760s half of the total mileage of turnpike trusts constructed between 1696 and 1836 was built, so that by the early 1770s there was an intensive network of roads around urban centres.[14] The inflation of the third quarter of the century and 'marketing flair' of the second half of the century, was one which professionals might exploit.[15] It was in this mid-eighteenth century that the ledgers, accounts and diaries of medical practitioners appear to become slightly more plentiful, although much depends on the accidental nature of documentary survival. However, this is only one element pointing towards a more commercial attitude to medical practice at this time. Commercialism was also apparent in the greater amount of travel being undertaken by surgeon-apothecaries in order to treat patients of all types, as Chapter 4 suggests. Although it is unwise to underestimate the extent of early movement, this mobility by practitioners seems to have differed from earlier epochs when it was either itinerant specialists (for example bonesetters, or cataract couchers) or

---

[10] N. McKendrick, 'The Consumer Revolution of Eighteenth Century England', in McKendrick, Brewer and Plumb, *Birth of a Consumer Society*, p. 9.
[11] H. C. Mui and L. H. Mui, *Shops and Shopkeeping in Eighteenth Century England* (Kingston, Canada, 1989), pp. 228, 235, 289, 291; P. S. Brown, 'Medicines Advertised in Eighteenth Century Bath Newspapers', *MH*, xix, (1975), pp. 152–68.
[12] Earle, *Making of Middle Class*, pp. 108, 118.   [13] Mui and Mui, *Shops*, pp. 38–41.
[14] E. Pawson, *Transport and Economy: The Turnpike Roads in Eighteenth Century Britain* (1977), pp. 137–40.
[15] Langford, *Commercial People*, pp. 449, 664.

patients who tended to do most of the travelling, whereas physicians or surgeons confined their journeys mainly to élite patients. This active pursuit of the medical consumer or patient by practitioners indicates their entrepreneurial orientation. Flexibility in relation to market opportunities was also shown by the way in which practitioners exploited the opportunities created by the very excesses of consumption, so that physicians such as Cheyne promoted a healthy regimen to counteract the high living of the affluent Georgian.

By the mid-eighteenth century three out of five men and two out of five women were literate. A more educated population might have been expected to increase medical custom, but whether a larger lay readership, a boom in Georgian advice books and a wider dissemination of information on health and sickness undercut or advanced the claims to expertise of doctors is uncertain.[16] Well-informed Georgian consumers showed marked scepticism about the remedies proferred by the medical 'profession' so that in many cases the household retained sovereignty as the consumer of its own physic. It also continued to patronise the medical fringe. In this competitive context at the end of the eighteenth and early nineteenth centuries there was a growing emphasis on professionalisation among physicians, surgeons and apothecaries. A significant part of its rationale was an attempt to restrict competition by demarcating the orthodox from the unorthodox. During the eighteenth century the decline and ineffectuality of licensing (whether ecclesiastical or by medical colleges) had contributed to vigorous competition in what historically was an unusually open market. The failure to establish a monopoly in medical practice for orthodox practitioners meant that empirics, quacks, and alternative practitioners competed successfully with them.

What was the impact on the medical market of industrialisation? From the late eighteenth century very rough estimates of national income are available. The period 1780–1820 covers not only the years of the industrial revolution, but the wars against France and an abnormal run of bad harvests, both contributing to an unprecedented rate of increase in prices, and over these years there was also an acceleration of population growth. Estimates suggest that money incomes per head of population during this period rose little more than prices, leaving little improvement in per capita real incomes.[17] Average real wages were rising at approximately the same slow rate, suggesting that these decades did not witness a significant redistribution of income from

[16] P. Laslett, *The World We Have Lost* (1983), pp. 132–3; R. Porter, ed., *The Popularization of Medicine* (1992), pp. 5–7, 33, 215–6.

[17] N. Crafts, *British Economic Growth during the Industrial Revolution* (1985).

workers to owners of land and capital. The net effect was thus that there was little or no change in the income available for the purchase of all medical services, although the rapid growth in population would have generated some increase in the size of the market.

In the remaining decades of the nineteenth century the position changed quite dramatically. From the 1830s there was a marked increase in national income per head (adjusted for changing prices). By the 1860s this series had expanded by over 50 per cent, and by the 1880s the level of average income was already about double what it had been in 1830s.[18] By the eve of the First World War there had been a further rise in real terms of some 60 per cent. The estimates of real wages rose broadly in line with this series for national income per head, again suggesting little change in the distribution of income between the main social classes. The steady advance in spending power revealed by these figures would gradually have raised more of the population over the threshold where they could afford to include in their occasional expenditure some contribution to the costs of medical treatment, and would further have increased the sums which the better-off could spend on doctors, and also on allied medical items. With the total population also expanding these trends implied a welcome and persistent rise in the potential demand for the services of the medical profession, even though this still only involved a minority of the population.

Offsetting this was the fact that, as Chapter 1 indicated, there was a continued inability by the profession to restrict its own numbers. A significant downward pressure on medical incomes resulted which was particularly acute for the GP during the second and fourth quarters of the nineteenth century, and at the beginning of the twentieth century, as Chapter 5 demonstrates. Open access to the profession led to acute competition at all levels. Thus, whilst publicity was increasingly frowned upon as commercial activity unbecoming to a profession, the importance Victorian surgeons or physicians attached both to publication and to honorary office in a medical institution hinted at their awareness that publicity was necessary to attract patients. In their attempts to shift the demand curve for their services upwards practitioners were aided by an English population which rose from five million to 34 million between 1721 and 1911. This meant that there was a pyramid-shaped age structure with a young population which had resulted from an increase in fertility (arising pre-

---

[18] Estimates by C. H. Feinstein in B. R. Mitchell, *Abstract of British Historical Statistics* (second edn, 1988), pp. 837–9.

dominantly from lower ages of marriage during the period from 1680 to 1820), and a birth rate which continued to rise until the 1870s. An expansion in medical practice in terms both of male midwifery and treatment of children's diseases was the obvious economic response to be expected if doctors were economically rational, and Chapter 9 analyses this development. This was also part of a Victorian trend to move into specialisms as a way of carving out new career possibilities in response to changing market opportunities.

Despite long term advances in real standards of living, only a restricted section of the population could afford to pay for the cost of their medical treatment. Even with a very exclusionist policy on admissions during the period of the industrial revolution, voluntary hospitals found that local demand outstripped their resources so that poor patients were turned away without treatment.[19] Chapter 8 indicates that medical altruism by individual doctors continued to be needed for poor patients. And a public system of free medical treatment that had flourished under the Old Poor Law continued to operate despite the economic retrenchments of the Poor Law Amendment Act of 1834. Indeed, the powerlessness of the medical profession to resist the imposition of local tendering for poor-law appointments during the early years of the New Poor Law suggests its own weak position in the market. A mid-nineteenth century changeover from pricing all kinds of medical treatment on the basis of medicines supplied, to pricing on the basis of services rendered to patients, is usually discussed in terms of the move from trade to profession. The economic rationale was to give doctors greater flexibility in pricing their services. However, attempts to introduce agreed price schedules for GPs at mid-century may also indicate that this very adaptability was leading to price competition and undercutting that was unwelcome to doctors.

At the end of the period a three-tier medical market was clearly operating. At the bottom was a group which obtained much of its care from the poor law, and the rest from a growing number of medical charities. These were the people who, in the late Victorian and Edwardian periods, would pay less than £10 house rental in cities, or £8 elsewhere, and who were excused the payment of poor rates because of poverty.[20] Despite increasing national wealth this was still over half the population. Earlier this bottom tier comprised up to two-thirds of

[19] C. Webster, 'The Crisis of the Hospitals during the Industrial Revolution', in E. G. Forbes, ed., *Proceedings of the XVth International Congress of the History of Science* (Edinburgh, 1977), p. 215.
[20] Poor Rate Assessment and Collection Act, 1869 (32 and 33 Vict. c41).

the population.[21] The middle group were those who, although better off economically, for the earlier part of our period paid medical fees infrequently, and then with difficulty. With increasing medical provision they could obtain some of their medical care through the free out-patient departments of voluntary hospitals or, alternatively, through subscriptions to clubs and friendly societies. This group included from one-eighth to one-quarter of tenants living in houses with rentals of £10 to £15 per year who were generally excluded from Victorian and Edwardian doctors' fee schedules which linked charges to income, and therefore to presumed ability to pay the practitioner. But this second group also extended into the lowest segment of patients in doctors' fee schedules – those in the £15 to £25 a year house rental category, who might be expected to pay fees, albeit small ones. The third and best defined group were the middle-class and upper-class patients who paid more substantial fees to the doctor. The fuller financial implications of this structure for practitioners' incomes are discussed in Chapters 5 and 6.

For the poorest part of the population the services of a practitioner were a matter of last resort to be reserved for cases of serious illness, or for more troublesome cases of childbirth. The poor law was the main source of medical help and it is significant that nearly three-quarters of cases of mid-nineteenth century pauperism concerned sickness.[22] Unfortunately, there is little surviving evidence from patients themselves of their independent attempts to finance the doctor's bill until the latter part of our period. However, it seems clear that doctors' bills took a long time to pay off, and might even involve pawning of possessions, whilst prolonged sickness could render even a comparatively well-to-do family quite destitute.[23] Practitioners' ledgers themselves indicate the difficulties that were experienced by showing the incidence of unpaid bills by working people, or through instalment systems of payment, particularly in cases of midwifery.

Official enquiries during the late nineteenth century indicated that expenditure on the doctor was not an item that was a matter for regular budgeting even by the better-off skilled aristocrats of labour who would have fallen into the middle band of our three-tier medical

---

[21] P. Colquhoun, *A Treatise on Indigence* (1806); G. King, *National and Political Observations and Conclusions upon the State and Condition of England* (1696); H. Perkin, *Origins of Modern English Society* (1969), pp. 20–1.

[22] A. Digby, *Pauper Palaces* (1978), p. 166.

[23] B. S. Rowntree and M. Kendall, *How the Labourer Lives* (1913), pp. 67, 115, 156; P. Johnson, *Saving and Spending. The Working Class Economy in Britain, 1870–1939* (Oxford, 1985), pp. 174, 206.

Table 2.1. *Medical expenditures of a working London cabinet maker,*
1850–1887

	Family income £–s–d	Medical expenditure £– s–d	Insurance incl. medical £– s–d
1855		6– 0–0	
1856		2– 0–0	
1857		2– 0–0	
1858		5–0	
1860		1– 1–6	
1861		1–12–6	
1862		– 5–6	
1864		4–11–2	
1867		1–19–0	
1874		1–11–6	
1875		1–19–0	
1883		15–0	
1886		1– 0–0	
Total	4781–0–0	25– 0–2	66–19–0
% of total income		0.5	1.9

Nots: The medical expenditure included nursing care in 1855, 1857 and 1861.
Source: Board of Trade Returns of Expenditure by Working Men, PP, 1889, LXXXIV,
p. 140.

market.[24] An enquiry by the Board of Trade in 1889 into long-term
expenditures by working men was instructive in this respect, even
though only 34 usable returns were received from 730 enquiries. The
returns indicated both a great variation in expenditures from year to
year, and the serious impact that illness had on family fortunes. A
London joiner, for example, earning good money of £80 p.a. lost five
weeks from sickness. (And, since time off work imposed an immediate
financial penalty this may be taken as a lower limit in interpreting
periods of sickness.) He incurred a doctor's bill of 3 guineas, wiping
out two years of savings. Table 2.1 shows the family medical expenditures from 1850 to 1887 of a cabinet maker, a labour aristocrat who
spent £25 on doctors, nurses and drugs and a further £67 on insurance.
Medical expenditures were incurred in only 13 out of the 38 years, but
on average amounted to only 0.5% of his annual income.

[24] *Report to the Board of Trade on British and Foreign Trade and Industrial Conditions*, PP
1903, Cd 1761, XVIII, pp. 209–258 gave data on the cost of food and cost of living of the
working classes in the U.K.

The time taken off work for sickness recorded in these Board of Trade returns accorded with the broader national experience of friendly societies and thus may perhaps be taken as fairly representative. The returns indicated that from one to two per cent of income only was usually spent on medical attendance, together with medical-related expenditures such as drugs, nursing care, and on contributions to insurance with friendly societies or clubs.[25] Significantly, more was spent on insurance contributions for sickness benefit from friendly societies and clubs than was spent directly on individual doctor's fees, although the former may well have benefited the doctor indirectly through the collective employment of a club doctor. (Interestingly, a later and more detailed survey for the years 1937–8 for working-class family expenditure gave a very similar result in finding that from one to three per cent went on medical expenditures, broadly defined as in the nineteenth-century return.)[26]

It is instructive to look at the top tier of the medical market. Although a few upper-class patients gave individual patronage to the physician, discussion of these is deferred to Chapters 6 and 7. Here we concentrate on the more substantial numbers of middle-class household budgets. Middle-class medical expenditures were rarely listed in manuals of household economy and when they were included they came into the budgetary afterthought or miscellaneous category. It is not surprising to find a well-known doctor lamenting that the public had a 'blameworthy' attitude to the medical profession. 'In calculating their annual expenses, many people do not reckon the cost of medical attendance [so] the doctor's bill comes on them with … [a] shock.'[27] In this context it is instructive to find that *A New System of Practical Domestic Economy* of 1830 listed medicine with entertainments and other incidents, whilst Walsh's popular *A Manual of Domestic Economy* of 1857 and 1879 included expenditure on illness with amusements and other residual items. The former expenditure comprised from 2.5% to 3.5% of expenditures in households with incomes from £150 to £750, whilst the latter rose from 5 per cent at £100 to 12.5 per cent of expenditure at an annual income of £1500.[28] In the expenditures of four professional single women published in 1898, *actual* spending on doctors and medicine amounted to between 0.7% and 2.3% on incomes

[25] *Board of Trade Returns of Expenditures by Working Men*, PP, 1889, Cd 5861, LXXXIV, pp. 100–2, 110.

[26] J. N.Nicholson, 'Variations in Working Class Expenditure', *Journal of the Royal Statistical Society*, (1949), p. 393.

[27] C. West, *The Profession of Medicine* (1896), p. 79.

[28] *A New System of Practical Domestic Economy* (1830) p. 434; J. H. Walsh, *A Manual of Domestic Economy* (1857 and 1879), pp. 606 and 677.

Table 2.2. *Middle-class medical expenditures and budgeting for 1898 and 1901*

	£ (i)	£ (ii)	£ (iii)	£ (iv)	£ (v)	£ (vi)	£ (vii)	£ (viii)
Annual Income	100	104	130	136	150	227	250	800
Medical Expenditures	2.0	0.7	0.9	3.1	3.0	2.5	3.0	30.0
% of income	2.0	0.7	0.7	2.3	2.0	1.1	1.2	3.8

Notes: 1 Columns (i) to (iv) and (vi) represent actual expenditures on the doctor and on medicine and columns (v), (vii) and (viii) recommended spending on the doctor.
2 Recommended medical expenditures for an income of £150 included those for dentist, chemist, charity etc so that my figure in columnn (v) assumes that one half of the total would go to the doctor.
Sources: C. E. Collett, 'The Expenditure of Middle Class Working Women', *Economic Journal*, VIII (1898), pp. 545–9; *Cornhill Magazine*, 83, 1901, April to May issues.

that ranged from £100 to £227 per annum.[29] These expenses, together with *recommended* budgeting for middle-class medical expenditures in 1901 are shown in Table 2.2.[30]

Table 2.2 indicates that under four per cent of middle-class expenditure went on the doctor and on medicine. (A later and more substantive enquiry into middle-class expenditure during 1938–9 gave a general confirmation of this order of magnitude by indicating total medical expenditures of 3.6% to 3.9% of income.)[31]

Since illness was unpredictable, there is abundant evidence to indicate that paying the medical costs incurred at these times was problematic. This was compounded by the fact that it was customary to send in the doctor's bill annually – well after the gratitude stimulated by the doctor's ministrations had waned. And there was evidence of patient resistance to the kind of bill that doctors used. An 'overwrought patient' wrote to *The Times* in 1878 asking why the practitioner

Never condescends to give me any items or dates on his bill, but fleeces me under the simple comprehensive heading 'Medical attendance'. If my tailor were to send in his account merely 'to clothes' I should have no scruple in

[29] C. E. Collett, 'The Expenditure of Middle Class Working Women', *Economic Journal*, VIII (1898), pp. 545–9.
[30] *Cornhill Magazine*, 83 (1901), January to July issues.
[31] Massey, '1360 British Middle-Class Households in 1938–9', *Journal of the Royal Statistical Society*, (1942).

having it out with him ... I cannot so treat my doctor ... If he would give me some details, were they only dates, he would greatly soothe.[32]

The medical profession's response was to suggest that motives of delicacy meant that it was 'in the interest of the patient rather than of the doctor'[33] to submit generalised accounts, in that the privacy of the patient-practitioner relationship might be endangered if too much information appeared on an itemised bill. However, there were other equally important matters pertaining to the doctor's self-interest: his self-perceived status as a member of a profession; the unpublicised custom of spreading costs so that the better-off patient effectively subsidised the less affluent; and the time involved in preparing more detailed accounts. *Punch* had earlier satirised the generalised bills of the medical profession and suggested what an itemised bill might look like![34]

--Esq

To------------------------------------, Surgeon, Apothecary etc

	£	s	d
Jan 13 To attending you at your own request at a distance of 5 miles	0	5	0
To listening for half an hour to a detail of your symptoms	0	4	2
To asking you to put out your tongue	0	1	0
To feeling your pulse	0	1	0
To inquiring whether you had slept well on the previous night	0	1	0
To replying in the negative, to your question whether oyster sauce was good for you?	0	6	8
To answer your question, Whether I considered you consumptive? by telling you to make your mind easy, for that your lungs were as sound as my own	0	6	8
To saying "Yes" when you inquired, Whether you were bilious	0	6	8
To telling you, in answer to your question, What I thought was the matter with you? "that you had got a common cold"	0	6	8
To recommending you to put your feet into warm water, and take a basin of hot gruel, going to bed	0	3	4
To calomel pill	0	0	6
To black dose	0	1	0
Total	2	3	9

[32] *BMJ*, 1878 (1), p. 57.
[33] *BMJ*, 1878, (1), p. 197.
[34] *Punch*, VI, 1844, p. 66.

With difficulties attached to fee income GPs sought appointments, especially the better-paid ones. Appointments were particularly associated with the middle and bottom tier of patients. The poorest patients on the lowest tier utilised charitable dispensaries, free outpatient departments in voluntary hospitals, and the facilities of the poor law – either the poor-law infirmary, or the services of the poor-law medical officer. The appointment of poor-law medical officer, although low-paid, was eagerly contested by local GPs. Doctors building up a practice were keen to become known through holding a public office, and well-established doctors would take a local office (however ill-paid), rather than see a stranger take it and begin to build up a competing practice.[35] As a result such salaries remained low. But the moans of the profession on this issue should not be taken at face value. For example, 'the work I do for a [poor-law] salary of £70 would bring me in £240 if charged at the ordinary fees of this district.'[36] Such public offices amongst the poor, if well done, allegedly led to practice opportunities amongst the better-off, although this probably occurred less frequently as the period advanced and class differentials sharpened.[37] It is arguable that of more importance financially was the hidden ancillary income from the performance of public vaccinations that compensated for the low formal salary of the poor-law doctor. And one also needs to remember that if such services had not been provided by collective means, the poorer members of society would have been unable as individuals to afford the services of a qualified practitioner. The 'charitable' offices of the doctor would then have received even less recompense.

The middle group of patients paid for their medical services less through individual fees than through subscription to friendly societies – thus providing for themselves mainly through collective action. This club or contract practice was an inflammatory issue for the medical practitioner, who disliked the collective muscle of consumers being used to force low rates of professional remuneration. Periodically, there were attempts by local associations of doctors to raise the payments received, of which the best known was that begun in the Midlands in 1868-9.[38] Moves to raise these payments from friendly societies had little permanent success since, in what by the late nineteenth century was an over-stocked profession, if one doctor refused a low-paid appointment another accepted.

---

[35] *BMJ*, 1892, (1), p. 795 and 1878, (1), p.470.   [36] *BMJ*, (11) 1907, p. 1095.
[37] Contrast *SC on Medical Relief*, PP, 1854, xii, Q 1568 with *RC on the Poor Laws and Relief of Distress*, PP, xl, Q 39391.
[38] *Lancet*, (1) 1868, pp. 17, 99, 202–3; *BMJ*, (1), 1868, p. 38.

Whilst clubs covered the breadwinners it was much less usual for them to do so for dependants. As a result a cheaper form of medical service was needed and the so-called 'sixpenny doctor' was the outcome. In 1907 the *BMJ* denounced the sixpenny practice as 'an attempt by underselling to obtain patients who cannot be obtained by merit.'[39] The proliferation of branch surgeries in large towns at the turn of the century showed the competitive nature of practice amongst this group of patients. So too did the bitter denunciations by the regular medical profession of the abuse of charitable provision by patients who, it was considered, could afford to pay for private attendance. For example, attendance at outpatient clinics in London hospitals increased by four-fifths between the 1860s and 1890s.[40] Also deeply resented were the 'pernicious profusion' of charitable agencies, the touting for custom by provident dispensaries in the midst of others practices, and the 'enormous abuse' of out-patients facilities at hospitals.[41] That there was such bitterness hints at the precariousness of some medical incomes and the diversity of status amongst GPs.

A revealing light was shed upon the heterogeneity of incomes by differential reactions within the medical profession to the National Insurance Act of 1911 with its new source of income for medical practitioners in the panel payments from insured working people. Those who had engaged in club practice considered that the higher insurance payments (seven shillings in comparison with from three to five shillings per head in clubs) were easily earned, that their incomes had benefited, and therefore thought favourably of the act.[42] (One disadvantage noted was that, in contrast to club practice, where a bottle of medicine was the desired outcome, under the new legislation an additional prescription was now required!) Those practitioners who were more socially established and financially secure had earlier been hostile to the so-called 'club' practice, and saw the panels as a continuation of this under a different name. They resented what they perceived to be the legislation's demeaning of the doctor's independence and professional status. Status was intimately related to educational attainment and to proficiency in practice.

---

[39] *BMJ*, (11), 1907, p. 480.

[40] G. Rivett. *The Development of the London Hospital System, 1823–1982* (Oxford, 1986), pp. 113, 140.

[41] *BMJ*, 1889, (11), pp. 900–1, letters from Hugh Woods, a 'Country Doctor' and a 'lover of the profession'.

[42] Special Inquiry by the *Lancet* in the autumn of 1913 and spring of 1914. See also B. B. Gilbert, *The Evolution of National Insurance in Great Britain* (1966), p. 438 and A. Digby and N. Bosanquet, 'Doctors and Patients in an Era of National Health Insurance and Private Practice', *Economic History Review*, second series, XLI (1989).

Education and later practice

During the eighteenth century surgeon-apothecaries entered medicine by apprenticeship, unlike physicians who laid claim to a book-centred university education. The benefits of apprenticeship in controlling entry (and thus reducing later competition) and guaranteeing competence outweighed, in Joan Lane's study, its alleged drawbacks in expense, inflexibility and lack of system, and thus ensured the system's survival into the nineteenth century.[43] An apprentice might promise, as the 14-year-old William Hey did in 1767 to his master, William Dawson, a surgeon-apothecary of Leeds, that for seven years:

> The said apprentice his said master well and faithfully shall serve, his secrets shall keep, his lawful commands shall do ... and the said William Dawson for and in consideration of the sum of thirty pounds of good and lawful money ... [promises to] teach, learn and inform his said apprentice ... in the arts trades or mysteries of an apothecary and a surgeon ... and shall also find, provide to and for his the said apprentice, sufficient and enough of meat drink and lodging.[44]

This kind of five- or seven-year apprenticeship might be supplemented by a later period spent walking the wards of a hospital in order to widen professional experience. Hey, for example, spent two years in London, with six months learning dissection, attending lectures in midwifery and medicine, and pupillage to William Bromfield at St George's Hospital. Hey's sojourn was much longer than that required for membership of the Company of Surgeons which at that time only required hospital experience of six months. Later, in 1813, it was increased to twelve months.

A system of apprenticeship was only as good as its personnel; in the hands of a conscientious master the apprentice did well. J. G. Crosse, later an eminent surgeon and an FRS, was the beneficiary of an efficient apprenticeship. He admired his old master. 'He was made up of affection and kindness ... my old, my earliest, my best instructor.'[45] This was Thomas Bayly, a Suffolk surgeon-apothecary, who had earlier studied under Percival Pott and Robert Young at St Bartholomew's Hospital. Crosse made careful observations of Bayly's work, and was not only interested in what he did and how he did it, but also

---

[43] J. Lane, 'The role of apprenticeship in eighteenth-century medical education in England', in Bynum and Porter, *William Hunter*, pp. 63, 100.

[44] Quoted in S. T. Anning and W. K. J. Walls, *A History of the Leeds School of Medicine* (Leeds, 1982), pp. 1–2. Hey was a founder of Leeds General Infirmary.

[45] Norfolk R. O., MS 476, Memoirs of J. G. Crosse, 21 October 1835. Crosse married Bayly's daughter.

in the reasons that informed his actions as a surgeon. Crosse observed a wide variety of surgery including the treatment of fractures, hernias, tumours and the performing of amputations, as well as the occasional lithotomy or autopsy.[46] In addition he had probably, like most apprentices, learned how to run the shop, keep the books, and make up the common medicines dispensed there. A century later a country doctor, J. Lynn Thomas, gave the same kinds of reasons for being 'always glad that ... I had the opportunity of witnessing operations which varied from arm-to-arm vaccination to amputation of the breast and ... removal of cataract ... Sometimes on wet days I was left at home to make pills and study pharmacy and pull out teeth on a few occasions.'[47]

Whether an apprenticeship was a useful way for an intending practitioner to spend time between the end of schooling and the start of an institutional medical education was debated during the first half of the nineteenth century. It was agreed that it gave a useful, broad experience of the practical realities of practice and an acquaintance with a range of patients unlikely to be encountered by walking the hospital wards. Indeed, the Apothecaries Act of 1815 strengthened the apprenticeship system since it required a five year apprenticeship for the licentiate's qualification – the LSA. This included formal courses in a variety of subjects, and six months of hospital practice, whilst the remainder was spent in the private practice of the master. But in the long run, the increasing demands of medical students' formal course-work undercut apprenticeship, whilst many thought it had become outmoded with a more efficient system of education in hospitals and medical schools. The outcome of this long-drawn-out debate was that apprenticeship was abolished by the Medical Act of 1858.[48] The act did not, however, end the practice of employing pupils, and a few prac-titioners continued to offer private pupillage until the end of the period.

During the eighteenth century, when apprenticeship was the norm, the more ambitious like William Hey would end their preparation for their chosen careers with a spell at a London hospital. The practical value of this experience was widely attested. Richard Kay recorded his satisfaction during 1746 when he studied under Benjamin Stead, the Apothecary to Guy's Hospital. 'Seldom a day but something remark-able happens', and 'the operations, [and] weekly anatomical lectures I

[46] Norfolk R. O., MS 5249, Crosse's descriptions and illustrations of Bayly's surgical cases. Thomas Bayly (1749–1834) practised in Stowmarket.
[47] *BMJ*, 25 July 1914, p. 170. [48] Loudon, *Medical Care*, pp. 176–80.

have here the opportunity of are very good and edifying.'[49] An assistant at the Westminster Hospital in 1786 stated that, 'the intention of
this diary is as a mirror to show me my transactions so that I may be
able to improve my time to the greatest advantage.'[50] Lettsom analysed the importance of his hospital training at St Thomas' where,
following a five-year apprenticeship under a Settle surgeon, he
became a surgeon's dresser. 'I continued to take notes of, and made
reflections upon what I saw, and thus acquired a method of investigation and decision, which ever afterwards proved of the highest use
in determining my medical conduct and practice.'[51]

By 1800 study at the University of Edinburgh was widely acknowledged to be the most prestigious medical training, with its useful
mixture of theoretical and practical instruction. Actual contact with
patients was not necessarily a prime consideration in students' selection of courses. Midwifery attracted only a small minority of the
student body, understandable perhaps since this was a low-status
option that was not required in order to graduate. But clinical medicine also recruited badly.[52] The utility of this second course may have
been more limited than its title suggests, as one frustrated student had
revealed earlier:

There is always such a crowd of students about the physician and surgeon,
that there is nothing either to be seen or heard, nor even a great deal of benefit
if both were to be had. A few superficial questions are asked and some
rudiments prescribed without saying why.[53]

This course was given at the Royal Infirmary, and the routine procedures performed on poor patients may also have reduced the
course's attractiveness, since one might speculate that the student
aspired to treat the rich. Adam Smith commented that, 'it is not so
much to extend their practice as to increase their fees, that they are
desirous of being made doctors.'[54] Additionally, despite an emphasis
by professors on the importance of clinical observation of patients,
students tended to prefer the clarity and simplicity of the printed

[49] W. Brockbank and F. Kenworthy, eds., *The Diary of Richard Kay, 1716–1751* (Chetham Society, vol. CVI, third series, Manchester,1968), pp. 70, 72.
[50] Wellcome MS 1856, Diary of Assistant Physician at the Westminster Hospital, 1786.
[51] Quoted in J. J. Abraham, *Lettsom, His Life and Times, Friends and Descendants* (1933), pp. 44–5.
[52] L. M. Rosner, *Medical Education in the Age of Improvement, Edinburgh Students and Apprentices, 1780–1826* (Edinburgh, 1991), pp. 53–6.
[53] Quoted in Rosner, *Medical Education*, p. 54 See also J. Langdon-Davies, *Westminster Hospital* (1952), pp. 110–13 for a similar view by a student of the inadequacies of clinical teaching in London in 1834.
[54] Adam Smith to William Cullen, 20 September 1774 in E. C. Mossner and I. S. Rose eds., *The Correspondence of Adam Smith* (Oxford, 1977), p. 175. I am grateful to Professor R. H. Campbell for this reference.

medical textbook to the ambiguities of symptomatic analysis. Both factors thus undercut the importance of the 'clinical gaze' that is often alleged to be a central feature of medical advances in this period, and which is discussed further in Chapter 3. The most popular courses, attracting more than three out of five students, were anatomy and surgery, chemistry, and medical practice. (The latter was a misleading title for what was a course in pathology and the nosology of disease.) All were correctly perceived as being central to successful later practice.[55]

At Edinburgh there had been some conflict of interest between the managers of the Infirmary, concerned to protect patients and thus restrict the access of medical students, and students who wanted to copy clinical notes and observe patients freely. The students argued against such restrictions in 1785, stating that 'The great object of a student's attendance at an infirmary is to examine the phenomena of diseases for himself and to see the method of treating the sick.'[56] In Georgian London not only the hospitals, but also the dispensaries and anatomy schools were important in medical education. William Hunter's famed Anatomy School, for example, pulled in large audiences to learn anatomy in the French manner, by dissection.[57] And the growing number of dispensaries also gave useful clinical instruction through lectures and visits to the homes of poor patients, although attempts to give more theoretical instruction in lectures were unsuccessful as students preferred those at hospitals.[58] By 1815 a transition was occurring at London hospitals in which pragmatism was giving way to a greater stress on underlying principles, and where there was a common core of instruction for intending GPs, surgeons and physicians. Pupils attempted to integrate the theory of the lectures to practical observation in the wards in discussing cases they had seen.[59] However, this close relationship between clinical teaching and ward visits was less well developed than in France.[60]

[55] Rosner, *Medical Education*, pp. 56–8, 67.
[56] Quoted in G. Risse, *Hospital Life in Enlightenment Scotland. Care and Teaching at the Royal Infirmary of Edinburgh* (Cambridge, 1986,), p. 248.
[57] R. Porter, 'William Hunter: a Surgeon and a Gentleman', in Bynum and Porter, *William Hunter*, pp. 22–3.
[58] Z. Cope, 'The influence of the Free Dispensaries upon Medical Education in Britain', *MH*, XIII (1969); J. E. Lane, 'Robert Willan', *Archives of Dermatology and Syphilology*, 13 (1926), p. 737; S. C. Lawrence, 'Private Enterprise and Public Interests: Medical Education and the Apothecaries Act, 1780–1825' in R. French and A. Wear, eds., *British Medicine in an Age of Reform* (1992), pp. 62–3.
[59] S.C. Lawrence, 'Science and Medicine at the London Hospitals: the Development of Teaching and Research, 1750–1815' (unpublished PhD thesis, University of Toronto, 1985), pp. 171, 179, 411–2.
[60] T. Hodgkin, *An Essay on Medical Education* (1828), pp. 17–8.

Paris was at this time a Mecca for graduate students from Britain and elsewhere, since clinical supremacy had passed from Great Britain to France. Not only Hodgkin, but Astley Cooper, J. Clark, Forbes, Farr, W. A. F. Brown and many others studied there.[61] The emergence of the Paris School after the French Revolution meant that medicine and surgery had become united in the medical school; a 'revolutionary school in the healing art'. Here practical training was to take on a new significance. Physicians had already begun to abandon their view that internal diseases were inherently unamenable to observation, and gradually replaced a speculative general pathology with exact observation and a localised pathology to decide upon the proximate causes of disease in the body. They learned to rely – rather as surgeons had done before them – on physical signs of damage and visualisation of local structural changes. Paris-trained clinicians thus had a 'pictorial-anatomical concept of disease'. The Paris school encouraged both physicians and surgeons to study pathological anatomy and experimental pathology. The consequent reorientation of medicine 'led to dramatic results in diagnosis and nosology.'[62] And, in unifying medicine and surgery, and thus instituting a common training, it also facilitated a growing domination of the medical market by trained personnel.[63]

Ascendant in the earlier years of formal medical education in Britain were the partial interests of students and faculty, but increasingly the public interest in medical education came to the fore. Adam Smith had suggested that a medical degree could be nothing but 'a mere piece of quackery' since it was not possible to guarantee the competence and good sense of those given such paper qualifications.[64] In his view medical education was a monopoly which needed to be eliminated in order to establish a free market.[65] His Georgian contemporary, William Cullen, had disagreed:

As the life and health of their fellow-creatures are so often entrusted to those practising medicine and depend so much upon their skill, it seems a matter of

[61] E.W. Ackernecht, *Medicine at the Paris Hospital, 1794–1848* (Baltimore, 1967), pp. 44, 192–3.
[62] T. Gelfand, *Professionalizing Modern Medicine. Paris Surgeons and Medical Science and Institutions in the 18th Century* (Westport. Connecticut, 1980), pp. 165, 178; O. Temski, 'The Role of Surgery in the Rise of Modern Medical Thought' *BHM*, 25 (1951), pp. 257–9.
[63] Gelfand, *Professionalizing Modern Medicine*, p. 189.
[64] Adam Smith to William Cullen, 20 September 1774 in Mossner and Rose eds., *Correspondence*, p. 177.
[65] J. Thomson, *An Account of the Life, Lectures and Writings of William Cullen*, MD (2 vols., Edinburgh, 1859), Vol. I, pp. 477–8.

no small importance for the public interest, that care should be taken to prevent any uneducated or unskilful persons from practising this art.[66]

Cullen's view was supported by a later Royal Commission which stated that, 'It does not appear to us that the principles applicable to a trade can with propriety be extended to the education of a country.'[67] But *laisser-faire* views were strong and the Medical Act of 1858 did not prohibit the practice of the unqualified, merely imposing penalties on those who were unqualified but who *falsely* pretended otherwise. It was assumed that 'if a statutory distinction was drawn between registered and unregistered practitioners the public would know how to protect itself against unqualified practitioners.'[68] And, despite the fact that professional development between 1815 and 1884 ensured that training had to take place in both surgery and medicine for the key qualifications in general practice of LSA (Licentiate of the Society of Apothecaries) and MRCS (Member of the Royal College of Surgeons), registered practitioners in 1858 had to be qualified in only one of them. It was not until the Amended Medical Act of 1885 that registered practitioners were legally obliged to have a dual qualification.

In line with this gradual growth in concern over the public interest came a need to ensure greater proficiency and hence a substantive growth in the medical curriculum during the second half of the nineteenth century. Intellectual developments meant that older subjects were subdivided, and new courses introduced. By the early twentieth century the laboratory and its inculcation of scientific skills was reinforcing and supplementing the traditional capabilities of bedside medicine in provincial medical schools.[69] At Sheffield Medical School, for example, developments in laboratory science were seen as the key to later consultancy practice.[70] Despite this, much criticism was directed at medical courses. Flexner wanted the clinical excellence of the British training informed by the scientific spirit then found in German medical education, so that practical training was infused by investigative science.[71] Trenchant criticisms also came from George Newman who considered that English medical education neglected preventive medicine, hygiene and public health; needed a more

---

[66] Thomson, *William Cullen*, I, p. 482.
[67] *Report of RC of Enquiry into Scottish Universities*, 1830, p. 12.
[68] *Report of RC on Medical Acts*, PP 1882, xxix, para 2.
[69] S. V. F. Butler, 'A Transformation in Training: the Formation of University Medical Faculties in Manchester, Leeds and Liverpool, 1820–1884', *MH*, 30 (1986), p. 131.
[70] S. Sturdy, 'The Political Economy of Scientific Medicine and Science: Education and the Transformation of Medical Practice in Sheffield, 1890–1922' *MH*, 36 (1992), p. 137.
[71] T. N. Bonner, 'Abraham Flexner as Critic of British and Continental Medical Education' *MH*, 33 (1989), p. 476.

intensive study of obstetrics and gynaecology and ignored a study of the initial stages of diseases that intending doctors would later find invaluable in practice.[72]

How medical students related their medical education to later practice is as yet unclear. Correspondence of practitioners with their erstwhile teachers suggests considerable respect and a strong sense of professional indebtedness. 'Tho' it is now twenty years since I had the happiness of listening to your instructions yet they have made such an impression on my mind', was a not atypical comment.[73] Whilst this source is by its nature likely to be biased both in selectivity and sentiment, it would be unwise to discount it entirely and, within the authoritarian ethos of medicine, to underestimate the intergenerational impact of teaching on practice. Contemporaries were clear that a formal medical education could only serve as a preliminary to a lifetime of further learning during practice. At the inauguration of the Leeds School of Medicine, Mr Teale, giving the presidential address, warned that 'so far from the act of receiving a diploma being considered the *completion* of your medical education you must regard it as being the very threshold – The whole life of a medical practitioner is one continued course of pupillage.'[74] Training increasingly focused on disease rather than on a Hippocratic view of a whole person in a given environment, and thus was of greater relevance to the creation of specialists than of GPs.[75] Social medicine – as practised by GPs in their later professional life – received decreasing emphasis, as doctors' training moved inexorably into its modern hospital setting.

The relationship of a medical education to a medical career was seen as not only a matter of intellect and practical experience, but as possessing an important social component as well. Obtaining a hospital appointment as the 'dresser' (assistant) of an eminent specialist was perceived as vital in securing later career prospects because of the force of private patronage. An élite medical education was also regarded not just as a technical training but one that prepared the

---

[72] Sir George Newman, *Some Notes on Medical Education*, PP 1918, Cd 9124, XIX, pp. 104–7, 114, 117, 150–3.

[73] RCPE, Cullen correpondence, Dr Clephan to William Cullen, 10 December 1779. This was one of many apparently very sincere professions of gratitude by Cullen's former pupils in his consultancy correspondence.

[74] Quoted in S. T. Anning and W. K. J. Walls, *A History of the Leeds School of Medicine* (Leeds, 1981), pp. 18–9. The speaker, T. P. Teale, lectured on anatomy, physiology and pathology, and gave the address in October, 1831.

[75] See, for example, the criticisms of the B. M. A. in BMA, *The Training of a Doctor. Report on the Medical Curriculum* (1948), paras 160–1, 340–59.

graduate to move in genteel society; a medical education at Edinburgh, Oxford or Cambridge opened doors to the wealthy patient. An appearance of gentility tended to reinforce medical authority, or alternatively to compensate for a lack of therapeutic success. It also reassured the patient that the practitioner had no overriding pecuniary interest in their treatment. In reality, the generality of medical men were not a learned profession in the sense of having had a good liberal education before acquiring their professional skills. In constructing a gentlemanly demeanour other means were therefore required and here the medical societies had a strategic role.[76]

Ethics and etiquette

In certain respects medical practice was an occupation rather than a profession, but did medicine have ethical components which differentiated it from other occupations? In an increasingly *laisser-faire* society in which earlier ethical considerations within a moral economy had been undercut, moral concerns of medicine might have become much more distinctive. However, the major discussion – Percival's *Medical Ethics*, of 1803 – confined itself mainly with intra-professional demarcation or medical etiquette, rather than standards of moral behaviour by doctor towards patient. Percival did suggest general guidelines in that the doctor should 'unite tenderness with steadiness' or 'condescension with authority' but there was little on specific issues.[77] In Percival's view difficult areas of medical etiquette were confined principally to the mode of conduct during consultations, where a seniority rule would ease the problem of reaching agreement. Rather than being concerned with safeguarding vulnerable patients, the thrust of the principal Georgian professional discussion of ethics was revealingly about regulating 'trade' within a bustling medical market. Within that market a vexed area of etiquette concerned relationships between surgeon and physician or, from the second half of the nineteenth century onwards, of consultants or specialists on the one hand and GPs on the other. Here the central issue was the undesirability of 'poaching' another practitioner's patient. Changing structures in the medical profession were one long-term explanation

[76] J. Rendall, 'The Influence of the Edinburgh Medical School on America in the Eighteenth Century', in R. G. W. Anderson and A. D. C. Simpson, eds., *The Early Years of the Edinburgh Medical School* (Edinburgh, 1976), p. 103; J. Jenkinson, 'The Role of Medical Societies in the Rise of the Scottish Medical Profession, 1730–1939', *SHM*, 4 (1991), p. 258.

[77] Quoted by I. Waddington, 'The development of medical ethics – a sociological analysis', *MH*, 19 (1975), p. 38.

of such disputes, but in the medium term were the result of an intensification of professional rivalries arising from growing competition in the medical market. From the second half of the nineteenth century these issues were increasingly dealt with away from the public gaze. As part of the process by which medicine became self-regulating disputes among medical personnel were seen as sensitive matters that should not be contested before a lay audience. This was intimately bound up with the attempt to increase medical expertise and authority. How effectively the profession safeguarded the public interest is doubtful, given the tiny numbers of those whom the General Medical Council found unfit to practise.[78] This concern with desirable privacy and confidentiality within a profession forms an intriguing counterpoint to the equal concern with undesirable secrecy in nostrums outside the profession, discussed below.

An interesting but little-noticed area in medical ethics and etiquette concerned the financial rewards that were appropriate for the practitioner. Here one may see a nascent profession grappling with the problems and tensions of a commercial society. Percival had warned that one issue in medical etiquette involved financial equity between practitioners. 'A wealthy physician should not give advice *gratis* to the affluent; because it is an injury to his professional brethren.'[79] More significant was the question of whether health was a commodity to be bought like any other, and whether doctors should be hustling capitalists or be influenced by a higher morality. The appropriateness of medical attendance, and hence the fees the practitioner charged the patient were thus of crucial importance. Percival's contemporary, John Gregory, warned that, 'The attendance given to a patient should be in proportion to the urgency and danger of his complaints ... But some delicacy is often required, to prevent such frequent visits as may be necessary, from being an additional expense upon the patient.'[80] Early Victorian medical students and practitioners were admonished by the eminent surgeon, Benjamin Brodie, that material reward formed, 'but a part, and a small part, of professional success' since otherwise an unworthy course of action might be pursued in which, 'you might be unscrupulous in your promises, undertaking to heal the incurable,

---

[78] For example, between 1881 and 1886 the numbers struck off each year varied between 0 and 5 (*Medical Register* (1886) p. 69.
[79] T. Percival, *Medical Ethics* (Manchester, 1803), p. 47.
[80] J. Gregory, *On the Duties and Qualifications of a Physician* (Second edn, 1820), p. 47. Gregory (1723–73) was Professor of Medicine at Aberdeen and then Professor of Physic at Edinburgh.

[and] making much of trifling complaints for your own profit.'[81] Aspirant doctors in the late-Victorian period were admonished that it was only 'unsatisfactory recruits' to medicine who saw it as 'neither more nor less than a means of earning a livelihood.'[82] It was acknowledged that practitioners owed their families a living, yet as members of more than a mere trade or occupation they had other (and by implication), higher responsibilities. Thus, by the end of the nineteenth century, Charles West could write confidently that, 'The duty of the practitioner is, first, to his patient; next, to his colleagues; and, lastly, to himself.'[83] Indeed, it is interesting to notice that one of the allegations against the National Health Insurance Scheme of 1911 was that it would make medicine into a mere money-making business, based on unscrupulous practitioners' attempts to maximise the number of patients on their insurance panels.[84]

That prescriptions about formal medical etiquette increasingly focused on the need for genteel rather than entrepreneurial behaviour is probably indicative of the ideal rather than real situation in which practitioners found themselves. In the earlier part of our period, advertisements for a practitioner's book might discreetly insert information about the author's practice, but by 1873 this was held by the Royal Colleges of Surgeons and Physicians to be below the dignity of the profession. In the same way, connections with money-making medical museums or pharmaceutical firms were frowned upon by élite bodies.[85] Self-promotion through advertising or the selling of medicine came to be seen as the attribute of the quack or those lower in status, such as the chemist. Thus, another important aspect of medical etiquette concerned the so-called 'secret remedies', which smacked of trade. In the late eighteenth century Monro outlined the orthodox view that, 'no man ought to be tempted by any view of private reputation or gain, to conceal what can be for the general benefit of mankind', whilst Percival argued that 'No physician or surgeon should dispense a secret *nostrum* ... if mystery alone give it value and importance, such craft implies either disgraceful ignorance or fraudulent avarice.'[86] The BMA was still holding to this line of argument during the early twentieth century, except that now these

---

[81] B. Brodie, *An Introductory Discourse on the Duties and Conduct of Medical Students and Practitioners* (1843), pp. 31–2. B. C. Brodie (1783–1863) was surgeon to Guy's Hospital and President of the Royal Society.

[82] J. de Styrap, *Practitioner* (1890), p. viii.

[83] C. West, *The Profession of Medicine* (1896), p. 21.

[84] *Lancet*, 4 July 1914, p. 64.   [85] Peterson, *Medical Profession*, pp. 252–4.

[86] *The Works of Alexander Monro, MD, published by his son Alexander Monro* (Edinburgh, 1781), p. 143; Percival, *Medical Ethics*, p. 45.

secret remedies were distanced from the profession and seen as the province of the quack. The stance over secret remedies of the *BMJ*, the official periodical of the BMA, was morally dubious, since although the BMA was loudly trumpeting its denunciation of these 'quack' remedies the journal continued to take lucrative advertising from the manufacturers of proprietary medicines until 1920, long after an equivalent journal – the *Journal of the American Medical Association* – had ceased to do so.[87]

Competition with the medical fringe

Quackery was inextricably bound up with secrecy; 'secret remedies' or nostrums were central to its entrepreneurial success. Secret remedies were criticised for hindering the advancement of medicine and encouraging the neglect of the known by enhancing the appeal of the unknown.[88] Yet the orthodox were not immune from this charge of secrecy. Buchan argued in his best-selling *Domestic Medicine* that,

No laws will ever be able to prevent quackery, as long as people believe that the quack is as honest a man, and as well-qualified as the physician ... the most effectual way to destroy quackery is to diffuse knowledge ... Did physicians write their prescriptions in the common language of the country, and explain their intentions to the patient, as far as he could understand them; it would enable him to know when the medicine had the intended effect; would inspire him with absolute confidence in the physician; and would make him dread and detest every man who pretended to cram a secret remedy down his throat.[89]

And regular medical practitioners in their dealings with each other (let alone with patients), were also accused of being less than open. In his lectures to Edinburgh medical students James Gregory indicted the Faculty for making assertions 'fabricated in the closet, with a view to establish some particular theory or remedy', and went on to argue against such practices since 'in clinical cases there is no room for quackery.'[90]

The previous chapter briefly discussed quackery in relation to the types of practitioner, and this one looks at it from the perspective of patients' relationships with practitioners. In the eyes of the profession

---

[87] P. W. J. Bartrip, *Mirror of Medicine. A History of the British Medical Journal* (Oxford, 1990), pp. 191, 198–9, 201.
[88] John Gregory, *On the Duties and Qualifications of a Physician* (second edn, 1820), p. 49.
[89] W. Buchan, *Domestic Medicine* (second edn, 1772).
[90] Wellcome MS 2596 Clinical Lectures by James Gregory.

patients' self-help was increasingly viewed as the real quackery.[91] Consumer independence was aided by self-help manuals: Wesley's *Primitive Physick* of 1747 and Buchan's *Domestic Medicine* of 1769 went through numerous editions. The empowerment of the patient reinforced an economic capacity to choose or reject an orthodox practitioner, and thus made so-called fringe or quack medicine its substitute or complement. In the Georgian age such 'quackery' was to a considerable extent assimilated within orthodox medicine, whereas by the Victorian age it became increasingly separated as alternative medicine.[92] The eighteenth century lacked the medical etiquette that later demarcated fringe from orthodoxy; what was proper or im-proper was still largely unformulated.

Members of the regular Faculty might warn against the risks involved in succumbing to quackery, but at the same time be fasci-nated by it and in the eighteenth century also be prepared to learn from it. Dr Richard Wilkes, a Wolverhampton physician, provided an apt instance of this. In 1739 he complacently retailed the sad story of a Coventry alderman, who took the nostrums of one of the Georgian age's most famous empirics – Mrs Stephens – but then died.[93] Wilkes's fascination continued, since three years later he again recounted a case of a Mr William Robins of Stafford who had spent more than one hundred pounds on Mrs Stephen's medicines, yet ended up being cut for the stone by a Bristol surgeon. Wilkes concluded 'I think it pretty evident that Mrs Stephen's medicines are not capable of dissolving the stone, but only of giving ease.'[94] Significantly, in relation to patient-power these cases cited by Wilkes showed patients employing both fringe and orthodox practitioners, and employing shrewdness in attempting to avoid the risks of lithotomy.

The extent of fringe medicine during our period is not known. Even the parliamentary *Report as to the Practice of Medicine and Surgery by Unqualified Persons in the UK* of 1910, was unable to quantify the numbers of practitioners, despite having the results of replies from Medical Officers of Health. Some found fringe practice decreasing and some increasing; in certain areas there was stated to be very little or

---

[91] M. Neve, 'Orthodoxy and Fringe: Medicine in Late Georgian Bristol', in Bynum and Porter, *Medical Fringe*, p. 44; S. W. F. Holloway, *Royal Pharmaceutical Society of Great Britain, 1841–1991. A Social and Political History* (1991), p. 61.

[92] R. Porter, 'The Language of Quackery', *Bulletin of the Society for the Social History of Medicine*, 33 (1983), p. 68.

[93] Wellcome MS 5006, Papers of Dr Richard Wilkes, fos. 18–19.

[94] Wellcome MS 5006, fos. 151–2.

none, whilst elsewhere it was large and increasing in extent.[95] Water casters, chemists, bonesetters, dentists, Christian Scientists, faith healers, herbalists, sellers of proprietary medicine, abortionists, old women and witches were amongst those surveyed. There were some tentative suggestions about the location of different types of practitioners: witches were said to be found only in outlying districts; wise women especially in rural areas; water casters retained their hold in the West Riding; abortionists flourished in the Midlands and the north of England; whilst bonesetters were still popular in northern mining areas. These tantalising glimpses reveal first that the consumer retained a variety of choice in what was a competitive market, and secondly that regional preferences differed. This second point is significant in relation to the regional doctor-patient ratios indicated in the previous chapter, where northern areas were seen to be less well provided for than the south. This suggests an interesting complementarity in the incidence of alternative and regular practitioners, although the dynamics are unclear in indicating which predetermined the other. (This also relates to the regionalisation in recourse to poor-law doctors where northerners were less prone to consult than southerners, indicated in Chapter 8.)

Where orthodox medicine was conspicuously unsuccessful in therapeutic terms, the patient might see the quack as at least no worse, whilst promising better. This was recognised by the regular practitioner as a basic cause of the success of the medical fringe. The Quaker physician, Dr Lettsom, in the course of his long tirades during the 1770s against the urine-caster,[96] Myersbach, in which he called him 'this adventurer, whose success in the chamber pot, has succeeded his own most sanguine hopes', nevertheless had to recognise that Myersbach's success was rooted in the regular Faculty's failures. 'When the skill of the best physician has been baffled by the obstinacy of some disease ... [and] When a man is disappointed of a hasty cure, he often flies to pretenders in physic.'[97] A Victorian doctor wrote with acute observation, if less sympathy of 'A desire to seek relief in medicine, a flying from one medical man to another ... and finally perhaps an

[95] *Report as to the Practice of Medicine and Surgery by Unqualified Persons*, PP 1910, xxxvii (Cmd 5422), p. 11.
[96] Water casting or conjuring was a popular form of diagnosis amongst fringe practitioners; they undertook to see what was medically wrong with clients through looking at their urine.
[97] Wellcome MSS 3246–8, J. C. Lettsom, 'Fugitive Pieces' (1776). See R. Porter, 'I think ye Both Quacks', in Bynum and Porter, *Medical Fringe* for a fuller account of this dispute.

entire surrender into the hands of a quack.'[98] Fields such as cancer, 'female complaints', venereal diseases, eye complaints, and consumption (TB) were profitable for those promoting medicine with the glibbest pen or tongue. At the end of the eighteenth century, the regular practitioner, Thomas Denman, was wise enough to see some good in this situation, although also inadvertently revealing the pressures this put upon the regular practitioner to promise more than could be delivered.

The credulity of patients renders them liable to the impositions of empirics ... If it be allowed, that regular practice despairs of giving assistance, when the disease is arrived at a certain state, ... empiricism ... may not only be permitted but encouraged, with the expectation of some casual good; and if, by the expenditure of money, hope, though of short duration, can be procured, the purchase is cheap at any rate. It is upon this principle that honest men are sometimes obliged to equivocate, or to promise more than they are able to perform.[99]

The Faculty was obliged to recognise reluctantly that quack or secret remedies could do good. After a crusade against secret nostrums the *BMJ* was forced to acknowledge in 1912 that, 'It would be folly to deny that quack medicines ever did good. It would be strange indeed if they did not sometimes, as for the most part they are made of materials in common use in medical practice.'[100] And instances of serious illnesses, cited at this time as being untreated because of a recourse to nostrums, revealed several – TB and cancer amongst them – where contemporary medical treatment could have had equally limited efficacy.[101]

Quackery had an appeal not only in therapeutic but also in economic terms; where expense limited access to orthodox medicine the door was pushed open to alternatives. Nostrums were a cheap and economical means to self-help by the putative patient. The quack reinforced this financial advantage with geographical and intellectual accessibility; itinerants brought their wares to the patient in a public market, whilst their handbills and newspaper advertisements spoke clearly to customers of cures for common afflictions. 'A fixed gout; dim eyes; asthma; the bile; the piles; a pain in the bowels; the scurvy; bad sore eyes; all are easily cured, and the small pox prevented.'[102] Quacks were skilful popular psychologists in so far as they exploited the desire for reassurance and privacy, advertising as 'the Private Medical

---

[98] A. B. Granville, *The Spas of England and Principal Sea-Bathing Places* (1841), vol. I, p. xxxiii.
[99] T. Denman, *An Introduction to the Practice of Midwifery* (second edn, 1794), p. 195. Denman was a Licentiate of the College of Physicians.
[100] *BMJ*, 13 July 1912.   [101] *Report as to the Practice by Unqualified Persons*, p. 20.
[102] L. James, *Print and the People, 1819–1851* (1976), p. 232.

Instructor', 'the Silent Friend', 'the Wife's Friend', or 'the Friend in Need'.[103] 'A Woman's Cure for Women's Ills' traded on women's reliance on female networks to advertise that 'Mrs Lydia E. Pinkham, was often called to help her neighbours and friends who suffered from the diseases and ailments of women', and was now making her expertise more generally available.[104] Those tormented with an affliction that they felt might bring shame upon themselves, such as impotence, venereal disease, or a pregnancy outside wedlock, were easy targets for these promises. Latent hypochondriacal tendencies were stirred into life by references to 'Nervous Debility', or 'Nervous Prostration' in advertisements for nerve tonics. 'Invigoroids', for example, targeted a substantial section of the population with its promises to help in cases of 'Back pains, brain fag, dejection, general weakness, head pains, hysteria, impotence, loss of flesh, lost vitality, nerve paralysis, nervous debility, senile decay, unnatural forebodings, weakness of generative organs.'[105] In many cases no great damage was done and some gain could occur, if only through a placebo effect, but in others the presence of noxious substances (opiates in infants' cordials was the most notorious instance) meant that actual harm resulted.

For the fringe practitioners skilful advertising was central to their success in attracting credulous consumers. Who could resist the collection of artefacts as testimonials that had been assembled at Mahomed's Baths in nineteenth-century Brighton, where crutches, club foot 'reformers', and spine stretchers hung on walls and apparently testified to the efficacy of the vapour baths and massage in curing disability?[106] When science was at a greater premium by the end of our period, the fringe adopted a scientific veneer in its claims. 'The remedy is declared to be the outcome of years of research in the laboratory.'[107] Fringe medicine might also appeal through the seductive simplicity of its monistic therapeutics: the water cure, for example, promised health in the mid-nineteenth century to those willing to bathe inside and out. And, a common ingredient in the appeal of the fringe to the prospective client, from the eighteenth to the twentieth century, was the testimonial or the example of esteemed clients. Joshua Ward, who promoted a strong antimonial pill and drops, (and left a large fortune when he died in 1761), had many famous patients, including George II, Lord Chesterfield and the novelist Fielding.[108] Others worked assiduously to get the recommendation of famous doctors in order to

103 Quoted in Rivington, *Profession*, p. 95.
104 BMA, *More Secret Remedies* (1912), p. 190.
105 BMA, *Remedies*, p. 51.   106 C. Musgrave, *Life in Brighton* (1970), pp. 203–4.
107 *BMJ*, 13 July 1912.
108 L. S. King, *The Medical World of the Eighteenth Century* (Chicago, 1958), pp. 51–2.

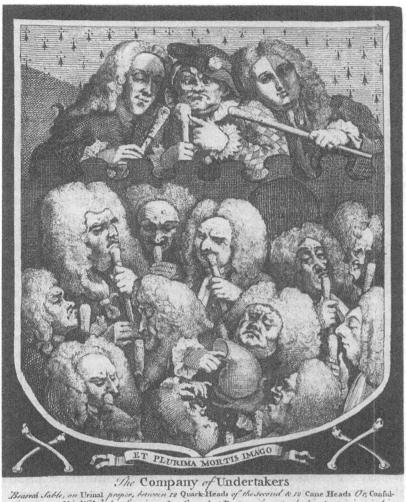

Plate 1   W. Hogarth, 'The Company of Undertakers' (1736)

promote their remedies. This was also true of those who did not see themselves as fringe practitioners, as in the case of the surgeon, Charles Broughton's promotion of his ointment, which was designed to combat cancerous tumours. He wrote letters to the Georgian consultant, Cullen, in an attempt to get Cullen's backing, 'I pride myself in adhering to plain facts and cultivating your confidence', and, 'I aim to make proselytes of respectable characters.'[109]

The activities of purveyors of proprietary medicines were not curtailed by government. Patent medicines were excluded from the Pharmacy Act of 1868 and the Sale of Food and Drugs Act of 1875. A Select Committee on the subject reported on the day that the First World War broke out, so that action was delayed for another twenty years. Equally, Parliament showed a reluctance to intervene to do more than guide democratic choice in the matter of the unqualified practitioner, through the creation of a *Medical Register* of the qualified in 1858. Promoters of patent medicines took advantage of this since they might add meaningless letters after their name, whilst some even used the presence of the government stamp on the medicine bottle's label to make it appear as an official authentication of its contents.[110]

Contemporaries were well aware that the medical profession was not immune from the deficiencies that it was highlighting among quacks, notably their partial therapeutic success. Hogarth's 'The Company of Undertakers' of 1736 depicted three famous 'quack' practitioners (Sarah Mapp, John Taylor, and Joshua Ward) in ironic juxtaposition with a group of physicians distinguished by their goldheaded canes. One of the latter is practising uroscopy – usually denounced by the regulars as the mark of the empiric 'piss-prophet'. (See Plate 1.) Proponents of alternatives, such as medical botany, were loud in their denunciations of orthodoxy which they termed medical despotism and which they alleged had led to a mystification of medicine that had weakened a more democratic system of care. In turn, the sceptical public perceived that both orthodox and fringe practitioners shared a concern to earn a living from medical practice, and hence that there existed a strong economic dimension of self-interest in the former's desire to limit competition. This must have acted powerfully to undermine the doctors' case. Equally, the members of the profession may have considered that alternative remedies and alternative practitioners undercut not only their incomes but, additionally, their pretensions to scientific authority over matters of health and sickness.

[109] RCPE, Cullen Correspondence 31/1, letter of 26 July 1774 and third letter (undated). Charles Broughton was a London surgeon (P. J. and R. V. Wallis, *Eighteenth Century Medics* (Newcastle on Tyne, 1988), p. 80).
[110] For example, BMA, *More Secret Remedies*, pp. 186–7.

3

Medical encounters

This chapter discusses medical encounters and focuses on the kinds of treatment doctors could offer patients. There are some problems in adopting this approach in the relatively meagre survival of archival evidence on rank and file – rather than élite – members of the medical profession. Also, the well-known drawback of prescriptive literature (of which medical teaching was a part) makes it is difficult to know to what extent admonitions were heeded in later practice. Some readers may also need to be persuaded that two centuries of medical treatment possessed sufficient thematic coherence to be treated as one period. To those whose view of the Georgian, Victorian and Edwardian periods is shaped by perceptions of the growth of scientific medicine, judgements may appear biased against the emergence of modern elements, and thus to over-emphasise continuity. However my research led to the conclusion that limitations on the scope of ordinary practice remained sufficiently strong for many traditional elements to survive into the modern era. The chapter broadly follows Shryock's interpretation that modern medicine did not suddenly arise in the 1870s, and that the gap between science and medical practice – more particularly general practice – remained wide until well into the twentieth century.[1] There were important scientific developments, notably in hospital-based surgery and in the development of germ theory, but therapeutics (i.e. the treatment of disease) changed much less dramatically than epistemology (i.e. the theory of the grounds of knowledge), so that the customary skills of bedside medicine remained important. The chapter begins, however, by surveying the framework of morbidity and mortality within which doctors practised.

[1] R. Shryock, *The Development of Modern Medicine* (second edn, New York, 1947), pp. 274–5, 314.

Morbidity and mortality

Improved mortality accounts for only one-third or less of the increase in English population between 1680 and 1820.[2] It is thus difficult to sustain earlier interpretations that medical advances of the eighteenth century, such as the opening of hospitals or the spread of inoculation, were significant overall since it now appears that these had no more than a limited and local impact.[3] The relative parts played by the medical profession, medical institutions, medical science, sanitary improvements, or by a more general improvement in living standards and thus more specifically by diet, have been contentious issues. Central to the debate has been McKeown's thesis that until the mid-twentieth century therapeutic medicine had relatively little to do with the decline in mortality, which resulted primarily from a 'silent revolution' in improved living standards from the late eighteenth century (arising from improved nutrition and hence improved resistance to disease), and secondarily from mid-nineteenth-century public health or environmental measures initiated by central government.[4] Subsequently more importance has been placed on public health measures, not so much those of the 'sanitary revolution' of the mid-nineteenth-century state, as on late-nineteenth century measures (1865–1914) at the local level.[5] Recent historical work on nutritional status (the state of the body as it balances food intakes against the demands made by growth, work and disease), suggests that in the second quarter of the nineteenth century rising real income did not lead to expected improvement in height, since its impact was offset by a poor mid-century disease environment.[6] Historians have also placed emphasis on the diversity of environments in which people lived and worked, with health being related to improvements not only in public hygiene – notably in water supply and sanitation – but in occupational

---

[2] E. A. Wrigley, 'The Growth of Population in Eighteenth Century England: A Conundrum Resolved, *Past and Present*, 98 (1983) p. 131.

[3] Compare the arguments in, for example, P. E. Razzell, 'Population Change in Eighteenth Century England: A Reinterpretation', *Economic History Review*, second series, XVIII (1965) and E. Sigsworth, 'A Provincial Hospital in the Eighteenth Centuries', *College of General Practitioners' Yorkshire Faculty Journal* (June 1966) with later work such as S. Cherry, 'The Hospitals and Population Growth', *Population Studies*, XXIV (1980) and Wrigley, 'Growth of Population'.

[4] T. McKeown, *The Modern Rise in Population* (New York, 1976).

[5] S. Szreter, 'The Importance of Social Intervention in Britain's Mortality Decline *c.* 1850–1914: a reinterpretation of the Role of Public Health', *SHM*, 1 (1988), pp. 1–38.

[6] R. Floud, K. Wachter and A. Gregory, *Height, Health and History. Nutritional Status in the United Kingdom* (Cambridge, 1990), p. 298; R. Floud, 'Standards of Living and Industrialisation' in A. Digby and C. H. Feinstein, eds., *New Directions in Economic and Social History* (1989), p. 128.

health where advances were much slower. Historically the occupational mix in the pre-industrial population differed substantially from that in the industrial one, so that health hazards altered during the eighteenth and nineteenth centuries. Advances in occupational health were slow since Victorian public health experts intervened where vested interests were least affected, and therefore preferred compensation to preventive health measures in the workplace.[7]

Historical gradients of mortality and morbidity are only partially explored. Pathbreaking work has indicated the intricacy of disease patterns in the eighteenth century, such that attention needs to be concentrated not only on a general mass of chronic, acute and epidemic diseases but on occupational-, age- and gender-specific illness, as well as on sickness influenced by distinctive ecological factors that was endemic to a particular geographical area.[8] Constructing an epidemiological pattern needs to take account of complex past demographic, climatic, social and experiential conditions that contributed to local variation. Seasonal fluctuations were important, with late summer peaks arising from enteric infection and late winter from airborne infections. These mortality peaks might occur differentially so that upland regions had spring peaks and marshland areas autumn and spring ones. Equally, the weather could impact on seasonality with varied results, not least in respect to age groups, since cold winters increased mortality for the old whereas hot summers did so for infants.

In years of mortality crises the death rate was more than forty per cent above the norm. During 1719–20 enteric fever (typhoid and dysentery) was prominent in the mortality peak; this followed a hot dry summer when it is likely that abnormal numbers of flies had bred in a poor sanitary environment and then contaminated food. During the 1720s the nutritional status of the English population came under strain in one of the most severe peaks of mortality. There was a probable connection between mortality peaks and poor harvest in 1728, as there was to be later in 1795. Dysentery and/or typhus was

---

[7] P. Weindling, 'Linking Self Help and Medical Science: the Social History of Occupational Health' in P. Weindling, ed., *The Social History of Occupational Health* (1985), p. 10.

[8] Wrigley and Schofield, *Population History*, pp. 670–92; M. Dobson, 'Population, Disease and Mortality in Southeast England, 1600–1800' (unpublished Oxford D.Phil thesis, 1982), pp. 283–295, 306; M. Dobson, 'Mortality Gradients and Disease Exchanges: Comparisons from Old England and Colonial America'; *Social History of Medicine*, 2 (1989), pp. 259–298; J. Walter, 'Famine, disease and crisis mortality in early modern society' in J. Walter and R. S. Schofield, *Famine, Disease and the Social Order in Early Modern Society* (Cambridge, 1989); J. Landers, 'Mortality and Metropolis: the case of London, 1625–1825', *Population Studies*, 41 (1987), pp. 72–5.

implicated in the 1741/2 peak of mortality, and it is possible that both an extremely hot summer and a poor harvest in 1741 contributed to a conjunction of poverty, hunger and disease. A major upsurge of mortality in southern England in 1780 was associated with fever but of an unknown variety. Given the indefinite nature of contemporary statements, retrospective diagnosis is highly problematic since fever might refer not only to typhus and typhoid but equally to malaria, influenza, relapsing fever, or scarlet fever. In mortality crises during 1831/2 and 1832/3 a succession of diseases were involved: diarrhoea (summer 1831), the first outbreak of cholera (summer and autumn 1832), and influenza (spring 1833).

Smallpox was a very important threat to health during the eighteenth century, but was endemic and not implicated in major peaks of mortality. It rarely struck the same person twice so that its targets were the young who had not yet acquired immunity. However, children had it in a relatively benign form so that even here it was not a major killer. Inoculation – introduced in the 1720s, popularised in an improved Suttonian form in the 1760s, and with parish initiatives in mass inoculation (later vaccination in the early nineteenth century) – diminished the threat of smallpox and therefore helped stabilise mortality. However, in south-west England and in Wales there were fierce epidemics from 1837 to 1840. Marsh fever or malaria continued endemically through most of the eighteenth century, and was the key variable in a sharp upward disease and mortality gradient in confined areas such as the Fens and Romney Marsh.

Crisis mortality was not universally experienced. Localities had their own rhythms of death and villages and towns a few miles apart might have diverse epidemiological experiences. Overall, the incidence of such local crises fell gently during the eighteenth century and sharply thereafter. Their occurrence was linked to geographical remoteness, which was progressively reduced by urbanisation and the growth of market towns during the eighteenth century. However, the concentration of larger populations in towns enhanced the possibility of disease, as did the impact of recent migrants who had not had the same exposure to endemic disease. Urban areas had more frequent and severe peaks of mortality than did rural ones, where only moderate increases in mortality occurred. Regionally, too, pre-industrial England had diverse experiences of crisis mortality, with the south-western counties worst off and south-eastern ones the most favoured. And within these patterns objective reality might be distorted by subjective appreciation of morbidity; for example, fevers were endemic and – particularly in the early eighteenth century – had a large impact on mortality peaks, yet attracted little comment from contemporaries.

With the beginning of civil registration in 1837 it becomes possible to analyse mortality patterns with greater confidence. Extensive migration from rural to urban areas had important consequences because of the gradients in mortality and morbidity between country and town. Urbanisation dramatically affected life chances: whereas one in five lived in towns in the early eighteenth century, three out of four did so two centuries later.[9] Life chances in large cities were poor whilst those in urban areas more generally were worse than those in small towns or in rural areas; regional and local variation therefore continued. During the 1860s, for example, expectation of life at birth was particularly good in country areas in the south and south-west of England, and particularly bad in urban, industrial areas in the northern counties of Lancashire and Yorkshire. What has been termed the 'urban penalty' had been particularly severe during the period of rapid industrialisation and urbanisation (*c.* 1750–1850), and one improvement in expectation of life towards the end of our period lay in the narrowing of the earlier gap between town and country. An intriguing – and as yet unexplained – difference also existed between areas in the east and west of the country with the former having relatively much higher mortality rates among infants than among adults. Complementing this attention to environmental influences, and thus to geographical variation in mortality, has been a concern by historians and demographers to tease out age-specific variations. It has been argued persuasively that certain age groups made a greater contribution than did others to the general decline in mortality. The importance of a cohort effect was evident in that from 1851 to 1901 this contribution was concentrated in children and young adults, whilst from 1901 to 1910 it was focused on those under one year old.[10]

Researching morbidity patterns in the past is even more complex than researching mortality patterns. The incomplete state of medical knowledge in the past makes historical statements on causes of death problematical. For example, typhus and typhoid were combined until 1869 in the Registrar General's statistics. Doctors' diagnoses were more symptomatically based than now, with powers of diagnosis so

9 R. Woods, 'The Effects of Population Redistribution on the Level of Mortality in Nineteenth centruy England and Wales', *Journal of Economic History*, XLV (1985), pp. 649–51.
10 R. Woods and P. R. Hinde, 'Mortality in Victorian England: Models and Patterns', *Journal of Interdisciplinary History*, XVIII (1987), pp. 39–41, 47.

imprecise that little confidence can be placed on their statements of cause of death in the certificates on which the Registrar General built up his returns. From these and other sources, however, a broad picture of the types of sickness that prevailed can be constructed for Victorian and Edwardian England. Infectious diseases that were spread through the air included: smallpox, diphtheria, respiratory tuberculosis, bronchitis, scarlet fever, pneumonia, measles, influenza and whooping cough. Those spread by water included typhoid, cholera, diarrhoea and dysentery. In addition there were a number of degenerative diseases such as heart disease and cancer, as well as a large residual category of unknowns. Four cholera outbreaks occurred between 1832 and 1866 whilst diphtheria was pandemic from the 1850s to the 1900s. The virulence of other diseases was subject to autonomous fluctuation: that of tuberculosis declined from the mid-nineteenth century onwards; conversely scarlet fever was in a very active form from the 1840s to the 1870s. Although the incidence of tuberculosis had halved during the second half of the nineteenth century, there had been a substantive increase in morbidity and mortality from 'flu, pneumonia and bronchitis. By the end of our period preventive health measures virtually eradicated cholera, typhoid and smallpox.[11]

Some evidence on morbidity is susceptible to quantitative analyis: first on an accurate basis from friendly society members' sickness records of the 1860s to 1890s; and secondly on a more limited basis from poor-law sources. Definitions of sickness in these two sources were distinctive but related; friendly societies defined sickness as inability to work whereas for the poor-law, although inability to work was central to relief for the able-bodied, relief in times of sickness was also given to other categories of individuals. In 1909 one-third of poor relief cases were stated to have arisen from sickness. Chronic sickness was particularly likely to be relieved by the poor-law authorities, with one-third of indoor cases and more than half of the outdoor cases.[12] However, the true extent of poor-law cases of sickness amongst certain groups was allegedly much larger. For example, three-fifths of men relieved under 50 years old were aided because of sickness. Where causes of medical treatment were concerned, one-quarter of cases were unclassified, with bronchitis and pneumonia the next most frequently treated category, followed by rheumatism and gout, pulmonary tuberculosis, heart disease, and ulcerated legs.[13] Chronic sick-

---

[11] S. Szreter, Mortality and Public Health, 1815–1914', *ReFRESH*, 14 (1992), pp. 2–3.
[12] *Majority Report*, 1909, Part 2, para 124.
[13] *Royal Commission on the Poor Laws*, PP 1910, LIII, pp. 543–5. This was a detailed return of 1907 that covered one in five unions.

ness was also of growing importance to friendly societies, with an increase from about one-quarter to one-third of their members' total sickness during the late nineteenth and early twentieth centuries. Friendly society records are invaluable in indicating the duration and frequency of sickness on an age-specific basis. Predictably, sickness expectation rose with age and there was an increasingly steep upward gradient in the duration of periods of sickness. The incidence of members experiencing sickness each year rose from one in five at 20 years of age to one in three by the age of 64. Sickness rates varied from up to one week per year for young adults before the age of 35, to a period of up to two weeks for the 35 to 55 year old range, and thereafter from two to four weeks until the age of 60.[14]

Overall, this evidence suggests that the incidence of sickness was somewhat less than the two to three weeks a year that the British Medical Association estimated to be necessary for each person insured, in their 1905 survey of contract (club) practice, and may therefore be taken as a lower limit.[15] These data on the extent of morbidity are problematical, however, in indicating that at a time when mortality was declining in the population at large, morbidity – as shown by members of friendly societies – was actually increasing. An interesting hypothesis suggests that what was occurring was the result of what is termed 'insult accumulation'. Susceptibility to disease might be related to past sickness; the earlier mortality decline had resulted in high-risk individuals surviving death, but being prone later to experience non-fatal diseases or other 'insults'.[16]

What impact did the endeavours of the medical profession make upon this complex pattern of morbidity and mortality? Medical expertise and theories of disease helped establish a case for an interventionist public health policy.[17] Medical interventions occurred in public health in four main ways: through the profession acting as a pressure group for health reforms (as in the *Lancet*'s campaign on poor-law sickness provision during the middle of the 1860s); through actions of individual doctors (for example, John Snow's work on the water-borne spread of cholera); through work as medical statisticians and demographers (for example, the Registrar General, William Farr);

[14] *RC on Poor Laws*, 1910, LIII, p. 851, 855 (evidence of F. G. P. Neison). See also, *Insurance Monitor*, March 1885, p. 125; *Insurance Age*, May 1896; *BMJ*, 13 August 1910, p. 391. It is important to appreciate that these are aggregate figures based on late-nineteenth-century figures from several societies.

[15] *BMJ* 13 August 1910, p. 391.

[16] G. Altier and J. C. Riley, 'Frailty, Sickness and Death: Models of Morbidity and Mortality in Historical Populations', *Population Studies*, 43 (1989), pp. 25–45.

[17] J. M. Eyler, *Victorian Social Medicine* (Baltimore, 1979), p. 198.

and through medical research and teaching.[18] In addition, a few medical advances had an important impact on both mortality and morbidity: smallpox inoculation and vaccination were for a long time the only elements here, but were joined at the turn of the twentieth century by other advances such as diphtheria antitoxin, insulin for diabetes, and liver extract for pernicious anaemia.[19] In the context of curative relationships between practitioners and their individual patients it would be useful to find a correlation between mortality and the ratios of doctors to population. As yet, there has been little testing of this hypothesis, although one study for England and Wales in 1861 found no statistically significant relationship.[20] However, because an effect is immeasurable in terms of mortality does not necessarily mean that doctors' efforts were unimportant in relation to morbidity. Until more is known of distinctive historical patterns of morbidity it is difficult to prove that doctors had a positive impact on health. A more accurate appreciation of the extent of untreated sickness is also an obvious precondition for any evaluation of the doctor's effectiveness. A large – though unquantifiable – amount of sickness went untreated by doctors; an informed contemporary estimate in 1910 put this as 'plainly enormous'.[21]

Did evolving patterns of morbidity and mortality cause changes in medical practice and medical income? For example, did success in curing acute and infectious diseases result in more chronic illness in an ageing population? A related area that is central to any attempt to answer this formidably difficult question is illness behaviour. By this is meant the varied ways in which people respond to their physical and/or mental state; perceiving it in some circumstances as an illness which may (or equally may not), need attention from a professional. Self-assessment, physical morbidity and psychological states influence decisions to become a patient. But the doctor's expectations about how the individual has made sense of the 'illness' do not necessarily match the historical situation. Was health perceived as merely an interval between sickness, or sickness a rare episode in a healthy life? Was a patient's self-perception that of being more- or less-well, when the doctor's diagnosis was one of serious malfunction and disease? His-

[18] R. Woods, 'Public Health and Public Hygiene: The Urban Environment in the Late Nineteenth and Early Twentieth Centuries', in in R. Schofield, D. Rehur, and A. Bideau eds., *The Decline of Mortality in Europe* (Oxford, 1991), pp. 244–5.

[19] S. J. Kunitz, 'The Personal Physician and the Decline of Mortality in the Late Nineteenth and Early Twentieth Centuries', in Schofield, Rehur, and Bideau, *The Decline of Mortality*, p. 255.

[20] Woods and Hinde, 'Victorian Mortality', pp. 50–1.

[21] S. and B. Webb, *The State and the Doctor* (1910), p. 246.

torically, expectations of health in the population as a whole may have risen so that the illness threshold has been lowered. Conditions earlier accepted stoically as part of, for instance, the menopause or old age, and hence untreated in the past may later be redefined as illnesses needing treatment. Financial incentives to adopt sick-roles were much less powerful than they have since become, but they may have been important at the margin in friendly society cases. Thus, in what is as yet a poorly conceptualised and under-researched subject, cultural contexts, socio-economic resources and individual needs may all have shaped perceptions of illness and decisions to seek treatment from the doctor.[22]

Social and clinical skills

In deciding whether to seek medical treatment the social personality of the doctor was one significant variable. Resourcefulness, adaptability, commonsense, and mental and physical resilience were amongst the vital qualities necessary to sustain a successful practice. Patience, sensitivity, and sympathy were necessary qualities in gaining insight into the patient's condition when taking a case history and listening to the patient's account of symptoms experienced and pains endured. In diagnosis the importance of clinical instinct was acknowledged; an unconscious process that informed a conscious application of the lessons of past experience. And sound clinical judgement needed to be backed up by other, more personal, attributes if a practitioner was to obtain the confidence of a patient. Decisiveness in making judgements, authority in imposing the treatment, and practical competence in adopting procedures, contributed to a professional 'presence' that induced trust in the patient. Since their therapeutic impotence in the face of many diseases remained, practitioners continued to need good personal qualities to retain the faith of patients; they sustained constitutions and relieved symptoms rather than administering a rapid 'magic bullet' having instant success.

The significance of a good bedside manner was recognised by other doctors as being particularly important in creating a practice among more affluent patients. Dr H. L. Thomas, who was a popular practitioner with the middle classes in London during the first half of the nineteenth century was praised for having had an elegant appearance. He habitually wore the 'black dress-coat, waistcoat and trousers,

---

[22] Editorial on 'The concept of illness behaviour: culture, situation and personal predisposition', *Psychological Medicine*, 16 (1986), pp. 1–2.

black silk stockings and pumps, and a spotless white cravat' of the traditional physician. Moreover, he was said to be 'perfect in the sickroom; cool, attentive and kind.' Effective too, in a more low-key way was Dr Pinckard of Bloomsbury Square, whose 'common-sense expression of face ... at once inspired the patient with confidence.'[23] Getting on with patients and putting people at ease in the sick room were seen as vital ingredients in building up a successful domiciliary practice. Dr Belcombe, with a mid-century practice in York, for instance, had 'that sort of open and affable manner which is calculated to win the confidence of patients.'[24] But his Exeter colleague, John Haddy James, was criticised for bringing a 'military discipline into the sick-chamber where he was feared and obeyed.'[25] And Dr Vincent of Lincoln's Inn Fields was less successful than his brethren since 'he was a minute and careful observer; but he wanted manner. He failed to inspire his patient.'[26] How did practitioners develop a desirable professional presence? Georgian practitioners, if of humble origin, acquired these public *personae* through adopting the manners of the gentry, perhaps studying general advice books in order to learn the rules of polite society, and thus polish off their rough edges. But those who entered the more competitive medical market in the late nineteenth century might study a specialist, professional handbook to develop the appropriate manner for a doctor. The young practitioner was told that 'There is an art ... in making the necessary examination, giving instructions, and then departing with a cheerful, self-satisfied demeanour that inspires confidence on the part of the patient and his friends.'[27]

Central to doctors' tasks were history-taking and diagnosis. The Georgian medical student was taught at the University of Edinburgh that the patient's testimony should be looked upon with a degree of scepticism. Cullen advised that 'From the patient's expression of his own feelings, and these from ignorance of language, and other causes are very uncertain ... our judgement of diseases ... is upon a very precarious footing.'[28] Orthodoxy continued to insist on the problem-

[23] J. F. Clarke, *Autobiographical Recollections* (1874), pp. 114, 120, 123.

[24] Granville, *Spas*, I, p. 145. H. S. Belcombe, a Quaker, was the son of the physician, W. Belcombe, and succeeded him as Visiting Physician to the York Retreat (A. Digby, *Madness, Morality and Medicine* (Cambridge, 1985), p. 52).

[25] Haddy James (1788–1869) was Surgeon to the Devon and Exeter Hospital (Plarr, vol. I, pp. 605–6).

[26] Clarke, *Recollections* (1874), p. 123.   [27] de Styrap, *Practitioner*, pp. 29–30.

[28] Brotherton Library, University of Leeds, MS 566, Mr James Tatham's Notes on William Cullen's Lectures, 1772–3. Tatham became a successful Leeds surgeon-apothecary (*Eighteenth-Century Medics*, p. 584).

atical nature of these activities. James Russell, later Physician to the General Hospital in Birmingham, wrote in 1853 that 'Much has to be taken on the testimony of our patient, and is disguised by his limited capacity for such observations ... The consequence is that we are frequently compelled to act upon probable evidence.'[29] The warnings about poor patients were even more forthright. James Gregory stated that 'The patient is often willing to deceive us, and one who has not been used to practice cannot readily detect him. In such cases we are often obliged to cross question him, as a judge would do a witness or a criminal.'[30] Thus, an additional element in making a diagnosis, although this did not receive explicit acknowlededment, was social class. A good medical education inculcated set procedures for making a diagnosis. Lettsom wrote during the late eighteenth century of how

I devoted my time incessantly to the hospital and the lectures which London afforded. As a small gratuity admitted me to see the books of the physicians, and to acompany them round the wards, I embraced as many opportunities as I possibly could ... In the morning early, before attendance was given I normally viewed many select patients, took down the symptoms and afterwards compared the recipes ordered by the physicians.[31]

In hospital practice there was a new emphasis on a systematic physical examination of the patient.[32] James Gregory demanded of his Edinburgh students that they attended to 'the causes of the disease, unusual and accidental symptoms, external appearances, state of the pulse, state of the skin, respiration, sleep, the different excretions, and the menstrual discharge in women.' And his own late eighteenth century cases at the Edinburgh Infirmary precisely illustrated these points.[33]

Diagnosis in Georgian and early Victorian private practice was based on a whole-person, symptomatic approach that was empirically rather than theoretically based.[34] The patient's physique as well as

---

[29] J. Russell, *The Character and Claims of the Medical Profession* (Birmingham, 1853), p. 19. James Russell (1818–85), was first Senior Physician to the General Dispensary and later General Physician to the General Hospital, Birmingham.

[30] Wellcome MS 2596, Clinical Lectures on Patients in the Royal Infirmary delivered in the University of Edinburgh by James Gregory, MD, 1783–4, fos. 4–5. James Gregory (1753–1821), the son of John Gregory, was a successful university teacher, and the author of the widely-read *Conspectus Medicinae*.

[31] Wellcome MS 3245, Lettsom Autobiographical fragment, ND. Lettsom (1744–1815) was a founder of the London Medical Society and of the Royal Seabathing Hospital, Margate.

[32] C. Newman, 'Diagnostic Investigation before Laennec', *MH*, 4 (1960), p. 328.

[33] Wellcome MS 2596, Clinical Lectures, fo. 11; RCPE, MS 4, James Gregory's Clinical Cases at the Royal Infirmary, Edinburgh, 1780–1.

[34] King, *Medical World*, p. 315.

factors in the environment – such as the weather – were acknowledged as being important in sickness, so that making a diagnosis was
a unique response to individual circumstances and not a routine
activity. Significantly for James Gregory, 'diseases are not substances
whose natures are perfect, permanent and uniform but differing
according to circumstances in the age, habit, or life of the patient.'[35]
Further, according to William Hey II, the Leeds surgeon, 'we are not
only to consider what will cure the specific diseases but also what will
best agree with our patients.'[36] The doctor's five senses, the accumulated insight of experience, and – at times – a dash of intuition or
inspired guesswork, were crucial in making a diagnosis. It was also
important for the practitioner's credibility that – whilst the diagnosis
was sufficiently sober to appear a realistic response to the case – the
prognosis still left enough hope to be reassuring to patients, relatives
and friends.

Traditionally, therapeutics had been individually based and
informed by humoralist perceptions. The four elements of fire, air,
earth and water embodied equivalent hot, cold, dry and moist qualities; food containing these elements then turned into bodily juices or
humours, blood, phlegm, yellow bile and black bile. An imbalance of
the humours in the body meant dis-ease or sickness, which the doctor
then remedied by appropriate counter-balances, warming, cooling or
purging the bodily system.[37] This Galenic tradition – informing concepts of health – still had life left in it during the Georgian, and to a
much more limited extent, the early Victorian age. Hence there was a
reliance on the one hand on regular emetics and purges to clean out
stomach and bowel, and on the other hand on bleeding by lancet,
cupping or leeches, thus purging the system of its impurities and
restoring a healthy equilibrium in bodily fluids.[38]

Another major element in practice was prescription. Most practitioners had a pecuniary interest here in that before the mid-
nineteenth century their remuneration was based to a significant
extent on payment for medicines. Georgian surgeon-apothecaries

[35] RCPE, MS/7, James Gregory's Lectures in Medicine, c. 1805; Wellcome MS 2598, James
Gregory's Lectures on the Practice of Physic, fos. 5–6.
[36] Brotherton Library, University of Leeds, MS 560, Medical Notes (1796). William Hey
the Second (1772–1844), part of a Leeds medical dynasty, became Surgeon of the
Leeds Infirmary, of which his father, William Hey I, had been a founder.
[37] O. Temkin, Galenism. The Rise And Decline Of A Medical Philosophy (Ithaca, 1973),
pp. 17, 179; L. J. Rather, 'The)Six Things Non-Natural: A Note on the Origins and
Fate of a Doctrine and a Phrase', Clio Medica, 3 (1968) pp. 337–47; L. S. King, 'George
Cheyne, Man of Eighteenth Century Medicine', BHM, 48 (1974), p. 536.
[38] See, for example, G. Cheyne, An Essay on Regimen (second edn, 1740), pp. v-vi; The
Medical Works of Richard Mead (Dublin, 1767).

were knowledgeable in the use of a growing range of medicaments. They made up mixtures into liquid medicines (electuaries, draughts, elixirs, tinctures and juleps), and manufactured large pills known as boluses or later rolled the small pills that replaced them. To patients complicated medication might seem to be a visible sign of apparent expertise; a perceived advance on the herbal simples that were available in their own household. The doctor's prescription thus appeared to underwrite the individual nature of the therapeutic intervention which had been skilfully adjusted by the doctor to the unique circumstances of the sufferer. The mixture, the dose, the interval at which it was taken, and the panoply of instructions as to regimen, all exhibited professional power. And besides the large – though diminishing – amount of dross contained in contemporary pharmacopoeias, there were very effective drugs coming into widespread use during the eighteenth century: bark (quinine) for reducing fevers, opiates for painkilling and use as a sedative, and digitalis which was deployed as a diuretic in the treatment of dropsy.[39] These were powerful weapons and conferred added mystique. Moreover, these drugs in themselves might also add to the vast amounts of medication consumed, since their side-effects had to be offset by yet more prescriptions; opiates, for example, led to costiveness which in turn led to purging doses of calomel. Georgian patients' desire for physic was seemingly inexhaustible; in an increasingly consumer age health came to be seen as a commodity, and drugs were a convenient way to purchase it. By the beginning of the nineteenth century an underlying scepticism, if not lay disillusionment about the heroic scale of dosing emerged, as Gillray, Rowlandson and Gillray graphically suggested. Even the perceived unpleasantness of physic (see Plate 2.) did not necessarily produce satisfaction. Not that this necessarily impeded the medical profession's practice of using many drugs as was the case in the Bristol Infirmary.[40]

To expect an individualised and complex prescription for every case undertaken was unrealistic so that in practice if not theory, resort to routine prescriptions was common. Cadogan wrote deprecatingly in 1771 of the 'precarious skill of prescribing doctors.'[41] Institutions such

---

[39] J. K. Crellin and J. R. Scott, 'Pharmaceutical History and its Sources in the Wellcome Collections, II, Fluid Medicines', *MH*, xiv (1970), p. 132; A. Rook, 'General Practice, 1793–1803. Transactions of a Huntingdonshire Medical Society', *MH*, 4 (1960), pp. 344–5.

[40] H. Alford, 'The Bristol Infirmary in my Student Days, 1822–1828', *Bristol Medical and Chirurgical Journal*, September 1890.

[41] J. Rendle-Short, 'William Cadogan, Eighteenth Century Physician', *MH*, 4 (1960), pp. 288–309.

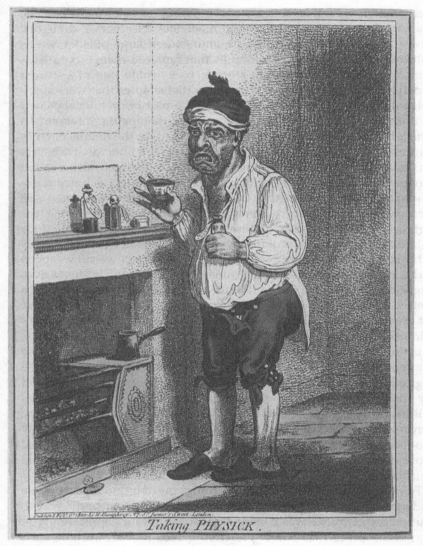

Plate 2   J. Gillray, 'Taking Physick' (1800)

as asylums were notorious for their routine medication whilst practitioners in private practice were not immune from the same failing. During the mid-nineteenth century Dr Darling of Russell Square, London, was described as being 'of the old school of blue pill and black draught, and treated most cases as bilious.'[42] A rather different set of circumstances might produce a similar outcome: fashionable early-Victorian doctors who pinned their reputation to one class of remedies, and attracted affluent patients with chronic conditions who sought relief in apparent infallibility, having tired of the constant variety earlier inflicted on them.[43] And, at the end of the nineteenth century the 'sixpenny doctors' practising in the poorest areas were criticised for an unthinking prescription of standard bottles of coloured medication.[44]

If pills for ills offered both comfort to the eighteenth-century patient, and a measure of prosperity for the practitioner, the same was equally evident in the range of surgical procedures. Percival Pott, the famed senior surgeon at St Bartholomew's Hospital lectured his students in the mid-eighteenth century as to the necessity of a surgeon possessing 'a competent knowledge of the anatomical structure of the human body, a close attention to the symptoms of diseases in the living, and a minute examination of the appearances of the dead.'[45] For the surgeon treatments ranged from the simple (such as bleeding, setting a broken bone, or opening abcesses), to more complicated interventions (amputation of a limb after a complex fracture, treatment of gunshot wounds, tapping for dropsy, and couching for a cataract). The more ambitious operator might cut for the stone (lithotomy), excise a cancerous breast (mastectomy), or undertake trepanning.[46] In viewing the Lancashire practice of his father the young Richard Kay commented that the variety of cases that a busy Georgian surgeon-apothecary encountered made professional life very taxing.[47] Not only were patients individuals but, precisely because of this, it was assumed that their surgical conditions were also differentiated.

Major surgery tended to be a matter of last rather than first resort for both surgeon and patient until the mid-nineteenth century. Patients were very reluctant to undergo surgery in an era without anaesthesia. Richard Snape deferred an amputation of the arm in 1759.

---

[42] For example, that given in the York Asylum by Dr A. Hunter (Digby, *Madness, Morality and Medicine*, p. 11); Clarke, *Recollections*, p. 123.

[43] Granville, *Spas*, II, p. 248.

[44] *BMJ*, ii, 1907, p. 480; A. Cox, *Among the Doctors* (1950), pp. 22–3.

[45] Wellcome MS 3958, Lectures on the Practice of Surgery by Percival Pott, taken down by J. Grigg, surgeon. Percival Pott (1714–88), MCS, FRS, was Surgeon to St Bartholomew's Hospital. This may have been J. Grigg (b. 1765) who later practised as a surgeon in Bath. (*Eighteenth-Century Medics*, p. 247).

[46] See A. Batty Shaw, 'Benjamin Gooch, Eighteenth-Century Surgeon' *MH*, xvi (1972), pp. 40–50 for an interesting account of the work of an able Georgian country surgeon.

[47] Brocklebank and Kenworthy, *Richard Kay*, pp. 63–4, entry for 27 June 1743.

'He would not consent to the operation till he is now in a very weak condition.'[48] Like patients, surgeons dreaded operations and William Cheselden stated that 'no one ever endured more anxiety and sickness before an operation.'[49] Many operations were undertaken reluctantly by the surgeon. Take, for example, a case of a strangulated scrotal hernia in 1785:

August 26 The operation was deferred as the surgeons did not think the symptoms sufficiently warranted the operation. An opiate was given. August 27 The surgeons saw him again in the morning and thought they could not with propriety operate ... In the evening he became considerably worse ... After making another fruitless attempt to reduce the hernia the operation was performed.[50]

When operations were performed on poor patients, and thus took place in the noxious atmosphere of a hospital, there were added anxieties. 'The termination of this case was considered as remarkably fortunate, for in this great and crowded hospital, it rarely happens that a compound fracture does well, or at best, not until after a tedious suppuration', wrote a surgical observer in St Bartholomew's Hospital at the beginning of the nineteenth century.[51]

Especially in the early part of our period medical limitations in the face of difficult disorders might lead to invocations of Providence. Disease could be seen as the punishment for sin, and good health be seen as God's work.[52] John Wesley expressed this well in his *Primitive Physic*. 'Above all, add to the rest (for it is not labour lost) that old unfashionable medicine, Prayer.'[53] The chaplain or priest thus played a vital role in the final moments of the patient, 'As her distemper has baffled all medical skill and assistance all we can do is by family prayer to recommend her to the Great Physician of Souls who alone can heal all our infirmities.'[54] Before hope had been abandoned, however, the doctor occupied a central position in the sickroom. Historians have seen the doctor as inheriting the mantle of the priest: the 'sacerdotalism' of psychological support for the patient was giving way to

[48] Brockbank and Kenworthy *Richard Kay*, p. 141.
[49] Z. Cope, *William Cheselden* (1953), p. 99. Cheselden was famed for his lithotomies, and took a minute to do the operation.
[50] Brotherton Library, Leeds, MS 560.
[51] Barnes Medical Library, Birmingham, MS 49, Cases of J. Badley in Surgery, 1802–3, Case 15.
[52] Wellcome MS 5006, Richard Wilkes's observation of 5 March 1743 on influenza outbreaks; Lincs RO, Flinders, 1, fo. 56, Matthew Flinder's observation of January 1782.
[53] J. Wesley, *Primitive Physic* (Epworth Press, 1960 reprint of second edn of 1791).
[54] Wilts. RO, uncatalogued Ailesbury papers, Robert Prichard (chaplain) to the Lord Bruce, 10 March 1794.

the 'rituals' (of professional procedures) and the 'mystical' words (of technical language).[55] In this context it is revealing that Abernethy – who was notorious for his brusque, arrogant manner with his patients – lectured on surgery as a 'god-like act.'[56] Increasingly, the patient's *faith* in the powers of the practitioner was seen by the profession as vital to recovery. 'Intercourse between physician and patient, in order to be successful, must be marked by candour, explicitness, straightforwardness, and the absence of all intentional delusion', admonished one early Victorian doctor.[57] And a late-Victorian professional handbook wrote that 'The faculty of keeping hope and confidence alive in the breast of the patient ... carries him with you on the road to recovery.'[58]

Limitations in encounters

Given the nature of these medical encounters what inferences may be made about the likely motivations and satisfactions of patients? Generalisations about the demand, rather than the supplyside of medical encounters are highly problematical. The sufferer's recourse to practitioners varied according to class, age and gender, as case studies in Part III indicate. The relative accessibility of regular practitioners was also relevant; the ratio of doctors to population was better in southern than northern England and, within this broad regional pattern, in urban than rural areas. Attitudes to doctors were conditioned by a multiplicity of influences including long-term changes in the force of religious as against medical explanations of illness. Perceptions of what constituted illness also influenced demand for doctors; the prosperous might discern an ague in an ache, whilst a poor person's stoicism in the face of severe bodily discomforts would have been hardened by penury. Fluctuating fashion in perceptions of health and sickness might constrain or expand demand for a doctor's services. In the longer term the development of a more scientific medicine enhanced medical authority, and thus raised demand for doctors. However, it is salutary to appreciate that awareness of iatrogenic risks is not a new phenomenon – as was shown by the poor's suspicion of early hospitals.

---

[55] M. Pelling, 'Occupational Diversity and the Trades of Norwich, 1550–1640', *BHM*, 56 (1982), pp. 485–6; F. B. Smith, *The People's Health, 1830–1910* (1979), p. 416.
[56] Barnes Medical Library, University of Birmingham, MS 51, Abernethy's Lectures on the Theory and Practice of Surgery, taken down by Bennett Dones. John Abernethy (1764–1831) succeeded Pott as Surgeon to St Bartholomew's Hospital.
[57] Granville, *Spas*, Vol. I, p. xxxix.   [58] de Styrap, *Practitioner*, pp. 19–30.

In a challenging study, Mary Fissell has argued that with the move from a traditional society to a class society, 'the bonds of a shared understanding of the body crack and break.' Poor patients, she suggests, were alienated from their bodies, and the distance from patient to practitioner widened. In the new infirmaries of the eighteenth century, she suggests, the patient's own narrative became increasingly faint within diagnostic case notes, and an accompanying change from the vernacular to Latin further limited accessibility. One objection to this interpretation is that the voice of the poor would not have been very familiar to the practitioner even before the advent of the hospital. More convincingly Fissell argues that the change in therapeutics from reliance on symptomatology and lay-patient narrative to mechanical reliance on measurement of the body's temperature, pulse or blood pressure shifted power from lay to professional. But despite this shift in power from patient to practitioner Fissell also indicates an increasing usage of infirmaries, such that 'a significant proportion of the population utilized the hospital' in the case of Bristol.[59] Whilst Bristol may have been unusual in that the traditional bonds between patients and subscribers were likely to have been stronger than in more industrialised areas, her conclusion on the take-up of hospital care does suggest that for poor consumers the utility of new hospital medicine outweighed its alienating properties. And as material in Chapters 8 and 9 suggests, some poor patients may also have empowered themselves by learning to manipulate the new institutions for their own purposes. Outside the hospital the language used by many practitioners in private practice was more patient-centred. Elite physicians took pains to acquire the conversational discourse of the gentry, whilst GPs acquired familiarity with local dialect. A general paucity of case notes in private practice may also indicate the continuation of much closer relationships between private practitioners and patients, with far greater reliance on oral than written communication, in contrast to institutional specialists concerned to make formal records.

The individual sufferer may have hoped that recourse to the practitioner would gain relief from insistently nagging pain, tackle the symptoms of acute illness, or help make sense of puzzling symptoms. Thus, desperation and fear in acute illness, or the need for reassurance over chronic ailments, might drive the sufferer to look beyond home-grown remedies or the medicines that could easily be purchased. In becoming a patient an invaluable commodity could be purchased:

[59] M. Fissell, *Patients, Power, and the Poor in Eighteenth-Century Bristol* (Cambridge, 1991), pp. 2, 108, 148–9, 159.

hope. In addition, the regular practitioner could usually supply more powerful weapons against the attacks of disease, and dull the ravages of pain, whilst an authoritative manner could allay the sense of help-lessness that beset patients and their family and friends alike. Medical explanations helped make sense of a mystifying illness, and the preci-sion of the steps laid down could suggest that a progression back to health was possible. There was a comforting sense that what might be done had been attempted. Not that all these ideals were necessarily realised. In cases of terminal illness in particular, officious medical interventions might compound rather than ameliorate the sufferer's problems. Finite therapeutic weapons made it easier for the prac-titioner to assume authority over illness than to subdue disease. (See Plate 3.)

Even with the confidence of their patients the prospect of recovery might be far from assured. In these circumstances how did doctors view their own limitations? Admissions of the finite healing capacity of medicine and of medical practitioners were more frequent in the eighteenth century, when frank disclosures of inadequacies were made. The eminent physician, Richard Mead (1673–1754), wrote that 'Our art is frequently obliged to rely on conjectures, nor is it to be expected that any one person will constantly hit the mark.'[60] Doctors had to come to terms with the fact that 'a great part of the practice of physic consists in alleviating urgent symptoms and in many cases nothing more can be done.'[61] In the privacy of their own casebook doctors frankly acknowledged the confines of their power to help their patient as did Richard Paxton. Reflecting on the death in 1759 of one of his female patients, he wrote

It is not easy to determine perhaps – whether this woman's life could have been saved under the treatment of a more experienced practitioner. No reflections were made by her friends ... to the disadvantage of the attendant surgeon; yet he did not feel that self-applause which is always to be desired after an unsuccessful case.[62]

Others also acknowledged the restricted effectiveness of medical intervention, as did Paxton's contemporary, Wilkes. 'I saw a poor woman at Hales Owen ... She was confin'd to bed and seem'd to be

---

[60] *The Medical Works of Richard Mead* (Dublin, 1767), p. 341. Mead (1673–1754) studied at Utrecht, Leyden and Padua, and became Physician to St Thomas's Hospital.
[61] Wellcome MS 2598, Lectures of James Gregory on Physic, vol. I, *c.* 1795, fo. 8.
[62] Wellcome MS 3820, Case book of Richard Paxton, Maldon, Essex, 1753–87, entry February 1759. Paxton (b. 1745) practised as a surgeon apothecary (*Eighteenth-century Medics*, p. 457).

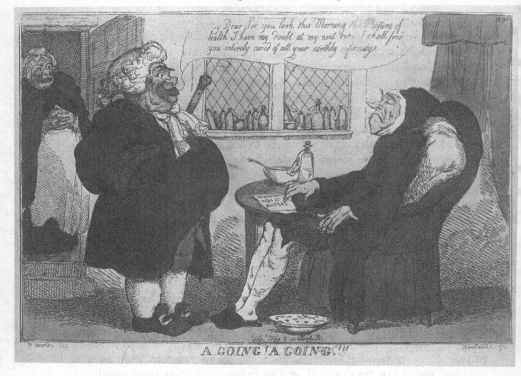

Plate 3   T. Rowlandson, 'A Going! A Going!'
The doctor says, 'My dear sir you look this morning the picture of health. I have no doubt at the next visit I shall find you intirely cured of your earthly infirmitys.' The patient holds a sheet with the words 'Prescriptions, bolus and blisters'

out of the power of medicines or art to relieve her.'[63] In contrast, for the Georgian optimist there might be a bright lining to every medical cloud, as was discerned by Alexander Monro I:

If practitioners in physic and surgery have sometimes uneasy minds on account of patients the nature of whose diseases they cannot judge with certainty, if they are disappointed now and then in the effects of medicines, and if they have the galling mortification of the sick dying unexpectedly, they have, on the contrary, frequently the comfort and pleasure of being surprised with the great relief which their patients, in very obscure, or even in diseases, which they are ignorant of, receive from medicines.[64]

[63] Wellcome MS 5006, Case book of Richard Wilkes, entry July 1739. Wilkes (1691–1766) practised in Wolverhampton as a physician and was the author of *A Treatise on Dropsy*.
[64] *Alexander Monro*, p. 637. Monro I (1697–1757), MD, FRS, was Professor of Anatomy at Edinburgh, and the founder of a famous medical dynasty.

Despite the eighteenth-century saying that 'the British kill their patients; the French let them die', a reputation for heroic dosing was not entirely justified.[65] Some British practitioners, including Cullen, adopted a much more moderate stance of therapeutic scepticism, as had Sydenham earlier. Cullen, characteristically, told a patient to rely not on physic but on a healthy lifestyle. 'A medical cure is not to be expected. It is not in the power of physic to give a new constitution. You must make the most of the one you have got.'[66] Heberden also gave a lead by advocating a simplified *materia medica*: 'Besides the few remedies here mentioned, it may be doubted whether ten others have upon any good authority been reputed specifics, or certain remedies for particular diseases.'[67] Less-well-known practitioners could also be unconvinced about the value of medication: 'I was not even certain that he received the smallest advantage from the medicine', and 'here as in many other cases nature performed the cure which we ascribed to medicines.'[68]

For the Georgian surgeon, cases that required major internal surgery were best avoided since they often led to death through shock or sepsis. John Hunter expressed the surgeon's dilemma incisively when he said 'with regard to operations, we should know when they will relieve, and when nothing but operations will relieve. We should know when the habit [of the patient] will bear an operation – this is sometimes almost impossible to ascertain.'[69] John Bell was one of the most skilled operators of his day but he acknowledged that cases involved risk. He referred to a surgeon reviewing a completed operation and, 'considering the danger that is over, he shudders at his hair-breadth escapes, and is conscious of having done what he can never venture to do again.'[70] Richard Kay reacted to a child dying of

---

65 Quoted in Ackerknecht, *Paris Hospital*, p. 129.

66 RCPE, 30/2. August 1770, advice to James Duncanson, suffering from a 'gravellish disorder'.

67 W. Heberden, *Commentaries on the History and Cure of Diseases* (New York, 1962), p. 6. Heberden (1710–1801), practised in London from 1748, attended such famous literary figures as Johnson and Cowper, and wrote several esteemed medical books.

68 RCPE, 31/16, Brandreth to Cullen, 2 May. Joseph Brandreth, MD (1746–1815) practised as a physician in Ormskirk, Liverpool (*Eighteenth-century Medics*, p. 73); Wellcome MS 5006, Case book of Richard Wilkes, entry May 1752, fo. 348.

69 Barnes Medical School, University of Birmingham, MS 1, Lectures on surgery by John Hunter, taken down by John Badley, ND. Badley, MRCS (1783–1870) later practised in Dudley, Worcs.

70 J. Bell, *Principles of Surgery* (1801–7) III, p. 219. Significantly, this was pasted into J. G. Crosse's correspondence (Norfolk RO, MS 20795). John Bell (1763–1820) was Professor of Surgery and Obstetrics at Edinburgh. Crosse (1790–1850) became Surgeon to the Norfolk and Norwich Hospital and was famous both for his lithotomy and for obstetrics.

rabies in the mid-eighteenth century, 'Lord, I pray thee help those that we are incapable of helping.'[71] Some were less resigned about the limitations of their power. A young assistant surgeon at the Norfolk and Norwich Hospital during the 1830s and 1840s, Benjamin Norgate, fulminated about the ravages of tetanus that caused 'the most horrible convulsions that can be imagined.' He expressed his feelings of impotence in his case book: 'This appalling disease, the treatment of which baffles the profession and shews how entirely ignorant we are of its pathology.'[72] From the mid-nineteenth century expressions of inadequacy increasingly gave way to greater professional self-confidence and a pride in medical advances.

Science and tradition

Medical practice was only gradually informed by more scientific insights. Amongst the important advances of the scientific revolution of the seventeenth century had been Harvey's discovery of the circulation of the blood and the creation of clinical bedside medicine by the 'English Hippocrates', Sydenham. In the growth of scientific medicine from the seventeenth to the nineteenth centuries, a new empiricism developed with an emphasis on observation and cautious inference, and with new standards of evaluation.[73] An upsurge of theory in the late eighteenth century, and a fresh awareness of critical standards, including those of statistical analysis, were also important.[74] In preventive medicine, particularly, there was a self-conscious spirit of scientific inquiry and experimentation. Percival wrote in 1776 that 'The rapid progress of science in this age of free inquiry, is a subject of gratitude and exultation.'[75] Prominent in investigating the nature of infectious diseases was John Haygarth who, in the same year, stated that:

I have long thought, that there is no subject on which a physician could employ his time and ability more advantageously for the benefit of his fellow-creatures, than in the investigation of the nature of febrile contagion, in order

[71] Brocklebank and Kenworthy, *Richard Kay*, p. 144, entry for 2 August 1749.
[72] Norfolk RO, NNH 49/1 Case book of Benjamin Norgate, 1830–1857, entry 11 August 1837. Norgate was Assistant Surgeon (1828–30) and Surgeon (1830–57) to the Norfolk and Norwich Hospital.
[73] L. S. King, 'The Development of Scientific Medicine' in L. S. King, ed., *Mainstreams of Medicine. Essays on the Social and Intellectual Context of Medical Practice* (San Antonio, 1971), p. 150.
[74] L. S. King, *The Growth of Medical Thought* (Chicago, 1963), p. 175.
[75] T. Percival, *Philosophical, Medical and Experimental Essays* (1776), pp. v-vi.

to ascertain the laws by which it is communicated, and by what means it may be prevented.[76]

Whilst Haygarth was sure that, 'truth will at last be certainly discovered',[77] weaknesses in methodology and techniques (notably inference through analogy, and the lack of a mathematics of correlation) impeded general progress in this social medicine.[78] In the case of vaccination the impact made by science was rapid.[79] Jenner wrote enthusiastically, 'I have at length accomplish'd what I have been so long waiting for, the passing of the vaccine virus from one human being to another ... I shall now pursue my experiments with redoubled ardour.'[80] A major change in medical practice ensued. 'All the surgeons here seem to practise it [vaccination] with the same regularity, they formerly practised variolous inoculation', confidently wrote a Norwich doctor in 1812.[81]

An important advance was made through morbid anatomy where a clinical view of specific disease linked to lesions observable at autopsy replaced an earlier interpretation of diseases as general physiological imbalance.[82] A surgeon wrote in 1792 of a dissection that followed a puzzling case. 'There was the cause of the symptoms and death, which without dissection must have remained an impenetrable secret.'[83] However, morbid anatomy also undermined old certainties and so might contribute to a therapeutic nihilism. Dissection might also underline the misdiagnoses that had been made earlier. At the beginning of the nineteenth century a post-mortem on a dropsical patient in St Bartholomew's Hospital produced this observation:

This case was supposed to be, dropsy of the peritoneum ... what was our surprise, to find the peritoneum healthy and one of the ovaries converted into a sac, and the source of the disease. How uncertain is medicine, or rather how

---

[76] J. Haygarth, *A Letter to Dr Percival on the Prevention of Infectious Fevers* (1801), p. 4. John Haygarth MD, FRS, was a physician first in Chester and then in Bath.

[77] Wellcome MS 91800, Haygarth to Lettsom, 16 October 1806, writing on pestilential fever.

[78] J. C. Riley, *The Eighteenth Century Campaign to Avoid Disease* (1987), pp. 148–9.

[79] G. Miller, *The Adoption of Inoculation for Smallpox in England and France* (Oxford, 1957); P. Razzell, *The Conquest of Smallpox* (Firle, Sussex, 1975).

[80] RCSL, Jenner correspondence, letter from Edward Jenner to E. Gardner, 19 July 1796. Jenner MD, FRS, (1749–1823) practised in Gloucestershire.

[81] RCSL, uncatalogued MS, letter from Edward Rigby to Charles Murray, Secretary to the National Vaccine Establishment, 13 January 1812. Rigby (1747–1821) was a leading local practitioner, Lord Mayor of Norwich in 1805, and the author of *An Essay on Uterine Haemorrhage* (1775).

[82] C. E. Rosenberg, 'The Shape of Traditional Practice, 1800–1875' in G. Rosen, ed., *The Structure of American Medical Practice, 1875–1941* (Philadelphia, 1983), p. 7.

[83] Wellcome MS 3820, fo. 193. Richard Paxton discovered a 'polypus' (blood clot) in the right ventricle of the heart of this twenty-two year old man.

defective is our knowledge of disease! Let this case stimulate us to greater exertions in pathology.[84]

And in the mid-nineteenth century the Physician to the Manchester Infirmary admitted that, 'the presence of mischief is often but obscurely indicated, and scarcely imagined by the medical attendant until, either it has developed itself by such signs as leave him no hope of remedy, or it is revealed by dissection.'[85]

Even before the Anatomy Act of 1832 had legitimated the study of anatomy through dissection, medical students managed to procure relevant experience. In the winter of 1767, for instance, William Stark wrote that he had 'attended with singular satisfaction and advantage Dr Hunter's anatomical lectures' in London, and at St George's Hospital had had 'excellent opportunities ... of examining those who die' and thus 'improved considerably in ... the anatomy both of the sound and of the morbid parts.'[86] At the turn of the nineteenth century, Edinburgh students were told of the importance of learning from the terminal stages of disease, and from the examination of the dead body.[87] At this time J. Badley, then at St Bartholomew's Hospital, commented that 'the body being almost immediately removed by the friends [of the patient], I was disappointed in my intention of examining it.'[88] Sir Astley Cooper, the most famous surgeon of his generation, emphasised to his early-nineteenth-century students the value of first-hand experience through observation at post-mortems.[89] J. G. Crosse described how at the Norfolk and Norwich Hospital in 1829 the surgeons took care that in any case of accident 'every dead body is examined ... in the presence of all ... pupils.'[90] It was above all the Quaker, Thomas Hodgkin, who in the 1830s argued that medical education was 'miserably defective' if it did not include morbid anatomy. He starkly counterposed the claims of traditional and scientific medicine, and vigorously stated the claims for a study of

[84] Wellcome MS 1145, Notebook of S. Berry.
[85] Manchester RO, M134/1/1/1/2, Miscellaneous papers of Edmund Lyon, fo. 1. Lyon (1790–1862) was Physician to the Manchester Infirmary from 1817.
[86] RCPE, MS 14, Miscellaneous correspondence, W. Stark to Professor T. Hamilton of Glasgow, 8 October 1765.
[87] Wellcome MS 2596, Clinical Lectures of James Gregory based on cases in the Edinburgh Infirmary.
[88] Barnes Medical Library, University of Birmingham, MS 49, J. Badley, Cases in Surgery, 1803–3, observation on case 42. See also, S. C. Lawrence, 'Desirous of Improvements in Medicine: Practitioners in the Medical Societies at Guy's and St Bartholomew's Hospitals, 1795–1815', *BHM*, 59 (1985), p. 99, for the typicality of Badley's view.
[89] Brock, *Astley Cooper*, pp. 109–10.
[90] Norfolk RO, MS 470, Diary of J. G. Crosse, 31 May 1829.

morbid anatomy. 'Those who are aspiring to become the worthy members of a profession which has for its object the restoration of health to our suffering fellow-creatures ... must see, that morbid anatomy ... constitutes a study the most essential to their art.'[91] Hodgkin thought that 'without morbid anatomy our nosology would be nothing but a catalogue of symptoms ... and all our attempts at diagnosis, except where the affection was literally external, would be mere empirical conjecture.'[92] His notes from post-mortem examinations of his patients showed very careful observations of diseased tissue made with a microscope and linked the dissection to the patient's case history. They are a fascinating conjunction of humanity towards the live individual and intense scientific curiosity towards the corpse.[93] Fearful popular attitudes to dissection are suggested by Cruikshank's depiction of the 'French' method of dissection as practised by Thomas Hodgkin. (See Plate 4.)

In *The Birth of the Clinic* Foucault analysed the significant change in medical discourse between the eighteenth and nineteenth centuries brought about by the 'clinical gaze' which marked a transition from the normal to the pathological, from the medicine of diseases to that of pathological reactions, and which thus began to focus on local states of disease. Foucault suggested that at this point in history the patient was no longer the subject, but rather the accident, of disease. Pathological anatomy, and particularly the part played by the clinician's eye – or medical gaze – of Bichat, opened up a new era of scientific medicine.[94] In oft-quoted words Bichat had written

For twenty years, from morning to night, you have taken notes at patient's bedsides ... and all is confusion for you on the symptoms which, refusing to yield up their meaning, offer you a succession of incoherent phenomena. Open up a few corpses: you will dissipate at once the darkness that observation alone could not dissipate.[95]

Despite the potential of scientific medicine, there were problems in its development and diffusion. Influential in England were social prejudices against dissection, and hence a difficulty during the late eighteenth and early nineteenth centuries of obtaining bodies to supply clinical material for systematic investigation of diseases.[96] Also,

[91] T. Hodgkin, *Lectures on the Morbid Anatomy of the Serous and Mucous Membranes* (2 vols., London, 1836, 1840), I, p. 2.
[92] Friends Library, London, microfilm 182, Hodgkin medical lecture notes, ND.
[93] Library of the Royal Society of Medicine, MS 165, Hodgkin Notes of Post-Mortem Examinations, 1845–52.
[94] Foucault, *Clinic*, pp. xi, 35, 59, 129, 141, 146, 191.   [95] *Anatomie Générale*, p. xcix.
[96] R. Richardson, *Death, Dissection and the Destitute* (1988).

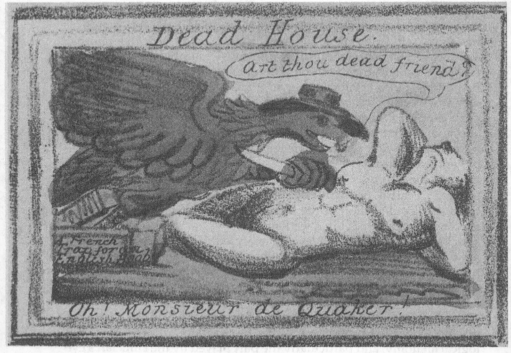

Plate 4   'Art Thou Dead Friend?' Detail from R. Cruikshank,
'The Seat of Honour or Servility Rewarded' (1830)

the professional bias against specialisms, and a continued tendency to
see them as quackery, militated against their development.[97] The
growth of what Maulitz has aptly referred to as 'a new grammar of the
body' was impeded by a continued separation of surgery and physic
in England, in contrast to the situation in France. 'To [English] surgeons the body was a mosaic of individual parts ... [and] For physicians the code of the body was different, involving an ecologic conception of interdependent regions.'[98] Thus, as Sir Anthony Carlisle
later commented it was not physic but rather 'surgery [that] has
advanced furthest as a rational and exact science.'[99] Surgeons by the
1830s were advancing into terrain formerly seen as the realm of the

---

[97] Shryock, *Modern Medicine*, pp. 50–1.   [98] Maulitz, *Morbid Appearances*, pp. 227–9.
[99] A. Carlisle, *Practical Observations on the Preservation of Health and the Prevention of
Diseases: on the Disorders of Childhood and Old Age* (1838), p. xiii. Sir Anthony Carlisle
(1768–1840) was Surgeon to the Westminster Hospital for nearly half a century and
twice president of the College of Surgeons.

physician. 'Can any definite line be drawn in practice between medical and surgical diseases?' asked Carlisle, and answered 'I think not.'[100]

Further significant advances in hospital surgery were made possible by the application of anaesthesia in the 1840s and antisepsis in the 1860s. The Scottish surgeon, J. Y. Simpson, commented that anaesthesia

both relieves [the surgeon] from the disagreeable necessity of witnessing such agony and pain in a fellow creature and imparts to him the proud power of being able to cancel and remove pangs and torture that would otherwise be inevitable.[101]

A ready acceptance of such a beneficial scientific 'discovery' as anaesthesia might appear obvious but its reception was problematical since it involved complex social and scientific forces.[102] Once this had been achieved major internal surgery was possible in which a new kind of relationship between surgeon and patient developed. There was a striking difference between the earlier operating theatre, grimed from long years of use and with surgeon dressed in frock coat, and that by the end of the century where hands, instruments, and patients' skins were awash with carbolic. The contrast between the operating styles of Astley Cooper (1768–1841), with his rapid and dexterous manner, and the systematic deliberation of Joseph Lister (1827–1912) several decades later, encapsulated the revolution in surgery that had occurred. Instead of rapidity on the part of the surgeon being of the essence in minimising shock to the body, lengthier operations were performed of a scale and complexity hitherto unknown. From the 1860s surgical gynaecology rapidly expanded, and in the 1870s and 1880s 'Surgical raids were made into abdominal territories hitherto sacred to pill, physic, blister, and the leech.'[103] Even the GP's 'kitchen-table surgery' in a patient's home could, with the help of chloroform, involve more complicated and lengthy procedures. For the surgical patient, however, septicaemia, erysipelas, and childbed fever remained real threats.

An optimistic view of the scientific transformation that was over-

[100] *SC on Medical Education*, PP 1834, xii, Q 5983.
[101] W.O. Storer, ed., *J. Y. Simpson's Obstetric Memoirs and Contributions* (2 vols., Edinburgh, 1855), ii, pp. 603–4. Simpson (1811–90) was Professor of Obstetrics at Edinburgh and introduced the use of chloroform in midwifery cases.
[102] A. Winter, 'Mesmerism and the Introduction of Inhalation Anaesthesia', *SHM*, 4 (1991), pp. 1–27.
[103] O. Moscucci, *The Science of Woman. Gynaecology and Gender in England, 1800–1929* (Cambridge, 1990), p. 108; J. Lynn Thomas, 'An Address on the Position of the Country Doctor in 1879 and To-Morrow', *BMJ*, 25 July 1914.

taking medicine was adopted by some surgeons. For example, 'the healing art is progressively becoming ever more certain [and] deserves public confidence' because of scientific advances that had revolution-ised 'the extent and rationality' of the healing art.[104] However, it is necessary to be aware of the polemical and selective use of the word 'science' at this time, both by practitioners and in medical period-icals.[105] Surgical advances gave a somewhat misleading picture of the scientific nature of Victorian medicine as a whole. Even in nineteenth-century hospitals the use of scientific instrumentation, such as the microscope, could be limited.[106] Lecturing on therapeutics in 1849, Professor John Hughes Bennett stated authoritatively that:

Whilst pathology has marched forward with great swiftness, therapeutics has followed at a slower pace. What we have gained by our rapid progress in the *science* of disease has not been followed up with an equally flattering success in an improved method of treatment. The science and art of medicine have not progressed hand in hand.[107]

This insight was not confined to the profession. A novel of 1852 commented that 'medical science is one of the things that makes little progress ... when it comes to curing you of a toothache, or a colic, or a fit of gout, my sure belief is that they made just as good a hand at it 200 years ago.'[108] Most doctors were more sanguine, although still making a distinction between progress in surgery and physic. A surgeon wrote in 1897 that in physic the advances were 'less striking ... [but] not less real.' Improved diagnosis resulted from advances in instru-mentation; the ophthalmoscope for eye diseases, the laryngoscope for windpipe and chest, the stethoscope for the heart and lungs, the sphygmograph and cardiograph for measuring heart beat, and the spectroscope or haematocytometer for the condition of the blood. An application of chemistry to diagnosis (as in diabetes or Bright's disease), and the use of Rontgen rays to survey the lungs and other internal organs, contributed to further range and precision.[109] But it is

---

104 Carlisle, *Practical Observations*, pp. ix-x, xi, xv-xvi.
105 J. Harley Warner, 'The Idea of Science in English Medicine' and C. Crawford, 'A Scientific Profession: Medical Reform and Forensic Medicine in British Periodicals of the Early Nineteenth Century' in R. French and A. Wear, eds., *British Medicine in an Age of Reform* (1992), p. 156.
106 T. J. Wyke,'Hospital facilities for, and diagnosis and treatment of, venereal disease in England, 1800–1870', *British Journal of Venereal Diseases*, 49 (1973), p. 80.
107 Quoted in J. H. Warner, 'Therapeutic Explanation and the Edinburgh Bloodletting Controversy', *MH*, 24 (1980), p. 241. Bennett was Professor of the Institutes of Medicine at Edinburgh.
108 Quoted in M. F. Brightfield, 'The medical profession in early Victorian England, as depicted in the novels of the period 1840–70' *BHM*, 25 (1961) p. 253.
109 M. Morris, 'The Progress of Medicine during the Queen's Reign', *The Nineteenth Century*, 41 (1897).

important to appreciate that this was the medical frontier of the specialist, and not the much more traditional terrain of the GP.

The important changes in physiology and in concepts of diseases did not immediately lead to a corresponding change in the doctor's power to treat them. In the 1850s Virchow had revealed the cell structures within tissues; work which was to be basic to later developments in pathology. From the 1870s the germ theory of diseases brought spectacular scientific advances in bacteriology that included Koch's identification of the tubercle bacillus in 1882. Replacing an earlier reliance on describing and classifying diseases came a new definition of disease specificity, the necessary causes of diseases, and disease-specific intervention. Although this was an epistemological revolution, it did not immediately result in a corresponding therapeutic revolution. With the exception of a few isolated breakthroughs, this took place in the mid-twentieth century.[110] Thus, when viewed from the perspective of the late twentieth century, the therapeutic advances of modern scientific medicine made by the end of the Edwardian period were still limited. Effective treatment was still lacking in a range of infectious diseases. For example, efficient therapy for scarlet fever was delayed until the advent of prontosil in 1935; puerperal fever until that of sulphonamides in 1935; and TB until the application of streptomycin in 1947 and BCG vaccination in the 1950s.[111] This meant that although the research scientist in the laboratory focused on diseases, the practising doctor remained patient-centred.

The influence of science on domiciliary medical practice remained limited so that there was continued reliance on traditional bedside medicine. In the seventeenth and early eighteenth centuries it has been suggested that there was 'a need by medical practitioners to be understood by patients, to relate to their expectations, and hence to attract their trade.'[112] This argument could also be extended – as far as general practice was concerned – to the rest of the eighteenth century, and well into the next century as well. Although a perpetual need to make sense of sickness and disease meant that newer, more scientific

[110] S. J. Kunitz, 'Personal Physicians and Mortality Decline' in Schofield, Reher and Bideau, *The Decline of Mortality*, pp. 252–4.
[111] T. McKeown, *The Modern Rise of Population* (1976), Chapter 5, *passim*; E. Shorter, *Bedside Manners. The Troubled History of Doctors and Patients* (New York, 1985), pp. 93–5.
[112] A. Wear, 'Medical Practice in Late Seventeenth and Early Eighteenth Century England: Continuity and Union', in R. French and A. Wear, eds., *The Medical Revolution of the Seventeenth Century* (Cambridge, 1989), pp. 294, 303–4, 320. See also, W. R. le Fanu, 'The lost half century in English Medicine, 1700–1750', *BHM*, 46 (1972), pp. 319–348, for the static nature of medical treatments in the early eighteenth century.

Table 3.1. *Medical treatment in the 1830s*

Scale of remuneration adopted by the Medical Practitioners of St Helens.

We the undersigned Medical Practitioners of St Helens agree strickly[sic] to adhere to the following as a minimum scale of charges.

To charge:
  1/od for each visit in the town
  1/6 for the first mile and 1/0 per mile afterwards
  2/6 for night visit and double mileage in the country. The night visit to be
      understood to commence after 10 o'clock p.m and before 6 o'clock a.m.

For every:
  Draught 1/6. zii Mixture 1/6, ziii + ziv Mixtures 2/0
              zvi 2/6, zviii 3/0, zxii 4/0, zxvi 4/6
  Bolus 6d. Pills 1d each. A Powder 6d. Powders 3d each
  Hj Lotion 2/6. Burn lotion 6/od a gallon or 1/6 a pint
  Embrocations and linaments to be charged as Mixtures
  Burn Linament 1/6 a pint, 2/6 a quart, 3/6 for 3 pints
  Blister and Ointment for an adult 2/0

  Dressing a wound 6d or 1/0

  Extracting a tooth 1/0. Bleeding 1/0

  Simple Fracture of the Arm 10/0
  Fracture of the Thigh or Leg 21/0
  Fracture of the Clavicle 10/6
  Child under seven years of age 7/6
  Dislocation of the Shoulder 21/0. Elbow 10/6
  Compound Fracture 21/0

  Introducing catheter 2/6
  Injecting an enema 2/6
  Vaccination 2/6

For midwifery 10/6 in the town and beyond the limits of the town mileage. For every consultation visit 5/0. For each consultation with a physician 5/0 exclusive of visit or journey. For every Midwifery case which is not paid for at the time of attendance 5/0 and over and above the usual charge. If a midwife has been in attendance to charge double.

It is understood that the deferred limits of the Town be as follows Hardshaw Hall, Parr Railway Bridge, Railway Station, Clare and Haddocks Colliery, Ravenhead Copper Works, Eccleston Glass Works, Crabfield Wall and Little Moor Flatt

Signed JOHN CASEY   THO. MERCER   JOHN BLUNDELL
       THOS. GASKELL   WILL GARTON   HENRY GREENUP

Note: I am grateful to Dr Jean Hugh-Jones for permission to reproduce this table of charges and to Dr Michael Bevan for drawing my attention to it.

explanations were invoked in medical lectures and specialist medical books, practical remedies showed more substantive continuity with the past. Table 3.1 shows the agreed charges for items of medical service in St Helens, Lancashire, *c.* 1839. Whilst a few items arise from the distinctive industrial nature of the district (notably the prominence of treatment for burns), the rest is probably not unrepresentative of the range of treatments commonly offered by GPs at that time.

The *Lancet* condemned the unscientific nature of medicine as it was widely practised during the 1840s. 'The information of the medical profession, generally, on matters of natural science, is very little greater than that of the people at large.'[113] Although the curriculum of nineteenth-century medical schools increasingly attempted to make room for a more adequate grounding in chemistry, physiology and pathology, it was harder to instil a more scientific mode of observation and thinking in aspirant doctors. In any case it took time for new cohorts to replace those trained earlier in a traditional mould. It thus remains problematic how soon a more scientific examination of patients, with attention to pulse, temperature and blood pressure, was generally established, rather than attention being concentrated solely on such external indicators as the tongue, eyes, urine and stools. GPs needed to be convinced that the use of instrumentation was linked to more successful outcomes. The bottom line for the busy GP, as distinct from the specialist physician, was that a ready recourse to prescription was less time-consuming than novel procedures. Medicines indicated to patients that something practical was being done and at least temporarily obscured the fact that in many instances the Victorian and Edwardian doctors had very limited weapons for fighting disease.

Diagnosis for the GP remained an inexact art rather than a precise science. In the 1890s an experienced Northumbrian GP gave his young colleague what he later found to be good advice, but found enigmatic at the time. 'You'll often find yourself puzzled about the nature of the complaint and about what you ought to prescribe for your patient. I find it is a good thing in such cases to find out what the patient likes most and *firmly knock him off it.'*[114] (Whether this was an epidemiologically informed view that excess might be implicated in disease or shrewd psychology in exercising professional authority is unknown.) The Registrar General commented in 1895 that one in twenty five of the total deaths certified by practitioners 'were stated so unsatisfactorily in the registers as to be worthless for the purposes of classification.' This total would have been far higher if further enquiries of doctors

[113] *Lancet,* I (1842–3), p. 127.   [114] Cox, *Doctors,* p. 37.

about 'deaths certified as due to tumour, dropsy, mortification, haemorrhage, and certain other indefinite conditions' had not reduced the total.[115] And, as late as 1920 there was a warning against the implementation of a proposal that National Health Insurance practitioners should insert diagnoses on their patient's 'Lloyd George' record cards since according to expert opinion medical work was based on probability, not certainty, in the vast majority of cases.[116]

Given the GP's restricted therapeutic power and reliance on psychological and social skills, why did Victorian and Edwardian society perceive an increase in medical authority? The credibility of the ordinary doctor was certainly enhanced both by the scientific successes of laboratory medicine and the achievements of hospital surgery. In addition, the growth of the Victorian state increased the number of medical offices, and this was both the cause and effect of doctors' increased influence. One late-Victorian observer noted 'As medical officers in parishes and unions, factory and prison surgeons, public vaccinators, medical officers of health, inspectors of nuisances, and very commonly as coroners, the doctors are daily assuming authority.'[117] Was this transformed into scientific legitimacy? The GP's task was made easier, and his authority enhanced, by an autonomous decline in the virulence of some diseases, by the major impact made by preventive measures in public health, and by therapeutic advances. In the 1890s there was effective treatment of diphtheria by antitoxins; in 1899 aspirin was developed for the relief of pain and fevers; and from 1910 the magic bullet, 'Salvarsan', was available to check the ravages of syphilis. How much the visibly accessible embodiments of this new science (such as even that humble example of instrumentation – the thermometer), were used or displayed in general practice is controversial. Shryock has stated that the clinical thermometer was coming into use in Europe during the second quarter of the nineteenth century, that pulse counts and hypodermic needles were found in the 1840s, the ophthalmoscope in the 1850s, blood pressure-measuring machines in the 1870s, and X rays in the 1890s.[118] In contrast A. J. Youngson has suggested that diffusion occurred slowly during the second half of the nineteenth century; available instruments, such as the thermometer and stethoscope, that would have established a more scientifically-based general practice were seldom used.[119] These scientific instru-

[115] *Report of the Registrar General*, PP, 1900, xv, p. 37.
[116] PRO, MH 62/130, Interdepartmental Committee, January 1920.
[117] F. B. Cobbe, 'Medicine and Morality', *Modern Review*, 11 (1881), p. 297.
[118] Shryock, *Modern Medicine*, pp. 168–9.
[119] A. J. Youngson, *The Scientific Revolution in Victorian Medicine* (1979), pp. 18–21.

ments had been introduced into London hospitals from the second quarter of the nineteenth century onwards.[120] One reason for historians' disagreement is that whilst it is clear that medical students would have become familiar with more advanced techniques during their hospital training, the rate of diffusion into general practice is uncertain. The lags following any innovation may have been intensified in general practice by caution about experimenting on patients, by financial reluctance to invest in instruments, and by a realisation that there was insufficient time to utilise any results obtained by their use. Reinforcing this in some practices was a traditionalist mindset which preferred to emphasise that healing was an *art*. The mid-Victorian James Russell encapsulated this. 'How limited, then, is that view which associates the practitioner in medicine only with his drugs or his instruments, which binds him down to his pestle and mortar, and deems his part ended with feeling the pulse or examining the tongue.'[121]

The GP personified a traditional 'whole-person' medicine rather than the disease-centred, impersonal medicine of the new science.[122] Helping to facilitate remission or recovery were the most effective reasons for patients to accept the authority of doctors, but in the theatre of the sickroom a confident manner in making sense of sickness by naming disease remained important. Equally impressive aspects of the doctor to the laity were the technical terms whose use conferred (or, on some occasions, appeared to confer) expertise. For inexperienced practitioners it was recognised that a little dissembling in this aspect of their work would pay dividends. One instance of this was the prescription, where the scientific mystique of the medicines prescribed could be made to seem complex and unintelligible to the lay person.[123] Whilst this advice was couched for the apparent purpose that 'you will debar the average patient from reading your prescriptions, and hampering you', its function may also have been to stop the laity penetrating professional knowledge. And was the notorious illegibility of doctors' handwriting also directed to this same end?

Implicit in this chapter's discussion of medical practice has been an attempt to evaluate the extent of continuity as against change. Charles West's *The Profession of Medicine* of 1896 is an apt illustration of the strength of customary views and practices. He saw the objects of medical education as inculcating 'keen observation, the calm judge-

[120] C. Newman, 'Physical Signs in London Hospitals' *MH*, 2 (1958), pp. 195–201.
[121] Russell, *Medical Profession*, p. 22.
[122] Loudon, 'Family Doctor', *BHM*, 58 (1984) p. 358.
[123] de Styrap, *Practitioner*, p. 197.

ment, the acute diagnosis, the skilful therapeutics', and the model given for the doctor's visit followed familiar lines since the doctor's manner with his patient should be 'natural, cheerful, gentle and sympathising.'[124] West's models were historically influenced, both because he self-consciously saw himself as operating in the tradition of Gregory and Percival, and because he wrote the book at the end of his career. This suggests how ideas that were current in medical schools in the early Victorian period could still be utilised forty years on, and their influence be prolonged still further through their impact on the future practices of the book's readers. Although new scientific methods of laboratory medicine quickly spread from their origins in Germany to leading universities in the USA during the late nineteenth century, they were much slower to penetrate British medical training and medical consciousness. This conservatism impeded the ability of the ordinary practitioner to make accurate diagnoses, and thus per-petuated a traditional form of bedside medicine. The strength of the medical hierarchy, with its accompanying authoritarianism also helped to perpetuate conservatism. So too did cultural traditions which might impede the reception and application of the new: the clearest case of this was the liberally-educated physician's slow take-up of manually-based medical technology. And there were more mundane reasons for lags in diffusion including the high cost of new drugs and the bulky inconvenience of some instruments which made them unsuitable for a mobile practitioner visiting the sickroom of a patient.

The social and healing qualities of West's practitioner were central elements in what has been termed 'traditional' medicine,[125] but these also need to be placed alongside the availability of the 'modern' – the new drugs, instruments and techniques whose use was informed by enhanced scientific understanding. This chapter has indicated that there were some real, if restricted, changes in ordinary medical prac-tice. Thus the traditional/modern dichotomy is one that appears to be too simple a demarcation; the balance of old and new was at any one time much more complex than that.[126] A situation obtained where there were overlapping layers of practice but with some interaction between conservative and progressive elements; the result sometimes

---

124 C. West, *The Profession of Medicine* (1896), Preface, pp. 12, 16, 23–6. West was Senior Physician to the Royal Infirmary for Children, and one of the founders of the Great Ormond Street Hospital.
125 Shorter, *Bedside Manners*, p. 26. Shorter discusses traditional medicine mainly in relation to the century from 1750 to 1850, and modern medicine from 1880 onwards.
126 See also Jordanova, 'The social sciences', p. 16.

appeared to possess internal coherence and at other times apparently consisted of a fortuitous amalgam of disparate elements.[127] This may be explained; first, by the time lag between the epistemological revolution and that in therapeutics; secondly, by the contrast between important advances in surgery and greater continuities in physic; thirdly, by the wide differences between the resources of the hospital specialist and those of the GP; fourthly by the differences in the practice of affluent and poor practitioners; and finally, by a cohort effect resulting from the date of initial medical training which was important in the slow diffusion of the 'modern' methods of the intellectual frontiers of medicine to the rank-and-file. One indication of the laggardliness with which general practice responded to scientific advances was the lack of basic equipment still clearly evident as late as the mid-twentieth century.[128]

This under-resourced nature of medical practice resulted from the low level of many medical incomes. The extent to which doctors had an unduly entrepreneurial orientation because of this, and the degree to which it influenced their treatment of patients was a matter of continued debate. Richard Kay remarked censoriously in 1740 that 'I cannot but observe that I fancy they thus put forward for the Get of Money' what he considered unnecessary medical interventions.[129] Half a century later, Lettsom wrote that 'our profession is prosecuted here more as a lucrative than as an honourable profession',[130] whilst another half century later, fellow Quaker, Hodgkin, wrote dismissively about colleagues who 'place the *summum bonum* of medical practice in converting the largest quantity of physic into gold.'[131] This economic dimension of practice is explored further in Part II.

---

[127] See the helpful chapter by M. Macdonald, 'Anthropological Perspectives on the History of Science and Medicine'.

[128] S. Collings, *Lancet*, i, 1950, p. 555; S. Taylor, *Good General Practice* (1954), pp. 453, 501.

[129] Brockbank and Kenworthy, *Richard Kay*, p. 34

[130] RCPE, MS 31/17 Cullen correspondence, Lettsom to Cullen, 3 August 1789.

[131] Friends Library, London, microfilm 182, Hodgkin medical lecture notes, ND.

The economic dimensions of practice

4

The creation of a surgical general practice

Georgian medical practice was characterised by its variety, and we have seen earlier that the regular or orthodox doctor operated against keen competition by irregulars – the so-called quacks and fringe practitioners. This chapter is concerned with the regular surgeon-apothecaries and surgeons of the Georgian period and their evolution into the general practitioners or consultant surgeons of the Victorian period. Following the Rose Case of 1704 apothecaries had been permitted to practise medicine rather than merely dispense it. This contributed to the merging of the role of the apothecary with that of other practitioners and, given the demand for treatment at modest cost, to the dominance before the end of the century of practitioners who described themselves as surgeon-apothecaries. John Abernethy commented that 'The diseases that fall under the care of surgeons are generally local and external.'[1] Traditionally the surgeon's work had focused on such external complaints involving manual treatment as the setting of fractures, the dressing of wounds and ulcers, the pulling of teeth, and the treatment of venereal diseases. Increasingly, the surgeon also moved from cases of abnormal to normal childbirth. And, in practice, if not in theory, some physic was also part of their daily routine since, as Astley Cooper later commented, 'The study of medicine is important to the surgeon; he should be able to prescribe with certainty.'[2]

Initially, there was a rise in the status of surgeon-apothecaries as was indicated by the increase in fees that they were able to command

---

[1] Brotherton Library, University of Leeds, MS 551, Notes on Abernethy's Lectures taken down by Thomas Teale, 1796.
[2] Brook, *Astley Cooper*, p. 111.

during the second half of the eighteenth century.[3] But the growth in their number meant that competition in the medical market intensified and their economic position deteriorated.[4] Equally, their social position could be ambiguous in the community with consequent social anxieties. They have been described as 'marginal men', occupying an uncertain position between a trade and a profession. This was both because they were 'members of a profession yet in the making' and were also socially insecure in the years before they forged contacts and social relationships with a cross-section of their local society through their activities in a range of voluntary associations.[5] There was more to gaining respect from the community than simply practising medicine; social diversity meant that professional marginalisation varied between communities.[6] Crucially, there was also differentiation for individuals in terms of their social status at birth and the marriages they were able to make; genteel connections assisted the practitioner in joining the local establishment. For the surgeon-apothecary or GP it was the locality – rather than the metropolitan élite and its attempts to control provincial practitioners – that was important.[7]

The experiences of GPs became increasingly differentiated as a result both of the growing number of registered practitioners and of the changing society in which they practised. In 1700 around one in five of the population lived in towns, whereas by 1851 more prospective patients lived in towns than villages, and by 1911 only one in five were country dwellers. The range of possible medical practices widened as a result. In seeking to elucidate the complex and changing situation of the surgeon, from surgeon-apothecary to GP, this chapter explores two themes: building a practice, and operating it with hope of expansion through assistants and partners.

Building a practice: territoriality and office

The concept of territoriality was implicitly understood as the basis of an economically viable practice. Practice had to be consolidated within

[3] I. Loudon, 'The Nature of Provincial Medical Practice in Eighteenth-Century England', *MH*, 29 (1985).
[4] Loudon, *Medical Care*, pp. 258.
[5] I. Inkster, 'Marginal Men. Aspects of the Social Role of the Medical Community in Sheffield, 1790–1850', in J. Woodward and D. Richards, eds., *Health Care and Popular Medicine in Nineteenth-Century England* (1977), pp. 128, 143, 148, 151.
[6] Marland, *Medicine and Society*, pp. 365–6.
[7] M. Durey, 'Medical élites, the general practitioner and patient power in Britain during the cholera epidemic of 1831–2', in I. Inkster and J. Morrell, eds., *Metropolis and Province. Science in British Culture, 1780–1850* (1983).

a limited diameter around the home of the surgeon-apothecary or GP. Fundamentally, this involved keeping out 'competition' whilst attempting to monopolise the growing range of public offices in the locality lest new entrants got a foot in the door. For most, territorial domination was thus an aspiration rather than an achievement.

Choosing the right area in which to practise was vital. Particularly in periods such as the post-war period after 1815 or that from the 1880s, when the doctor-patient ratio improved and competition for practice increased, a location with the right kinds of patients and with as few rivals nearby as possible was crucial for economic survival. Yet fundamental axioms such as this went unmentioned in medical training. A young doctor complained in the *BMJ* in 1907 that, 'Many a man of good qualifications and fair capital starts in life with most of his capital sunk in his education, never receiving a hint as to how to obtain a recompense for his services, and with no helping hand from his seniors in the profession.'[8]

As the pace of urbanisation and industrialisation increased so the choice of type of practice increased, and pressures intensified on the young doctor to make a shrewd choice as to where and how to operate. At the bottom end of the market was a cash surgery in a large town or port, perhaps supplemented by a branch surgery, and with club appointments. A more respectable option would have been a mixed working- and middle-class practice supplemented perhaps by a poor-law appointment. Above this would be either a suburban, middle-class practice with a range of appointments, or an unopposed country practice, preferably situated in good sporting country, and with a monopoly of local offices. And at the top would have been a well-established practice in a hospital town where there was the hope of prestigious appointments and a consultancy practice. Alternatively, there was a fashionable practice, with affluent patients in a seaside or watering place. As practices improved in terms of income so the asking price increased, so that a young doctor would have needed to have private means to afford the substantial premium.

During the eighteenth century practices were less differentiated and surgeon-apothecaries usually operated practices with a mixed clientele. Country practices were of considerable importance numerically, and it is therefore instructive to look in more detail at the preoccupations of a rural surgeon-apothecary. The correspondence of the surgeon-apothecary, Matthew Flinders, is particularly illuminating on the subject of fear of competition from rival practitioners.

---

[8] Letter from 'Fair Play', *BMJ*, (11), 1907, p. 480.

Flinders practised from 1775 to 1802 in Donington, in south Lincolnshire. His first entry on the subject came in 1789 and was relatively
restrained:

A Mr Wrangle from Boston of the Faculty has just now thought proper to fix in
the parish as my opponent – what the consequences may be to me, time must
develop – have determined to avoid chagrin – had I a less family, [I] would
gladly give up part of my fatigue, but as it is [I] am obliged under providence
to all exertion.[9]

Fortunately for Flinders, the upstart Wrangle found it impossible to
find sufficient patients to make a viable income. The real extent of
Flinders's earlier anguish was only revealed in his almost audible later
sigh of relief, 'blessed be to God the coast is now clear.' Unfortunately,
even in the less competitive Georgian period 'opposition' was a constant threat. Seven years later he again wrote in metaphorical letters of
blood:

It is an unpleasant circumstance to note that I have again an opponent in
business in Mr W[illia]m Ayliff who was apprentice with Mr Vise of Spalding
– he is a civil young man – & we are upon good terms … I have offered him
terms to resign all business but Don[ington] and a retail trade – but he has not
acceded to the terms so we must each do as we can for ourselves. I apprehend
the business is very limited for two.[10]

This entry is revealing both in indicating that a practitioner might find
it worthwhile to buy out opposition, and that he might contemplate
ceding the bottom end of the practice – retailing drugs – to a rival. The
eventual financial outcome for Ayliff in practising in the Donington
area was not recorded but Flinders must have found the situation, if
not desirable, at least surmountable, since we find him in 1800 complacently estimating his estate as worth £4000.[11] Flinders also contemplated taking an apprentice but was careful to think through the likely
consequences and thus ensure (as did others of his contemporaries)
that this engendered no future competition. He wrote, 'If I take him I
intend to have some form of writing to prevent his fixing over near
me.'[12]

Opposition was a hard fact of professional life for the urban practitioner but in the countryside this might fluctuate, as with Flinders.
That a practice was 'unopposed' was a highly desirable characteristic

[9] Lincolnshire RO, Flinders correspondence, ii, fo. 40, entry 7 November 1789. Wrangle
was born in 1770 and apprenticed in 1794 (*Eighteenth Century Medics*, p. 21).
[10] Flinders correspondence, ii, 1 February 1796. Ayliff was born in 1775 and apprenticed
in 1795 (*Eighteenth Century Medics*, p. 21).
[11] Flinders correspondence, iii, 23 November 1800.
[12] Flinders correspondence, i, December 1775.

to be able to state, and it was thus a prime selling point. Examining the nature of what was meant by an unopposed practice is possible for a later period through late nineteenth or early twentieth century advertisements of practices for sale. These revealed the slippery nature of the concept. Its ambiguity reflects the flexible concept of territoriality. How far away did the competition have to be before a practice could legitimately be described as unopposed? Usually, advertisers got round the problem by merely stating categorically that their business was unopposed. These assertions were more common in the 1870s than two decades later when there was a more cut-throat market. Evidence from the end of the nineteenth century shows how competitive conditions had become. Occasionally the term 'unopposed' was used in relation to a given distance: 'Unopposed country practice ... the nearest opposition is five and a half miles distant.' Whilst other advertisements did not state that they were unopposed, they clearly thought that they were in an advantageous position in stating: 'nearest opposition 3 1/2 miles distant', or 'nearest opposition 2 miles.'[13]

Georgian and Victorian doctors were deeply concerned about 'their' territory, in a way that perhaps had not characterised their predecessors in a less entrepreneurial age. During the seventeenth century patients had usually travelled to all but itinerant practitioners from a 'hinterland' of up to ten miles in extent, although the distances travelled might be very much greater when sufferers were sufficiently desperate or when the practitioner was sufficiently renowned.[14] From about the middle of the eighteenth century a more commercial attitude meant that practitioners travelled not just to the noble or genteel patient but to those from a much greater occupational range. Doctors attempted to gain as much as possible not only of a 'home' territory which they monopolised, but also to extend into a 'borderland' territory by pushing out their practice frontier into intermediate areas covered by colleagues. Success in practice probably extended the distances these practitioners might travel, as had been the case at the end of the seventeenth century.[15] And at the end of the nineteenth and beginning of the twentieth centuries technological innovation also expanded the doctor's hinterland, notably with the arrival of the telephone and the car.

[13] *BMJ Advertiser*, 7, 10, 21 October 1899.
[14] R. C. Sawyer, 'Patients, Healers and Disease in the Southeast Midlands, 1597–1634', unpublished PhD thesis, University of Wisconsin-Madison, 1986, pp. 196–200; M. MacDonald, *Mystical Bedlam* (Cambridge, 1981), pp. 54–61.
[15] F. N. L. Poynter, *The Journal of James Yonge, 1647–1721* (1963), pp. 186, 204.

The town-centred development of numerous turnpike trusts resulted in a vastly improved transport network by the mid-eighteenth century and an intensive network by 1770.[16] This was very important in extending the potential range of doctors' practices and hence in expanding the medical market. Indicative of this were an increased number of country practitioners and of town-based practitioners with rural practices (whether apothecary, surgeon or physician) by the mid-eighteenth century.[17] Even with these improvements, and with favourable topography and weather, not much more than four to five miles an hour could be attained on horseback so that the hinterland of a practice could not be infinitely extended.[18] Two late eighteenth-century surgeon-apothecaries, William Goodwin and William Elmhirst are taken here as useful exemplars since, whilst they practised at the same time, the spatial characteristics of their practices had both similarities and differences.

William Goodwin was a Suffolk surgeon who practised in Earl Soham at the end of the eighteenth century. His journeys, recorded in his diary for the years 1787–9, indicated quite clearly the extensive area that such a practitioner might expect to cover in treating his patients.[19] (See Map 3.) The 'home' territory comprised the regular extent of everyday practice; the locality round home where the surgeon might expect to be either the sole surgeon available or, if the practice was opposed, perceived by prospective patients as one of the main options available if medical treatment was required. In Goodwin's case this more limited area covered about 10 miles by 15, or 150 square miles. In estimating the extent of Goodwin's practice it is illuminating to see the much larger area – the 'borderland' territory – in which patients might *occasionally* call on his services. He made single journeys from Earl Soham to places that were nearly 20 miles away – such as Southwold on the Suffolk coast, or Bungay, on the Norfolk border. In its entirety Goodwin's practice embraced a region ten times larger than the immediate area of practice – this being 30 miles by 35, or over 1000 square miles in extent. One may speculate that some of these more distant visits could involve a consultation

[16] J. Chartres, 'Road Transport and Economic Growth in the Eighteenth Century' in A. Digby, D. T. Jenkins and C. H. Feinstein, eds., *New Directions in Economic and Social History II* (1992), pp. 52–4.

[17] J. Lane and A. Tarvner, 'Henry Fogg (1707–1750) and his Patients: the Practice of an Eighteenth Century Staffordshire Apothecary', *MH*, 37 (1993), p. 189; Wyman, 'The Surgeoness', p. 41.

[18] E. Hobhouse, *The Diary of a West Country Physician* (1934), p. 26.

[19] E. Suffolk RO, HD 365/1–3, Diaries of William Goodwin of Earl Soham, 1785–1809.

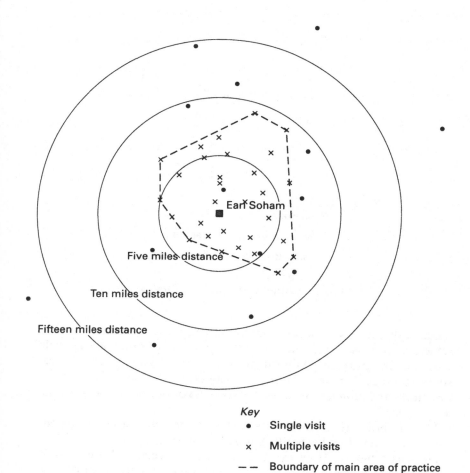

Key

• Single visit

× Multiple visits

− − Boundary of main area of practice

Map 3   William Goodwin's practice

with a colleague in a difficult case. Alternatively, a surgeon might build up a reputation in a particular speciality and thus draw on patients from a wider area in this particular type of malady. Goodwin's more distant cases concerned lues, scrofula, consumption, the drawing of teeth, and also varied female disorders. As such it is not easy to see any obvious rationale relating to Goodwin's specialist skills. Rather it appears likely that Goodwin had a very good general reputation which encouraged patients to call him in, even within the everyday treatment area of his professional rivals. Contemporary

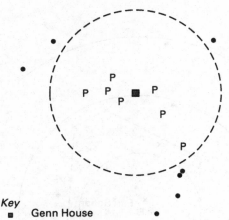

Key
■ Genn House
— . Five-mile limit of main practice
P . Parishes to which charges are made
● Occasional visits

Map 4   William Elmhirst's practice

medical directories indicated that Goodwin had a reasonable area in which to practise, since he had five opponents within a five mile radius of his practice. Only on the fringe of his main practice area, some 10 miles distant, were there clustered more than a dozen rival practitioners in the towns of Stowmarket, Saxmundham, Woodbridge and Yoxford.

Map 4 shows that Goodwin's total territory was larger in extent than that covered by his South Yorkshire colleague, William Elmhirst, a few years before. How can this contrast between a diffuse and a concentrated practice be explained? Elmhirst's home territory was more densely populated, having about one-third more inhabitants than that of Goodwin, according to the 1801 *Census*. Also important was the differing socio-occupational profile of the two areas; Goodwin's 'patch' had villages and small market towns surrounded by fertile agricultural land, whereas Elmhirst served an industrialised area where textiles and wire-drawing provided more substantial income for the working population, and thus a more buoyant medical market.

From his surviving ledger of 1779–83 it is apparent that Elmhirst's 'home' territory for practice was within five miles of his home base at Genn House, one mile south of the centre of Barnsley, comprising a total of 25 square miles. And, since the bulk of this practice was to the south of this, his practice was even more concentrated. He went beyond this much more rarely as, for example, to Ecclesfield (seven miles away), or even to Rotherham or Sheffield (about ten miles distant). Thus his 'borderland' territory stretched to an area roughly 15 miles by 12, or 180 square miles. This was little more than Goodwin's 'home territory'. However, from the evidence we have (admittedly fragmentary in each case), it would appear that Elmhirst cultivated his smaller professional patch much more intensively than did Goodwin, charging up patients to the accounts of no less than seven sets of local parish overseers.[20] His private patients also covered every social class, from gentry to servant. Since he charged differentially according to their perceived ability to pay, he managed to exploit the market efficiently, whilst tempering business acumen with personal humanitarianism. For instance, for curing an abcess on the arm, a Miss Allen was charged three guineas whereas a Widow Morton paid only five shillings for this.[21] Interestingly, Elmhirst left it to his patients to reimburse him for his travels, as they thought fit. His accounts show 'for riding charges and attendance what you please', rather than the standard set of charges for a day or night journey found in other surgeon-apothecaries' accounts.

For both Goodwin and Elmhirst such distances could be covered on horseback during a hard-working day; the immediate area of practice being influenced by the topography and state of the roads, with Yorkshire being less amenable for travel than was Suffolk. William Elmhirst died as a result of a riding accident; the local paper reported that he 'by some means fell or was thrown from his horse and kill'd on the spot.'[22] The nature of rural practice and the travelling demands it made on the country doctor were notorious. The earlier diaries of Richard Kay indicated an even worse situation, since fewer turnpike trusts had by then improved road surfaces. 'My riding today upon account of visiting has been upwards of 20 miles or near 30. Lord bless me and the beast I ride upon.'[23] The entries described four serious riding accidents encountered by the diarist's father, Robert Kay, in his practice as surgeon and physician in the Lancashire neighbourhood

---

[20] E. Sigsworth and V. Brady define the practice area slightly more broadly at 11 miles by 3, or some 30 square miles and also suggest that Elmhirst had accounts with only 6, rather than my estimate of 7 (*The Ledger of William Elmhirst, Surgeon and Apothecary, 1769–1773*, Humberside Polytechnic, ND, p. iii).

[21] Sheffield City Archives Em 888, Medical Ledger, 1768–73, entries May 1768 and 1772. This has now been edited – see the preceding footnote.

[22] Sigsworth and Brady, *Elmhirst Ledger*, p. ii.

[23] Brocklebank and Kennedy, *Richard Kay*, entry 3 August 1745.

near Bury, and an equal number experienced by his son. Their horses stumbled or fell, depositing their riders on muddy roads or swollen rivers and, on one occasion, Robert was even pulled off his horse by the force of other traffic jostling for passage in a narrow road.[24] But even without mishaps the wear and tear of travel continued to be daunting, particularly for the more ambitious surgeon with a growing consultancy practice. A Norfolk surgeon recorded wearily in 1836 that '5 times within 10 days I have seen a patient 33 miles off and each day attended to an extensive practice in and about Norwich – and ... such occupations are usual with me.'[25] In the 1840s a Hanworth surgeon was described as being 'so much engaged in practice that he is never to be seen except either mounting or alighting from a horse, and always equipped in top-boots and spurred.'[26] Even the advent of the railway did little to help the ordinary practitioner, in contrast to the eminent consultant who went on fewer – but better-paid – journeys.

Decent modes of transport were an important element in constructing the appropriate professional demeanour for successfully winning and retaining patients. 'A medical man can often ride into a practice more quickly than he can walk into one' commented a professional guide incisively.[27] Advertisements of practices for sale in the medical press were illuminating about the locomotive methods of doctors – a horse, or a horse and dogcart were by the 1880s and 1890s being supplemented by the cycle. The latter was seen as ideal for the urban practitioner, and more particularly for summer use.[28] In this case a tweed coat and knickerbockers replaced the frock coat and top hat.[29] Choice was expanding and the rapid changes in transportation may themselves have been a potent factor in the severe competition that practitioners faced at the turn of the twentieth century. In country districts the horse might be replaced by a gig, as in a Welsh practice covering a district six miles by eight.[30] The car had begun to be utilised although the *BMJ* did not feel able to endorse it as a sound investment for doctors until 1904.[31] The kind of transport transitions effected by

[24] Brocklebank and Kennedy, *Richard Kay*, entries 10 April 1738, 3 July 1738, 22 September 1742, 8 March 1746, 27 December 1748, 2 August 1749, 12 March 1750. The Kays, Robert (1684–1750) and Richard (1716–51), practised at Baldingstone.
[25] Norfolk RO MS 471, correspondence of J. G. Crosse, (1835–45), letter to Dr John Forbes, 21 December 1836.
[26] Granville, *Spas*, I, p. 206.   [27] de Styrap, *Practitioner*, p. 16.
[28] *BMJ Advertiser*, 7 October 1899.
[29] J. Pemberton, *Will Pickles of Wensleydale* (1970), p. 30.
[30] J. Lynn Thomas, 'An address on the position of the country doctor in 1879 and to-morrow', *BMJ*, 25 July 1914.
[31] Bartrip, *Mirror of Medicine*, pp. 152–3. And until the Finance Act of 1925 wear and tear on a doctor's car could not be claimed against income tax.

the GP were well illustrated by a rural Yorkshire practitioner, Thomas English, who walked his rounds at first, then – when he could afford to do so – bought a gig with two horses, using one each day. Finally, no doubt rejoicing, English bought a car in 1911. The irony was, however, that his patients viewed the latter with disapproval since it limited the accessibility of 'their' doctor. 'We have expected to see you pass, which we have, but in a flying machine.'[32] Indeed, the quite extraordinary affection given by local people to another Yorkshire practitioner – Dr Speiers of Swaledale – may well have reflected their gratitude for his continued accessibility since, even in the interwar period, he continued his rounds on horseback.[33]

Medically and socially practitioners seized every opportunity that their geographical territory offered to them. The financial accounts of eighteenth century surgeon-apothecaries are interesting in indicating the very wide range of patients treated – from servants through tradespeople, publicans and artisans to the gentry. In traversing the full range of these socio-economic groups the doctor was operating within a hierarchical society of ranks and orders. Accessibility to patients was a notable feature of Georgian country practice and it is significant that depictions of country doctors in contemporary cartoons indicated a more benign recognition of their hardworking life. (See Plate 5.) These contrasted with those depicting the self-centred mercenary concerns of their élite colleagues. Rural GPs in the Victorian and Edwardian periods still treated quite a wide social range of patients but the constraints of a more class-divided society meant that the poorest patients were now more obviously demarcated as paupers, whose treatment by the doctor was sanctioned by the more obtrusive bureaucracy of the New Poor Law.

Officeholding was another key feature of territoriality, and the clearest example of this principle was appointment under the poor law since this was linked to a geographical area. Under the Old Poor Law this area was the parish, and under the New Poor Law the medical district within the poor-law union. Under the Old Poor Law surgeon-apothecaries sought to maximise the number of parishes for which they acted as surgeon. Those who were conspicuously success-ful included Elmhirst, as well as McGrath with seven parishes in Bedfordshire, and Wilmer with a dozen in Warwickshire.[34] Joan Lane

[32] B. H. English, *Four Generations of a Whitby Medical Family* (Whitby, 1977), pp. 108–10.
[33] Swaledale Folk Musem, Reith, North Yorkshire has an informative display on Dr Speiers.
[34] J. Lane, 'Eighteenth-Century Medical Practice: a Case Study of Bradford Wilmer, Surgeon of Coventry, 1737–1813', *SHM*, 3 (1990), p. 378; Loudon, *Medical Care*, p. 232.

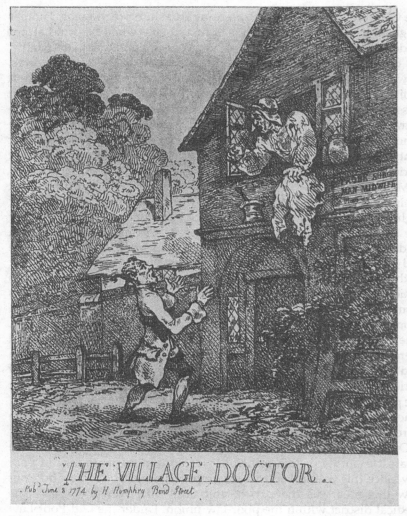

Plate 5   T. Rowlandson (after H. Wigstead), 'The Village Doctor'
(1774)

has suggested that as many as three out of four late-eighteenth
century practitioners in Warwickshire worked for various parishes.[35]
Under the New Poor Law the potential number of poor-law appointments shrank since some 15,000 parishes were gradually replaced by

[35] Lane, 'Bradford Wilmer' p. 372.

some 600 unions, each with several medical districts. In Norfolk, the fourth largest English county, the numbers of surgeons employed in each union in the first years after 1834 varied from two to eight, and their medical districts from as little as 1,000 acres to as much as 33,000. The worst inequalities were reduced as numbers of district medical officers in the county gradually rose from the 108 employed in 1844 to the 122 by 1861.[36] Nationally, numbers of district and workhouse medical officers grew from 2680 in 1849 to 4728 by 1906.[37] Poor-law office was therefore a major source of salaried office for the medical practitioner. Irvine Loudon has estimated that one in five provincial practitioners held a poor-law office at any one time, but that perhaps twice that number were involved with the poor law at some point in their career.[38] Although the stereotypical image of the poor-law medical officer was that of the young surgeon struggling to make a living, it is important to appreciate that the reality was somewhat different, since throughout their careers many practitioners continued to find it both a means to consolidate their territory, and a useful source of income.

Competition for poor-law office was variable; in remote areas it was difficult to get anyone to apply, whereas in more populous ones there was keen competition. In some rural areas it proved difficult to replace a district medical officer, however unsatisfactory his performance, because of the lack of a better alternative. A good illustration of this occurred in the Norfolk Unions of Henstead and of Forehoe in relation to the medical officer, R. J.Tunaley, who incurred numerous complaints of neglect of duties in the 1840s and 1850s, but was never dismissed from office.[39] Elsewhere, competition for union office was keener. For example, there were as many as eight applicants when the post of surgeon to the number 6 district of the Market Harborough Union in Leicestershire came up in 1866. One young applicant was Thomas Macauley, who possessed 'more than ordinary ability', according to his referees. He thought it necessary to go to the trouble to provide eight testimonials in a printed booklet, a procedure normally only adopted for more prestigious hospital appointments. This was not the result of ignorance of the realities of the situation since he

36 Digby, *Pauper Palaces*, pp. 166–7.
37 M. A. Crowther, *The Workhouse System* (1981) p. 136.
38 Loudon, *Medical Care*, p. 239. This is based on a small sample for 1848 and probably underestimates the proportion of rural doctors who held such office.
39 Digby, *Pauper Palaces*, p. 168.

had had prior experience of union duties as assistant to the Cosford Union Medical Officer.[40]

By the mid-nineteenth century a range of attitudes towards poor-law office was becoming apparent. It was valued because, although offical payment was low the poor law at least gave some recompense for what otherwise would have gone unrewarded in essential medical and surgical treatment of the poor. Equally powerful in its operation, however, was the principle of territoriality. 'Such is the fear of strangers being introduced into the [geographical] practices of the established medical men that duties will be undertaken.'[41] Another mid-nineteenth century commentator argued that 'They must take it to save their other practice.'[42] It was also suggested that poor-law practice might lead on to other practice since the medical officer knew 'that the eyes of all non-paupers are upon him, and that if he establishes a good character, he can make it pay among the farmers and small tradesmen.'[43] But not all were so happy about the workhouse connection. A successful London practitioner, for example, wrote with a breezy condescension of a 'country cousin' who practised in Hovingham, Norfolk, 'I bade adieu to my kind and intelligent ... brother practitioner, heartily wishing him better luck in his laborious and ill-regulated office, of surgeon to a Union of sixteen parishes, for which he receives the paltry sum of twenty pounds a year.[44] And, by the early twentieth century, such élite social attitudes were stiffened by economic anxieties. Some medical men – probably the better-established ones – were unwilling to take such office, fearing that their contact with the diseased poor would rebound adversely on their well-paid practice with the more affluent. The British Medical Association baldly asserted that 'people avoid calling in the parish doctor because he is the parish doctor ... no question of it.'[45]

During the nineteenth century there was increasing variety in the opportunities for making a medical income from salaried appointments, whether private or public, full- or part-time. The complexity of this array has been brought out clearly in a useful study by Dupree

40 Leics. RO, DE 513/500, Testimonials of Thomas Macauley.
41 *SC on Medical Poor Relief*, PP 1844, ix, p. 1044, communication from the BMA.
42 *SC on Medical Relief*, PP 1854, xii, Q 1545, evidence of Rev. C. Oxenden of Barham, Kent.
43 *SC on Medical Relief*, Q 1568, evidence of Charles Kingsley.
44 Granville, *Spas*, p. 206.
45 *RC on the Poor Laws*, PP, 1909, xl, Q 39391.

Table 4.1. *State officeholders in medicine, 1918*

Types of offices	Numbers
(1) Poor-law	
(a) Institutions	1080
(b) District MOs	3761
(2) School medical services	1300
(3) Certifying factory surgeon	1300
(4) General Post Office, MO	3360
(5) Army, navy & colonial service	3000
(6) Sanitary services,	
(a) MOH	1600 [FT 285]
(b) TB	238
(7) Lunacy Acts and Board of	
Control for Feeble-Minded	324
(8) National Health Insurance	16,392
Total	31,055

Note: The table involves double-counting since many GPs would have held more than one office.
Source: Some Notes on Medical Education by George Newman, PP, 1918, XIX.

and Crowther of Scottish medical appointments in 1911.[46] In England doctors were employed in Victorian and Edwardian public service in the army and navy, the colonial service, the police, the post office, and the school medical service. A range of public institutions had medical officers, including asylums, prisons and workhouses. Doctors also found posts in industry; public employment as certifying factory surgeons, and private employment in mining and railway companies. Table 4.1 indicates the very large numbers of medics in the major forms of state employment by 1918, with a highly significant doubling of the total having come about under the National Health Insurance legislation of 1911. The list is not exclusive, for example, district medical officers under the poor law also usually held an office as public vaccinator.

The vast majority of such public appointments were part-time, the major exceptions being those employed in the army, navy and colonial service, and those in asylums.[47] In 1912 fewer than one in four

---

[46] M. W. Dupree and M. Anne Crowther, 'A Profile of the Medical Profession in Scotland in the Early Twentieth Century: the Medical Directory as a Historical source', *BHM*, 65 (1991), pp. 223–9.

[47] See A. Newsholme, *The Ministry of Health* (1925), pp. 145–7, where Newsholme provides a breakdown of part- and full-time public medical appointments in 1917.

of those holding the important appointment of Medical Officer of Health had full-time posts.[48] MOHs had a high public visibility. Newsholme, who had been a very active MOH in Brighton, described them somewhat ambitiously as 'ministers of health each in his own area', but others – such as Winkfield in Oxford – were much less active.'[49] Such paid private and public appointments offered a secure and relatively easy source of money to the GP and were usually seen as valuable, so that doctors became increasingly entrepreneurial in pursuit of them. In addition, GPs might achieve an honorary appointment in a hospital or dispensary: during the early Victorian era around one in ten GPs had honorary appointments, mainly in dispensaries, since office in hospitals was much more competitive and increasingly reserved for an élite.[50] Later, cottage hospitals and children's hospitals offered GPs more accessible opportunities for hospital practice.

Some appointments were the exceptions to the rule in being regarded with ambivalence by the medical profession. By the end of the Edwardian period the better sorts of English practices made it a point of honour that they had no clubs. 'Clubs' were friendly societies that had contracted with a GP for a year's supply of medical care for their members and sometimes for their dependants as well. The open-ended nature of the commitment was less important in causing practitioners' disapproval than the very low payments per head that the clubs were able to impose on doctors in what had become a very competitive medical market. Also important was what was perceived as the undesirable strength in patient-power that clubs represented. Such consumer-controlled health insurance was becoming widespread in early-twentieth-century Europe, whilst a study of doctors in the State of Victoria, Australia during the early twentieth century also indicated a similar tussle of strength between doctors and clubs.[51]

What kinds of part-time medical offices could be combined with private patients in general practice? Two examples of Victorian country practices serve to elucidate the diverse ways in which public office could expand a practice. Charles Pitt took over a static Malmesbury practice in 1870. Within a few years he had become a poor-law district medical officer and public vaccinator to number 1

[48] *41st Report of LGB, 1912–3*, PP 1912–13, xxxv, Cd 6331, p. 398.
[49] Newsholme, *Ministry of Health*, p. 30; J. Parfitt, *The Health of a City: Oxford, 1770–1974* (1987), pp. 56, 132.
[50] Loudon, *Medical Care*, p. 225.
[51] T. A. Pensabene, *The Rise of the Medical Profession in Victoria* (1980); B. Abel-Smith, 'The Rise and Decline of Early Health Maintenance Organisations: Their International Experiences', *SHM*, 2, 1989, pp. 239–46.

district of the Malmesbury Union, and was also responsible for public health as the MOH to Malmesbury Urban Sanitary Authority, and later to the Rural Sanitary Authority as well. In addition he was called in under the provisions of the factory acts when accidents occurred, he provided medical assistance to the local police force, examined recruits to the local yeomanry, and did life assurance work for the Prudential. As the opportunities for medical work expanded, his territorial instincts and entrepreneurial flair meant that he capitalised on them; later examples included school medical inspections and the examination of milk in the local premises of the Ailesbury Dairy Company. From the 1880s onwards he performed such a wide range of work with local friendly societies that it became a major source of his income. His private practice was no doubt assisted by his high profile in these part-time paid offices, and also by his surgical work at the Malmesbury Cottage Hospital.[52] A similar experience was that of J. S. Taylor who practised in Thorne in South Yorkshire from the 1880s. Like Pitt he did work for the poor-law guardians, but also gave medical assistance at Thorne Grammar School, performed inspections for the West Riding Constabulary, and was paid for his medical services to the Manchester, Sheffield and Lincoln Railway. He later worked for Thorne District Council in the notification of contagious diseases. Finally, Dr Taylor had club appointments with no fewer than three friendly societies (the Oddfellows, Foresters and Royal Oak) as well as a further eleven sick clubs in Thorne and neighbouring Stainforth.[53]

In each case pluralism resulted from energetic practitioners attempting to monopolise public appointments in their territory. This dynamism was needed since, in the closing decades of the nineteenth century, the profession increased in size even more rapidly than did opportunities to hold office. This was revealed by advertisements of medical practices for sale. Table 4.2 indicates that for those fortunate enough to gain appointments, whether in town or country, such remuneration remained fairly constant at between one-fifth and one-quarter of gross income from the 1870s to the 1910s. Of much greater significance was the fact that over time such appointments became the province of only a minority of the profession. Whereas in 1877 two-thirds of country doctors and one-half of urban ones had appointments, forty years later the proportions had declined to one-half and one-fifth respectively. This deterioration in the towns had arisen from

[52] Wilts. RO, 1269/7–8; Pigot's and Kelly's *Directories*.
[53] RCPL, MSS 597–602, ledgers of Dr J. S. Taylor.

Making a medical living

Table 4.2. *Income from appointments in 1877–1909*

	Per cent of income from appointments of those holding such offices			Per cent of doctors having income from appointments		
	1877	1899	1909	1877	1899	1909
Rural	23	26	25	67	67	50
Urban	22	22	21	51	22	22

Source: Figures calculated from practices advertised for sale in the *BMJ Advertiser*, 1877, 1899, and from April to June 1909.

the greater expansion in numbers of practices, whereas country practices were both more stable in number and cushioned by the existence of comparatively more poor-law appointments per head of population. My estimate of one-fifth to one-quarter of practice income from appointments is a higher estimate than the 16 per cent given in 1911 in the Plender Report.[54] The latter sampled 171 urban practices, where it was predictable that the proportion of income from appointments would be smaller, because town medical incomes were higher and appointments more competitive.

The role of office in the career of a practitioner – and thus its function in creating a remunerative practice – varied. Above the more accessible foothills of offices that offered modest remuneration in a growing variety of posts were peaks of officeholding to be surmounted only by the well-qualified and the well-connected. For those aspiring to élite status the rewards came later than in general practice, and achieving office was much more crucial to success. Upward progress depended not only on ability but also on connection, since lay patronage – not to speak of nepotism – was usually important in gaining such office. There was contemporary anxiety about the manner in which patronage was exercised; the Select Committee on Medical Education of 1834 voiced the suspicion that it was not so much ability as social connection that determined hospital appointments.[55] In several hospitals – including those at Hereford, Exeter, Norwich, Lincoln, Huddersfield and Liverpool – more than one generation of a medical family benefitted from such prestigious offices. In these circumstances, contests for posts were sometimes acrimonious, being

[54] *Report of Sir William Plender on Medical Attendance and Remuneration*, PP 1912–13, 78, Cd 6305.
[55] *SC on Medical Education*, PP 1834, XIII, part 2, p. 98.

dependent on 'money, family influence and intrigue.'[56] Bitter contests surrounded elections as, for instance, with appointments of surgeons to the Sea Bathing Infirmary, Margate in 1792, or to the Bradford Dispensary in 1825.[57] Whilst waiting for election to such prestigious office, junior practitioners worked as assistants, afterwards termed residents or house surgeons, for which they later received a small salary or honorarium of £50 to £100.[58] An aspirant for a career as a general surgeon in a mid-nineteenth century hospital might reasonably expect to have been elected as an assistant surgeon in his early thirties, waiting another decade before reaching an appointment as a full surgeon.[59] Although hospital appointments allegedly had the drawback that medical autonomy and independence was infringed because of the amount of lay control, typically such considerations were subordinate to the necessity for the individual surgeon to achieve a good livelihood. Hospital posts enhanced public visibility and increased social contacts; the more prestigious usually having the potential to increase private practice. The careers of two contemporary surgeons will be taken as illustrative but contrasting examples of high-fliers since both Crosse and Haddy James achieved a 'place in the sun'.

John Haddy James (1788–1869) studied under the famous surgeon, John Abernethy, and for a time was House Surgeon at St Bartholomew's Hospital. The son of a retired Bristol merchant, Haddy James had attended Exeter Grammar School and been apprenticed for two years to Robert Patch, a surgeon at the Devon and Exeter Hospital. He was advised by Abernethy in 1812 that there were then only 'precarious prospects' in medicine, a verdict with which Haddy James concurred after assessing the prospects of achieving a hospital appointment in towns offering a reasonable opportunity of creating a successful practice. Deciding – like many of his generation[60] – that an army appointment was preferable in the short term he was gazetted Assistant Surgeon with the 1st Life Guards. But with the peace of 1815 he went back into civilian practice and decided to try his luck in Exeter where he had good lay and medical connections. With the help of excellent testimonials Haddy James was fortunate enough to be appointed almost immediately as one of the Surgeons at the Devon

[56] J. F. Clarke, *Autobiographical Reflections* (1874), p. 298.
[57] Wellcome AL 67615, Correspondence of John Anderson, letter May 1792; E. Wilmott, ed., *Journal of Dr John Simpson* (Bradford, 1981), p. 4.
[58] B. Abel Smith, *The Hospitals, 1800–1948*, p. 21; Peterson, *Medical Profession*, pp. 150–2.
[59] Peterson, *Medical Profession*, p. 137.
[60] Between 1790 and 1810 one in eight Edinburgh medical graduates entered the Army Medical Department (Rosner, *Medical Education*, p. 137).

and Exeter. That this kind of unpaid but prestigious post was the key to success in private practice, and also to further income from teaching and consultancy, was exemplified in Haddy James's career, since he rapidly built up a general private practice, began teaching at the hospital, and became one of the original 300 Fellows of the Royal College of Surgeons.[61]

Another of this band of 300 was J. G. Crosse (1790–1850), a surgeon with a general practice, and a reputation in obstetrics. His slower ascent in the profession was more typical than that of Haddy James. He started a practice in Norwich in 1815, the same year as had Haddy James in Exeter, but success did not come so swiftly to Crosse, who had to wait eight years before being appointed as Assistant Surgeon to the Norfolk and Norwich Hospital. Crosse had served an apprentice-ship with a Suffolk surgeon-apothecary, Bayly, studied in London at St George's Hospital and at the Windmill School of Anatomy, and then pursued further surgical studies in Paris. Unsuccessful in gaining a permanent hospital appointment in Dublin, he then pinned his hopes on Norwich. In deciding on Norwich as the centre of his professional life, he appears to have been reasonably confident of success there, having a written introduction to Edward Rigby, Physi-cian at the Norfolk and Norwich. Crosse wrote that 'Rigby's partiality to me increases and *I think I have got hold of him* – but there is no being certain of anything in times like these ... and although it be the common talk that I am called hither by Dr Rigby, I must not build too much on this foundation.[62]

The uncertainty of private patronage meant that doubts beset him. Four months after placing a brass plate on his door in May 1815, he was pessimistic about his future, 'Pretty miserable, advancing in years – going backward in knowledge and doing nothing in the way of practice to get a living.'[63] Private practice for Crosse increased with frustrating slowness, and that which did accrue was in part through the local recommendations of Bayly. Meanwhile, Crosse studied at the hospital and sought to improve his surgical skills, particularly in lithotomy (for which the Norfolk and Norwich Hospital was esteemed), and for which there was a steady demand, given the high incidence of 'the stone' in East Anglia.[64] His book on the subject, *The*

---

[61] Devon RO, 64/8/8/7 and 10, 73/12/1/1–9, letters of John Haddy James; Plarr, *Lives of the Royal College of Surgeons of England*, vol. I, pp. 605–6.

[62] Norfolk RO, MS 470, diary entry of 8 May 1815.

[63] Quoted in V. M. Crosse, *A Surgeon in the Early Nineteenth Century. The Life and Times of JG Crosse, 1790–1850* (1968), pp. 95–6.

[64] A. Batty Shaw, 'The Norwich School of Lithotomy', *MH*, xiv (1970), pp. 221–2.

Formation, Constituents and Extraction of the Urinary Calculus, was to win the Jacksonian Prize in 1833. Crosse's later reputation in obstetrics stood even higher. The growth of that private practice was some compensation for his failure in 1819 to be elected as Assistant Surgeon to the Norfolk and Norwich Hospital. Four years later he *was* successful, however, receiving three-fifths of the votes of the 500 lay governors who participated in the election, and three years after that he was appointed Surgeon.

Operating a practice: assistants and partners

For the surgeon-apothecary, later the GP, success had to be built up and maintained in a geographically more diffuse area than that of the institutional operating theatre. The range of medical functions performed by the GP, together with the geographical extent of practice, meant that a principal needed assistance. Infrequently, this professional situation might suggest a partnership, more often apprentices (in the early part of the period) or assistants (during the later part). Increasingly, however, the infirmary appears to have creamed the market for able aspirants to the medical profession, as was the case in Bristol by the 1770s,[65] so that a successor to the apprentice had to be found. Assistants, as successors to apprentices, fulfilled not only the same functions, but also more demanding ones. They were thus of greater importance in the dynamics of practice growth.

How many assistants were there? A guesstimate would suggest that numbers in mid-nineteenth century Britain were between three and four thousand, and this would have meant that one in every fourth or fifth practice employed one.[66] Assistants were likely to have been more common in larger practices or partnerships, as well as in country practices. If a public office such as that of poor-law district medical officer was taken by a GP it was essential to have an assistant to keep the 'shop', take messages during the absence on rounds of the principal and, if necessary, to deputise in giving medical care. It is instructive to see that the central poor-law authority – when faced with

---

[65] Fissell, *Patients, Power, and the Poor*, p. 134.
[66] The *Census* is not very helpful since it aggregated assistants with other categories of medical personnel. *Census* figures for medical assistants and students together were: 1851, 3655; 1861, 3566; 1871, 4514; 1881, 5992. Numbers of registered medical students in 1871 were 902, and in 1881, 1631. Such an estimate receives some corroboration from a much later survey for 1935–7, which indicated that fewer than one in five of all practices had assistants. Their use was heavily concentrated in larger practices; only one out of fifty in smaller practices but two out of five in the largest ones (A. Bradford Hill, 'The Doctor's Pay and Day', *Journal of the Royal Statistical Society*, CIV (1951), p. 23).

evidence of any neglect by district medical officers – instructed them to employ an assistant.[67]

The stereotypical image of the assistant was that of cheap labour. In 1847, for instance, a 'country practitioner' considered £30 a reasonable salary for an assistant.[68] However, a period as an assistant was more than merely sweated labour. Indeed it was recommended for those who wished to go into private practice, both in order to gain valuable practical experience, and with the hope of being taken on as a partner later on.[69] However, growing numbers of medical students, and increasing numbers of qualified doctors relative to viable openings for the newly-qualified, appear gradually to have transformed the meaning of assistant during the second half of the Victorian period. The late nineteenth-century and early twentieth-century advertising columns of the *BMJ's Advertiser* indicated a complex picture.[70] There were few references to assistantships as avenues to partnerships, so that it is likely that upward mobility from assistant to partner had become more difficult. And, where a partnership was not in prospect, principals might safeguard themselves in the traditional manner used with apprenticeships. They would specify that, on leaving, their assistant must practise elsewhere, in yet another application of the principle of territoriality.

During the 1870s individual advertisers in the *BMJ* who wanted assistantships ranged from the first-year medical student to the qualified practitioner. Revealingly, one of the few agencies that dealt with assistantships was warning by the 1880s that 'no assistant shall be recommended till direct inquiries have been made as to his antecedents.'[71] From this one might surmise that assistantships had traditionally been seen as a last refuge by the professionally or personally inadequate. The litany of requests for steady, sober or abstaining applicants, who were also God-fearing church or chapel attenders, would tend to confirm this view, since they hinted at the inadequacies of the usual applicant for a vacant assistantship. So too would the occasional admission by qualified doctors, who sought an assistant's post for themselves, that they had recently sold their own practice; having failed as a principal they were now reduced to an assistantship.[72]

---

[67] A. W. Greer, *Tubbs. A Nineteenth Century G.P.* (King's Lynn, 1988), pp. 55–6, 62 Norfolk RO Forehoe Minutes, 9 July 1849.

[68] *Lancet*, 13 November 1847, p. 528.   [69] Keeteley, *Students' Guide*, p. 31.

[70] The following have been consulted: 1877, 1899 and 1909 in complete sets, and 1876 and 1885 for incomplete sets.

[71] *BMJ Advertiser*, 3 January 1885, warning from the Scholastic, Clerical and Medical Association.

[72] For example, *BMJ Advertiser*, 9 December 1876.

Typically, an ability to ride a horse (later a bicycle) was seen as a near essential requirement for an assistant; a good, neat hand was useful for keeping the books; so too was maturity, and some advertisements specified that only those who were over twenty-five years of age need apply. Vacancies were geographically varied and were offered in rural, suburban, and urban locations. There were, in addition, conspicuously frequent openings for assistants advertised by colliery companies in mining districts, especially in Wales, where ability to speak Welsh was as mandatory as the applicant's good intentions towards alcohol consumption. These were demanding posts (as A. J. Cronin's later depiction showed so vividly), in which relatively good salaries of £120 to £160 were offered for outdoor posts where the assistant did not live with the principal. However, the attractiveness of the money was more than offset by the onerous duties demanded.[73] Generally, assistants were required to keep the books. Less frequently their duties involved dispensing, and sometimes also visiting patients. Individuals wanting positions might promise more than this: adverts in 1877, for example, boasted of abilities to vaccinate, perform minor surgery, dress wounds, extract teeth, or even conduct a branch practice.[74] Usually those advertisements offering medical skills came from students, then some way towards having gained a medical qualification, who wanted time off for study or for hospital duties, whilst in the rest of their day agreeing to perform an assistant's duties for a small salary of £25 to £30 per year. Full time salaries at this time were around £50 for an unqualified, and £60–80 for a qualified, indoor appointment; with £120–150 the going rate for a qualified outdoor post.[75] A few appointments promised to give a percentage on midwifery fees in addition.[76] The social character of the patients that the assistant might expect to encounter was occasionally indicated; predictably, it was the most humdrum or lowly part of the principal's practice. The assistant as medical workhorse could look forward at this point only to dealing with cases of ordinary midwifery, seeing members of clubs, or attending to poor-law patients. And, like prime candidates for the boxing ring, applicants were advised to include details of weight, age, and height. Later, even a photograph might be specified.[77]

[73] See the vivid portrayal of such a post during the 1920s in A. J. Cronin, *The Citadel* (1937).

[74] For example, *BMJ Advertiser*, 26 May 1877, 28 July 1877, 11 August 1877, 22 September 1877.

[75] For example, *BMJ Advertiser*, adverts by Mr J. R. Wilson, Medical Agent, 18 March and 10 June 1876.

[76] For example, *BMJ Advertiser*, 13 October 1877.

[77] For example, *BMJ Advertiser*, 13 October 1877.

The impression given by these advertisements was substantiated by the record left by a young and unqualified assistant, Alexander Blyth. He went to a London agent, a Mr Wilson of Charles Street where, having submitted testimonials, 'I wrote my name and he promised to get me a situation in a few days.' For a fee of 45 shillings, the agent succeeded in getting Blyth the offer of an indoor position in a busy practice run by the Ceely brothers in Aylesbury, Buckinghamshire. The wife of one of the partners wrote to him to describe the practice:

You will like to know the practice is for an agricultural neighbourhood – [a] large one parish district and the union [workhouse] included. Mr Ceely is also surgeon to the county prison and both belong to the county infirmary. Thus you will see that there is ample time for improvement in the profession. There is full occupation, but I think I may tell you nothing that an active and intelligent young surgeon cannot actively accomplish.[78]

The Ceelys were disappointed that Blyth had not yet attended medical lectures and reduced the salary proportionately. He was paid at the rate of £40 per annum for the first six months and £45 thereafter.

The realities of everyday practice during the 1860s and the discipline enforced by principals in a competitive medical market meant hard work, and Blyth found that he had succeeded two other short-lived assistants. On arrival he was given a room at the top of the house overlooking the market square where the practice was located. He began his duties in the surgery the evening he arrived. Normally, his routine was to dispense in the surgery from 8 am to 1 pm, and again in the evening after dinner. He was assisted by a boy who ran errands and delivered medicines. The practice was a flourishing one with wealthy private patients that included Benjamin Disraeli, the Duke of Buckingham and Lord Carrington. However, Blyth was confined to seeing the poorer patients whom he attended during the afternoon. He described how the paupers were 'most of them old people', and that he was 'as kind and affable as I well know how.' Here he was perhaps exhibiting some fellow-feeling for their lowly station in life. In a bleaker moment however, he described how his lot was 'to see a lot of wretched sick paupers in the union, or in the back slums, or any other dirty stinking place that generates disease.' He viewed busy market days with particular loathing, 'of all the days in the week I hate this day ... all the country louts for miles around drive their pigs and their ailments together at the same time.'[79]

Yet at the end of a hard day his desire for self-improvement led him

---

[78] Bucks RO box 5, diary of A. W. Blyth, letter of Mrs E. P. Ceely to A. W. Blyth.
[79] Diary of A. W. Blyth, 5 November and 17 and 22 October 1864.

to benefit from the small library in the practice's surgery; here he read Paget on pathology or Watson on physic. On occasion he became depressed, 'It is a great pity for my [sic] to be wasting my time as an assistant, when I ought to be studying up for the London University – but I suppose I must be patient.'[80] However, his inauspicious early years in medical practice did not prevent him later becoming MOH for Marylebone, and may indeed have given him invaluable experience for the post. He also became an authority on poisons, and his book, *Poisons, their Effects and Detection*, went through five editions.

After the Medical Act of 1858 the General Medical Council gradually tightened up on assistants' qualifications so that unqualified people could no longer practise with a registered doctor, unless they were bona fide medical students. In 1883 the General Medical Council decided that infamous conduct by a registered GP included the employment of an unqualifed assistant, and in 1888 the first practitioner was struck off for this offence.[81] Practice by the unqualified assistant lingered on, but in the medical press vacancies advertised were for qualified people only.[82] Advertisers now demanded details of experience, also stated that they required testimonials, and might even demand the 'usual bond'. This was a standard agreement drawn up by a lawyer for an agent's use, and was designed to 'protect principals'.[83] Also changed at the turn of the century was the state of the medical market, now endowed with an abundance of qualified doctors. This meant that the type of person being sought as an assistant was an informed and hard-working second-in-command, who would take an energetic part in a practice, and thereby earn a higher salary. Typically, this was of the order of £90–100, or more exceptionally up to £120 for an indoor post and a minimum of £150 for an outdoor one, rising to £200 or occasionally even more.[84] A decade later posts for indoor assistants were being advertised with remuneration varying from £120 to £150, and outdoor ones were typically in a range

---

[80] Diary of A. W. Blyth, 17 October 1864.
[81] R. Smith, 'The Development of Guidance for Medical Practitioners by the General Medical Council', *MH*, 33 (1993), p. 60.
[82] *Report as to the Practice by Unqualified Persons*, p. 29. This prohibition of the unqualified working with the qualified practitioner continued to be controversial. It is important to appreciate, however, that the Medical Act of 1858 had not prohibited unqualified practice; it merely stated that the unqualified should not pass themselves off as registered.
[83] See for example the statement by Percival Turner on his services to the medical profession, *BMJ Advertiser*, 27 November 1909.
[84] For example, *BMJ Advertiser*, advert by Scholastic, Clerical and Medical Association for assistancies, 7 January 1899.

from £180 to £250.[85] By this time, as Figure 1.1 indicated, the numbers of graduating medical students had levelled off, so tending to drive up the market rate for qualified assistants.

This was more especially true of the larger practice, and here the organisation might be that of a partnership. In the late eighteenth century only one in twelve English practices had partners.[86] A century later I would estimate that one in seven practices were partnerships, a figure that had increased to one in five by the end of the Edwardian period.[87] Advertisements indicated that there were several reasons for this. An expanding practice might seek to take on an additional doctor to sustain the load, as in 'a share in a large mainly surgical practice is offered to a young unmarried man for £1000 after one year's preliminary assistantship at a salary of £200 outdoor.'[88] In some cases this was a 'partnership with succession', whereby a doctor coming to the end of a working life wished to convert a single-handed practice into a temporary partnership, with the expectation that the entrant to the practice would then buy out the older partner in a couple of years. For example, 'Partner wanted with a view to succession in two to five years in well-established mixed-class dispensing practice.'[89] More common was when one of two partners wished to retire and a replacement was wanted. Typically, in these circumstances, a two-fifth share of the practice was offered with the option of bringing this up to one-half in a short time. There was an emphasis on the social qualities of the aspirant. For example, in 1909 'S. W. Co[unties] Partnership. Hospital town. Young well-qualified man used to good society required as Junior Partner in a really nice practice'.[90] Or, for a less imposing practice, 'Partnership with succession ... Only those who are energetic, tactful and of good character need apply.'[91] More generally, there might be a specification as to age (not under 30), marital status (married usually preferred), or occasionally on income (private means preferred). Premiums for partnerships were on average one and a half times the annual income, reckoned on the prior three years' receipts.[92]

Partnerships tended increasingly to employ more ancillary staff in

[85] For example, *BMJ Advertiser*, adverts by Scholastic, Clerical and Medical Association for assistancies, 9 and 16 January 1909.
[86] Lane, 'Bradford Wilmer, p. 371.
[87] *BMJ Advertiser*, analysis of practice advertisements for 1877, 1899, and 1909. The figure of one in five accords with that in PEP, *Report on the British Health Services* (1937), p. 143, where it indicated that a fifth of practices in London were partnerships.
[88] *BMJ Advertiser*, 19 June 1909.   [89] *BMJ Advertiser*, 7 October 1899.
[90] *BMJ Advertiser*, 12 June 1909.
[91] *BMJ Advertiser*, 2 January 1909.   [92] PEP *Report on Health Services*, p. 143.

order to economise on the principals' time. These were most often for dispenser and book-keeper appointments, but a less common variant was that of dispenser and surgery attendant, or even occasionally for chauffeur and dispenser. Whereas there had been very few such opportunities in the 1870s, such openings were more common by the 1890s and 1900s. One reason may have been that these were the unqualified assistants now presented under a different – and more acceptable – label. The post of lady dispenser and book-keeper, some-times with typing in addition, was also found, and reflected the contemporary expansion of white-blouse work.[93] But for single-handed practices the doctor's wife was more representative of female ancillary help. Only exceptional practices employed numerous ancil-laries. Harry Roberts' large East End practice of five partners had a dentist, medical masseuse, and two dispensers, as well as secretaries.[94] Expenditures on increased numbers of staff made good economic sense since their cost was likely to be more than offset by fees from the extra numbers of patients that could be treated, so that there would be a more than commensurate increase in net income.[95]

How large were practice expenses? Data are scattered and hard to collate,[96] and no precise figure can be reached before an authoritative estimate for 1913–14. For this date, there were returns from GPs, from which the BMA commissioned calculations by Bowley, the eminent statistician. He estimated that 25 per cent of gross receipts of good practices went on expenses, and 16 per cent in working-class ones.[97] Bowley calculated that travelling costs constituted 50 per cent of expenses, surgery expenses another 40 per cent, and the remaining 10 per cent was spent on rent, rates and fuel. He made the liberal assumption that one-third of all household rent, fuel and rates expen-diture was the appropriate share of the doctor's practice expenses. (This was likely to have been an over-estimate since at this date few practitioners had more than a surgery for their patients.) Once expenses had been deducted from gross receipts the net income of the practitioner was then liable to income tax; in 1913 this stood at 1s 2d in

[93] Based on advertisements in *BMJ* 27 January 1877, 28 January and 11 March 1899, 23 January and 30 January 1909.

[94] W. Stamp, *'Doctor Himself'. An Unorthodox Biography of Harry Roberts, 1871–1946* (1949).

[95] For a slightly later period, this was certainly the case. (Digby and Bosanquet, 'Doctors and Patients', p. 83).

[96] Expenses of from 7 per cent to 60 per cent were given in 1878, and with middle estimates for good practices of from 25 per cent to 33 per cent. (*Report on Candidates for the Army Medical Department*, PP 1878–9, XLIV, pp. 259–305).

[97] *BMJ Supplement*, 5 January 1924. Bowley's lower figure was for panel patients created by the national health insurance provisions of the 1911 act.

the pound.[98] The expenses of 1913–14 were possibly greater than in preceding years since certain items in practice expenditure – notably salaries and rates[99] – had risen steeply in the late Victorian and Edwardian era. At the same time, as the next chapter indicates, the income of the GP had become more precarious.

[98] B. R. Mitchell, *Abstract of British Historical Statistics* (Cambridge, 1962), p. 428.
[99] C. Feinstein, 'A new look at the cost of living, 1870–1914' in J. Foreman Peck, ed., *New Perspectives on the Late Victorian Economy* (Cambridge, 1991), p. 167.

5

The GP and the goal of prosperity

An American historian of medicine commented in 1977 that 'the economic history of medicine, especially before the twentieth century remains entirely to be written.'[1] Since then there have been several studies which have done a good deal to shed light on this hidden dimension of medical practice in England and Wales.[2] This chapter focuses particularly on the late nineteenth century and is thus complementary to these two studies. Although the business of medicine was vital to the doctor's survival open discussion was inhibited by professional custom and the prevailing gentlemanly ethic. There was none of that forthright discussion of medical entrepreneurship that was to be found in some other countries. In the USA, for example, the period closed with a spate of publications with titles like *The Physician as Business Man, How to Succeed in the Practice of Medicine, Building a Profitable Practice*, or even, *Dollars to Doctors!*[3] Whereas in America doctors were seen as individual entrepreneurs,[4] in England this was an alien concept. This reticence about the business aspect of medicine made life difficult for the practitioner, who usually discovered the economics of medical practice the hard way. It also creates problems for the historian, so that sources must be used innovatively in order to elucidate this hidden dimension.

[1] P. Starr, 'Medicine, Economy and Society in Nineteenth Century America,' *Journal of Social History*, 10 (1977).

[2] Notably, Peterson, *The Medical Profession*, Loudon, *Medical Care*, Marland, *Medicine in Wakefield and Huddersfield*.

[3] J. M. Taylor, *The Physician as Businessman* (Philadelphia, 1891); J. M. Mathews, *How to Succeed in the Practice of Medicine* (Louisville, 1902); T. F. Reilly, *Building a Profitable Practice* (Philadelphia, 1912); N. F. Wood, *Dollars to Doctors* (Chicago, 1912).

[4] G. Rosen, *The Structure of American Medical Practice, 1875–1941* (Philadelphia, 1983), p. 16.

Medicine as a business

'Even if I should begin practice on my own account it would be several years before I could expect any established business', wrote a newly-qualified surgeon in 1810.[5] How to acquire such business was a neglected topic in formal medical education, although it figured in the correspondence columns of medical journals, and doubtless was also the subject of anxious enquiry by juniors to their senior colleagues. One of the few systematic discussions of the financial side of British medical practice was a short chapter in de Styrap's *The Young Practitioner* of 1890:

As a medical practitioner you will hold two positions in relation to your patients: first, during illness you will have to render them your skilled professional aid. Later, when your skill is no longer needed, you will enter upon the second or business relation, which entitles you to claim a just remuneration for your services.[6]

This volume offered much useful information on topics such as fees, billing and debt collection. It warned that 'it is almost impossible to become rich by the practice of medicine' since, whilst it was 'comparatively easy to get practice among the moneyless poor', it was 'relatively hard to do so among the wealthier classes.'

Irvine Loudon has argued convincingly that the second half of the eighteenth century was a 'golden age of physic' when there was a buoyant medical market.[7] He suggests that the average rural surgeon-apothecary could earn £400 a year in mid-career.[8] Yet even at this time it took very hard work to create a flourishing practice. A rural surgeon-apothecary wrote in 1800:

I have by industry, rigid economy and painful application to a laborious profession – stooping to the lowest offices, among the lowest of the people, after many hundreds of watching nights and wearisome days – and for the modest hope of *sometime* arriving at independence doing things for the sake of saving, that not one in 20 of my profession would demean themselves to do ... I say after going on in this manner for 30 years I find myself ... worth about £4000 ... It will not maintain myself, wife and six sons and daughters as gentlemen and ladies.[9]

GPs' charges in early-nineteenth century practice were kept within relatively narrow limits with surprisingly little variation based on the status of the patient; thus a lot of patients had to be seen to acquire a

[5] L. Woodford, 'A Medical Student's Career in the Early Nineteenth century', *MH*, pp. 90–6.
[6] de Styrap, *Practitioner*, p. 200.   [7] Loudon, 'Provincial Medical Practice', pp. 25, 29.
[8] Loudon, *Medical Care*, p. 113.   [9] Lincs. R. O. Flinders III/3 letter to son, Matthew.

modest income.[10] And from 1815 to the mid-nineteenth century there was a notorious over-supply of doctors leading to low professional rewards.[11] For the early nineteenth century Loudon concluded that 'From 1800 to 1850 it became increasingly hard to become established in general practice, and income for the first few years was often very low indeed.'[12] He suggests incomes of £150 to £250 in the country and £300 to £500 in the town for those GPs attended with a 'fair degree of success'.[13] At the start of the Victorian period a leading surgeon, Sir Anthony Carlisle, commented that because 'the wants of the public require a great number of medical practitioners, ... the majority of them must necessarily be scantily paid.'[14]

For the more successful, income from teaching was a significant supplement. Considerable sums could be earned in apprenticeship premiums: provincial surgeon-apothecaries earned a few pounds upwards, those with hospital appointments got as much as 200 guineas, whilst for influential London medical masters the premium could be as high as 350 pounds.[15] Surgeons' interest in the infirmaries grew because it provided an important source of income through pupils and lecture fees, even if their actual posts in surgery were honorary unpaid ones.[16] Occasionally, teaching could be a business in its own right, as was the case with the partnership of Sharpey and Thomson, who offered extramural teaching in the Universities of Edinburgh, Glasgow and London during the 1830s and 1840s.[17] Thus teaching was, for most who practised it, a useful adjunct to other income. In 1873 it was thought that successful consulting surgeons (with additional income from lecturing to medical students and from a large number of pupils) could make £5000 annually after ten years' practice. And at the very top of their profession they would double this income.[18]

Data on élite surgeons' incomes from teaching, general practice, and specialist consultancy are more accessible than those for the ordinary practitioner, and suggest that rewards for a few were considerable. The estate values of those who were either President or Vice-

---

[10] Loudon, *Medical Care*, pp. 249–51.
[11] I. S. L. Loudon, 'A Doctor's Cash Book. The Economy of General Practice in the 1830s', *Medical History*, 27 (1983).
[12] Loudon, *Medical Care*, p. 258.   [13] Loudon, *Medical Care*, p. 261.
[14] A. Carlisle, *Practical Observations on the Preservation of Health* (1838), p. xxviii.
[15] J. Lane, 'The role of apprenticeship in eighteenth-century medical education' in Bynum and Porter, *William Hunter*, pp. 69–71.
[16] Fissell, *Patients, Power, and the Poor*, p. 136.
[17] L. S. Jacyna, ed., *A Tale of Three Cities. The Correspondence of W. Sharpey and A. Thomson* (Medical History Supplement 9, 1989), pp. xiv-xv.
[18] *Lancet*, 4 January 1873, p. 29.

President of the Royal College of Surgeons suggest a higher earning capacity among surgeons than physicians.[19] London surgeon-princes might command very high annual incomes at the peak of their careers: Henry Thompson made £8000, Benjamin Brodie £8–10,000, John Abernethy and James Paget each earned £10,000 and Astley Cooper £15,000 to £21,000.[20]

In their earlier years surgeons had to be content with smaller sums. Brodie, Assistant Surgeon to St George's Hospital made less than £300 from his private practice in 1809, although supplementing this with fees from pupils. Private practice income then increased incrementally by £200–250 per year so that by 1816 he made £1530 from fees and lecturing, and was able to afford a carriage. In 1819 publication of *Diseases of the Joints* contributed to a large increment of £1000, while appointment as Professor of Comparative Anatomy to the College of Surgeons gave his name further public prominence. Four years later Brodie made £6500 from his practice and more from pupils and teaching.[21] Acquiring a baronetcy, a country estate, and a life style of conspicuous consumption he remarked in later life that 'Prosperous as I was in my profession, I had always felt that I was overworked, and that what I gained in income was counterbalanced by the loss of comfort.'[22] But provincial surgeons, even those of considerable professional standing, made more modest fortunes. For instance, Crosse of Norwich, who achieved considerable reputation as a lithotomist and obstetrician, made only £47,000 from the first twenty-three years of a practice that had begun in 1815. On average this was only slightly more than the £500 per year estimated as the average earnings of the mid-century GP.[23] Crosse comforted himself with the reflection that he was not:

ambitious of very great earnings – not the least of possessing much wealth – fortunate matters to be able honestly to avow since I follow a profession which, in proportion to the labour done and the time given to it, and the powers of mind requisite, makes the acquisition of wealth impracticable.[24]

Later in the century, James Paget's largest annual medical income during his first seven years of practice was only £23, and he did not make £100 until he had been practising for 16 years. Once he had decided to make the transition from hospital to private practice,

[19] Peterson, *Medical Profession*, p. 208. The figures are for deaths from 1856–1928.
[20] I. Waddington, *The Medical Profession in the Industrial Revolution* (1984), pp. 31–2.
[21] *Autobiography*, pp. 77–8, 85, 97, 116, 127, 141, 166–7.
[22] *Autobiography*, pp. 167, 183.
[23] Thomson, *Profession*, p. 169.
[24] Norfolk R. O. MS 476, Memoirs of J. Crosse, fos. 62, 134.

however, his income steadily increased from £700 to £10,000 annually.[25] Henry Thompson's career revealed a more rapid progression. Qualifying in 1850 as a surgeon, he put up his brass plate as a consulting surgeon in Wimpole Street in the following year. From private fees – including those from both general and consultancy practice – he made only £162 in 1852 and £135 in 1853, but with a rise to £254 in 1854, following the award of the Jacksonian prize for his book on strictures. Within the next decade he became one of the best known consulting surgeons in London, and by 1865 was making £6645 from patients' fees. At the height of his career Thompson was able to charge £1000 for foreign consultations (such as that on Napoleon III), and make £8000 a year from only nine months' work, the other three months being taken as holiday. He left a fortune of £226,000.[26]

As to the comparative advantages or disadvantages of the profession, prescriptive literature gave useful general advice. H. B. Thomson suggested in 1857 that 'a fair average man, rather above the average standard in most of his qualities, and with no particular defects may reasonably expect to succeed in the profession of medicine.'[27] He was unusual in giving a precise indication of expected incomes and cited an average of £500 gross income per year in general practice. Later, a less sanguine eye was cast on the prospects of the young medical man; medical education was a 'costly' business and 'no one should embrace it who is not able to spend pretty freely for some years, in the hope of being able, at some future day, to make a good position and a good income.'[28] In 1875 it was stated that 'all GPs are underpaid',[29] whilst three years later came a series of warnings about the difficulties and financial pitfalls likely to be concealed in an advertised 'splendid opening for a young medical man' in general practice.[30] These ranged from the genuinely desirable (commonly either well-established practices in residential suburbs or those country practices in good sporting country) to the unappealing downside of the market – the practice nuclei usually located in inner city areas which gave a derisory net income. Whilst the former often indicated a voluntary leisure preference, with their 'no night work undertaken', 'midwifery declined' or 'no clubs', the latter suggested enforced idleness or underemployment.[31]

[25] S. Paget, ed., *Memoirs And Letters of Sir James Paget* (1901), p. 184.

[26] Z. Cope, *The Versatile Victorian, Being the Life of Sir Henry Thompson, Bt, 1820–1904* (1951), pp. 24–8, 47, 141, 153.

[27] *The Choice of a Profession* (1857), p. 145.   [28] *What Shall My Son Be* (1870), p. 55.

[29] *The State of the Medical Profession in Great Britain and Ireland* (Dublin, 1875), p. 12.

[30] *The Student's Guide to the Medical Profession* (1878), pp. 32–4.

[31] *BMJ Advertiser*, 1875–7, 1885, 1899, 1909.

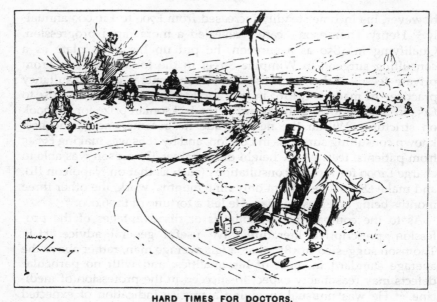

HARD TIMES FOR DOCTORS.

THIS IS NOT A POLICE TRAP, BUT ONLY UNEMPLOYED MEDICAL MEN WAITING ALONG THE BRIGHTON ROAD ON THE OFF-CHANCE OF A MOTOR-CAR ACCIDENT.

Plate 6 'Hard Times for Doctors' (*Punch*, 1907)

The large extent of medical underemployment (see Plate 6) towards the end of the nineteenth century and beginning of the twentieth century was the product of a number of factors. One was the increased supply of late-nineteenth-century entrants to the profession from medical schools (see Figure 1.2). Entry into the English medical market by those who had qualified in Scotland or Ireland exacerbated the problem, as did an abundance of alternative practitioners, druggists, and chemists. Patients could also turn to a number of free institutions, and it was in this period that there was a notable expansion in out-patient care in the voluntary hospitals. In these unpropitious circumstances what kind of income could the qualified practitioner expect?

For the late nineteenth century and early twentieth century little information exists on medical incomes. According to a recent study of the subject a broad stability in medical incomes existed during the late nineteenth and early twentieth centuries, although this conclusion was based on what was acknowledged to be a paucity of empirical evidence.[32] Peterson speculated that:

[32] Peterson, *Medical Profession*, p. 214.

The rank and file of the GPs were attempting to live as 'professional gentlemen' on incomes that were at least marginal and often well below the income of the £700 defined by Banks as required in order to sustain the 'paraphernalia of gentility'. Conceivably, a majority of all medical men were trying to maintain a gentleman's household on half that amount.[33]

Was this in fact the case? Because this issue is so important for an understanding of the structure and amount of medical earnings a special investigation was undertaken in order to resolve this issue. New estimates of medical incomes were compiled using advertisements of practices for sale in the *BMJ Advertiser*.

This is a rich source, but an unusual one, since most libraries ripped out this part of the journal before binding the year's issues. I have been fortunate in tracking down a limited number – sets for 1877, 1899, and a few years in the Edwardian era.[34] How reliable a source are these for medical incomes? Since the *BMJ* catered for the GP rather than for the small élite of consultants, this distribution may be taken as a broad indication of the incomes of the bulk of the medical profession. Clearly, certain caveats must be borne in mind, since advertisements would cast a rosy glow on the incomes and prospects of the practices. Nevertheless, there was a trend towards substantiating the accuracy of the figures in advertisements. Agencies recommended that vendors selling through them should have the practice books checked by an accountant, with a report available to prospective purchasers.[35] However, this was clearly a counsel of perfection. And given the semi-chaotic state of many practice ledgers it is unsurprising to find that the advice fell on deaf ears. Only a small minority of sellers included statements such as, 'certified returns about £600', 'accountant's audit over £700', 'books have been examined', 'books certified correct', or even, 'books open to accountant's investigation.'[36] In these circumstances agencies counselled caution. 'Before concluding arrangements the books should be examined and the numerous necessary inquiries as to bona fides made by a medical accountant, specially versed in such matters.'[37] This was presumably because of complaints by purchasers that the practice had failed to deliver the income specified in the advertisement. To take one instance, Dr Pooler complained that his Birmingham practice yielded only £412 during his

---

[33] Peterson, *Medical Profession*, pp. 219–20.
[34] These were found in the Countway Library at Harvard University, Boston and the Wellcome Institute for the History of Medicine, London.
[35] See, for example, the form issued by The Scholastic, Clerical and Medical Association Ltd for colonial practices in *BMJ Advertiser*, 3 July 1909.
[36] *BMJ Advertiser*, 3 June and 15 July 1899: 24 July, 4 September, and 11 December 1909.
[37] For example, advertisement of Mr Percival Turner, *BMJ Advertiser*, 24 July 1909.

first year's practice as a GP in the 1890s, compared with the £700 that had been predicted.[38] There could have been a number of reasons for this, so that fraudulent intent on the part of the seller should not necessarily be assumed. Any appointments held may not have been transferable ones, whilst the qualities of the incoming doctor may not have been such as to retain the confidence of patients. In addition, if the practice was a so-called 'death vacancy' then the practice may have been run down during a period of failing health. And, where partnerships were concerned, the personality and habits of the remaining partner(s) were also crucial in maintaining income. It may have been the case, for example, that the retiring partner was the 'power-house' of the practice, whilst the ongoing partner liked the bottle too much. Of course, the boot might be on the other foot as the earlier experiences of the Maldon surgeon, Richard Paxton indicated: he was saddled with an 'imperious and rude' newcomer who dishonestly never paid his full premium.[39] Purchasers needed to think hard about the size of the premium or purchase price sought in relation to the advertised income, since young practitioners might need to saddle themselves with a mortgage or loan. Premiums in the late Victorian and Edwardian eras varied from less than one-third (for a dubious practice nucleus) to one and a half times or even twice the annual practice income (for desirable, unopposed country practices or old-established urban/surburban ones).[40]

Agencies wished to sell practices in order to win commissions, and the higher the income advertised for the practice the larger the commission that was earned. Individuals who advertised also wished to display their practice in the best light so that the advertised figures on income should be taken as an *upper* rather than lower set of estimates. How far figures for a small sample of years may be taken as representative is a difficult issue, but in my judgement there is no reason to think that they were not. The assumption has been made that the same proportion of practices out of the total number of medical practices were advertised in this way in the years sampled. However, it must be acknowledged that an increasing number of medical agents advertised during the period: seven in 1877; nine in 1899; and twelve in 1909.[41] This is likely to have expanded the market, although it may have done so differentially, since more new agencies later operated

---

[38] H. W. Pooler, *My Life in General Practice* (1948). It isn't clear whether this was bought through an agency.

[39] Wellcome MS 3820.   [40] *BMJ Advertiser*, 1877, 1899, 1909.

[41] I have identified nineteen agencies in all, only three of which survived the four decades.

Table 5.1. *Estimates for medical incomes in 1878*

Period after Qualifying	Gross income £	Net income £
Immediately[a]	150–400	–
1 Year	25–150	–
1–5 Years	400–500	300
8 Years	[600][b]	—
10 Years	450–1500	200–1400
25 Years (age 50)	1000–1700	800
35 Years (age 60)	600–1200	470–1000

Notes:
[a] These were men from St Bartholomew's.
[b] £500 plus appointments.
Source: Report on Candidates for the Medical Department, PP, 1878–9, XLIV, pp. 259–305.

from the provinces rather than London. When evaluating the data below this fact must be borne in mind so that, for instance, there is a recognition that an increased number of small practices advertised *may* have been influenced by growing entrepreneurial activity rather than by an actual trend to smaller practice nuclei. As against that there is evidence of a greater expansion of numbers than in comparable professions. Between 1881 and 1911 numbers of doctors increased by 63 per cent, as against barristers and solicitors whose numbers rose by only 23 per cent.[42]

One source that can be used as a comparison is contemporary estimates given to a parliamentary inquiry into the relative incomes of civilian and army medical men in 1878, one year after the first set of calculations. The committee concluded, 'Taken one year with another, a young man obtains in civil life a net income of £300 a year within 5 years of commencing practice. After 10 years he is unlucky if he does not net £500 a year, and hence his income gradually rises to an average of £800 to £1000.'[43] Table 5.1 summarises the results of this enquiry.

Since much of this evidence came from top medical schools the range of earnings of their élite graduates was on the high side for the rank and file. Unfortunately, there was no indication of the distribution of medical incomes as a whole in this source (or indeed in any

[42] H. J. Perkin, 'Middle-Classs Education and Employment in the 19th Century: A Critical Note', *Economic History Review*, 14 (1961–2).
[43] *Report on Candidates for the Medical Department*, PP 1878–9, para 8.

Table 5.2. *Structure of general practices by gross income, 1877, 1899 and 1909 (per cent)*

	Country			Urban			All practices		
	i 1877	ii 1899	iii 1909	iv 1877	v 1899	vi 1909	vii 1877	viii 1899	ix 1909
<£300	2	17	4	4	19	11	3	18	9
£300–399	13	24	11	13	14	11	12	17	11
Nucleus/small	15	41	15	17	33	22	15	35	20
£400–599	41	33	40	25	31	31	34	32	33
£600–799	18	19	21	22	19	19	20	19	20
Standard	59	52	61	47	50	50	54	51	53
£800–999	13	2	14	12	8	15	13	6	15
Good	13	2	14	12	8	15	13	6	15
£1000–1499	12	4	9	18	7	12	15	6	11
£1500+	1	1	1	6	2	1	3	2	1
First class	13	5	10	24	9	13	18	8	12
N	127	208	170	119	534	408	246	742	578

Notes: These figures are for single-handed general practices, not partnerships. The 1909 figures are for 3 months only. A deduction of between 16% and 25% should be made to convert to net incomes.
Source: Calculated from advertisements in the *BMJ Advertiser*, 1877, 1899 and 1909.

other source for the period). This is the omission that I have attempted to rectify in Table 5.2, by analysing the *BMJ* advertisements for 1877, 1899 and for three months of 1909. (The three months are for April, May and June and constitute a quarter of practices advertised over the year. There is no reason to think that their composition and numbers differed significantly from those advertised in the other three quarters of 1909.) The figures are for ordinary practices and exclude partnerships. They show gross annual incomes and there would need to be a deduction of between one seventh and one-quarter from them to get net incomes. Taking medical incomes for 1877 (col. vii, Table 5.2), these show a lower range and median than those published in the parliamentary estimates in Table 5.1.

When contemporary perceptions are used to categorise them, the practices fell into four income groups. At the bottom of the range, with incomes of under £400 per annum, were those seen as merely a 'nucleus' for a practice or, if a little bigger, as a 'small' practice. Above these were those earning £400–£800 per annum, and those I have called standard, since no adjective appeared alongside them. The third category were the 'good' practices making £800–£1000, and at the top were the 'first class' practices of £1000 a year or more. In addition, it is possible to further subdivide them according to location. On the one hand, there were what were described as 'country' practices, and on the other a variety of 'city', 'suburban' and 'residential' ones, which I have aggregated together as 'urban' practices.

Taking country practices first, Table 5.2 cols. i, ii and iii, shows that in 1877 three-fifths were standard practices with gross money incomes of from £400 to £800 a year. The remainder were fairly evenly divided between small, good and first class practices. There were very few at the very top of the range with incomes over £1500, or at the bottom of the range with only a struggling nucleus of a practice giving an income of under £300 per annum. The figures for 1899 show a downward shift in the distribution of nominal incomes, mainly as a result of more practices falling into the £300–399 category of small practices rather than the marginally higher income band of £400–499 that characterised the standard practice. The rural sector of practice was economically precarious in that patient density was likely to be lower and expenses higher than in urban areas. This sector might thus be expected to show very markedly the effects of professional overcrowding during the 1890s that was highlighted in Chapter 1. But by 1909 the distribution in monetary terms was almost back to that in 1877. Interestingly, the 1911 *Census* commented that there had been a 'considerable decrease in numbers at the earlier ages'[44] in medicine which suggests that the overcrowded state of the medical market had by this time inhibited those without connection or capital from trying to establish a practice nucleus. With a declining population in the countryside, and a recognition that in any case lower incomes had traditionally been the norm there, the rural sector was not seen as a promising venue for a young doctor seeking his fortune. (There were, of course, other non-monetary compensations for rural practice,

---

[44] *Census*, PP, 1913, LXXVIII, p. 340.

notably the lifestyle and the country doctor's local prestige and reputation.) It was the city, however, that allegedly had the proverbial
streets of gold.

Urban practices do show that there was a greater potential for larger
earnings. (See cols. iv, v and vi of Table 5.2.) In 1877 nearly one-quarter
of practices were in the top bracket with incomes of over £1000 a year.
However, there were decreasing opportunities for making this kind of
money, since between 1877 and 1909 these first class practices almost
halved as a proportion of the whole. The possibility of making £1500 a
year was apparently eliminated but it is likely that, as the market place
grew more competitive, these very profitable practices changed hands
on word of mouth rather than by formal advertisement. (Also, the
trend to partnership would tend to take some of these more remunerative practices out of these figures for single-handed practices.) And
urban practices having an income of under £300 and thus trembling
on the brink of economic insolvency almost tripled from 4 to 11 per
cent. As with country practices, urban ones in 1899 showed a downward dip in the distribution of incomes at the top and bottom of the
range, when compared to either 1877 or 1909.

Reviewing the overall distribution of incomes from general practice
in the estimates in Table 5.2 (cols. vii, viii and ix), the median gross
income was about £600 in 1877 and again in 1909, and somewhat lower
– about £500 – in 1899. The corresponding net figures were of the
order of £480 and £400. The mean gross income was rather higher –
about £700 in 1877. This was higher than one would have expected
given Peterson's speculation that half of the medical profession were
living off £350 or below in this period. However, my estimates for 1909
fall between three others made for this period: first the Plender
Report; secondly, those given in unpublished estimates by the Inland
Revenue; and thirdly, Routh's calculations.

My estimates were lower than the average incomes given for GPs in
five towns in the Plender Report for 1910 and 1911, where average
gross incomes of £832 and £838 (net incomes of £717 and £725) were
indicated.[45] Since from the doctor's perspective these selected towns
had an unusually favourable ratio of practitioners to patients the
returns can hardly be taken as representative.[46] My estimates are also
considerably lower than Inland Revenue figures for 1914 in a sample

---

[45] *Report of Sir William Plender in Respect of Medical Attendance and Remuneration in Certain Towns*, PP, 1912–13, Cd 6305, LXXVIII, p. 679.
[46] The towns were Darlington, Darwen, Dundee, Norwich and St Albans, which had a practitioner to patient ratio of 1:1568 compared with a British average ratio of 1:2420 (Peterson, *Medical Profession*, p. 218).

of 280 metropolitan and provincial practices, where net income of £687 was recorded.[47] It is reasonable to infer that this sample comprised *all* medical practitioners and thus included élite high-income specialists, since 29 per cent of the sample had incomes of more than £1000. This contrasted with only 12 per cent of my 1909 sample of 'rank and file' GPs who had 'first-class' incomes of more than £1000. The difference between my estimates and those of Routh is small. The median income for a GP in my estimates for 1909 – of around £600 gross and £480 net – was higher than Routh's 1913–14 net income estimates of £395 for both rural and urban GPs, which was based on income tax returns.[48] My estimates, being based on practice advertisements, may give too buoyant a view of medical incomes, since the tendency of advertisements was to indicate what a seller hoped to get rather than what the practice was actually worth. It is possible that Routh's estimates may be more inclusive in giving a slightly lower range of medical incomes than practice advertisements, the former would cover incomes above the limit of exemption from income tax of £160, whereas there was a cut-off point of about £200 in advertisements.

The fall in nominal incomes between 1877 and the end of the century, and the subsequent recovery, indicated by practice advertisements, need to be considered in the context of the strong fluctuations in prices during these years. Between the early 1870s and the mid-1890s retail prices fell by about a quarter (23 per cent) so that the *real* income of the average GP may have increased slightly notwithstanding the squeeze on money incomes. Between 1899 and 1913 retail prices increased by about 15 per cent.[49] This would have reduced, but not eliminated, the benefits of the recovery in average medical incomes over this period.

Table 5.2 suggests that there had been a compression of monetary income *within* the period 1877 to 1909. This is significant in giving some credence to public anxieties shown in the *Lancet* and the *BMJ* at this time. The condemnation there of the slum 'sixpenny doctor', whose disreputable trade was held to undercut the fee structure of respectable members of the medical profession, is more readily appreciated given the growth in practice nuclei. So too is the fear of organised patient-power in medical clubs, highlighted in the *BMJ* enquiry of 1905, which emphasised the clubs' hated power to drive down still further their contract fees of three or four shillings per

[47] PRO, T 171/70, Chancellor of the Exchequer's private working papers for 1914 budget.
[48] G. Routh, *Occupation and Pay in Great Britain, 1906–1979* (1980), p. 63.
[49] Feinstein, 'A new look at the cost of living', pp. 170–1.

head.[50] And in the competitive medical market at this time, GPs regarded four-figure incomes with awe.[51]

The advertisements are also of interest in that they facilitate information retrieval on different sources of doctors' incomes. These sources comprised appointments, midwifery, and individual patients' fees. Income from appointments has been dealt with elsewhere (see Table 4.2). Estimates there indicate that midwifery made up about 10 per cent of income, and appointments – for those fortunate enough to hold them – from 21 to 26 per cent of income. Fee income had thus to provide about two-thirds of the doctors' income.

Fees

Fees were thus the most important component in doctors' medical incomes. For most of the nineteenth century there were attempts by GPs to relate their fee schedules systematically to the income of their patients. At first this was done through dividing up patients into broad occupational categories. Not all practitioners were in favour of this, the *Lancet* 'entertained very strong doubts' about the scale given in column (ii) of Table 5.3, and fulminated against 'an endeavour to estimate the value of mental acquirement and skill, by the gross, inefficient test of a metallic standard.'[52] Later, house rentals were taken by many doctors as a rough proxy for patient income and ability to pay fees. The three-fold classification of the Shropshire BMA table[53] was the best known, and the most widely adopted from the 1870s to the early twentieth century. It was, however, a matter of recommendation rather than prescription since the profession continued to entertain doubts about scales: the BMA asserted as late as 1909 that 'there is a strong feeling that it should be left to each medical man to put his own price on his own brains.'[54]

The first edition of the Shrewsbury table of 1870 recommended rental bands of £10–£25, £25–£50 and £50–£100. But the second edition of 1874 raised the bottom level from £10 to £15, since it was alleged that 'the great majority of £10 householders are professionally cared for by sick clubs.'[55] Whether doctors tried to get standard fees from the lower £10 to £15 group might have serious implications for their income. In

50 *RC on the Poor Laws*, PP 1910, LIII, p. 814 (evidence of T. G. Akland).
51 H. W. Pooler, *My Life in General Practice* (1948).
52 *Lancet* (1830–1), p. 532.
53 *A Tariff of Medical Fees Recommended by the Shropshire Ethical Branch of the BMA* (Shrewsbury, 1870, 1874, 1889).
54 *RC on the Poor Laws*, PP, XLI, Q 39,200, evidence of BMA.
55 *A Tariff of Medical Fees* (Shrewsbury, 1874).

Table 5.3. *Nineteenth-century fees: ordinary visits, excluding medicine*

Patient Income	1819 (i)	1830/1 (ii)	1842 (iii)	1870 (iv)	1874 (v)	1879 (vi)	1889 (vii)
< £25	3d	fee range from 5/0 to 10/0	1/6	1/0–2/6	1/0–2/6	2/6–3/6	1/0–2/6
£25–50	6d		2/6	1/6–3/6	2/0–3/6	2/6–5/0	2/0–3/6
£50–£100	6d		3/6–5/0	2/6–5/0	2/6–5/0	5/0–7/6	2/6–5/–
> £100	–		–	–	–	7/6–10/0	–

Notes:
(a) Most scales were recommended ones in the sense that they had no legal force. But (i) had been agreed as a standard enforced by fines.
(b) Most scales were promulgated by groups but (iii) is of interest in having been advocated by an individual surgeon.
(c) Some scales were local: (i) applied to Blackburn, (ii) to Newcastle, (vi) to Manchester. However, the Shrewsbury scale, (iv, v, vii), began as a local scale but became accepted as a guide in most areas.
(d) The Blackburn schedule, (i), had a two class division of labourer, servant and weaver, and the rest, which I have subdivided. The Newcastle schedule, (ii), operated a sliding scale between 5/– and 10/– for all classes of patients. For (iii) I have aggregated pauper and labourer into the smallest income category, small tradesmen and a grade higher into the second income category.
Sources:
(i) *Rules and regulations agreed and entered into by the medical gentlemen of Blackburn, 5 November 1819* (Blackburn, 1819).
(ii) *Lancet* (1830–1), p. 536.
(iii) *Provincial Medical and Surgical Journal* (1842), iii, p. 168.
(iv) *A Tariff of Medical Fees recommended by the Shropshire Ethical Branch of the BMA* (Shrewsbury, 1870), Cols. (v & vii) are later editions.
(vi) *Lancet* (1879), ii, pp. 621–2.

1871 this group rented one in eight houses but by 1901 this had risen to more than one in four. Table 5.4 shows that without them doctors were targeting their hopes of fee income on only about one in four of the population in 1870 or three in ten by 1900. The extent of the loss of income from poorer patients depended on the extent to which an individual doctor compensated for this by income from clubs (and thus in treating and getting income from the same patients by different means). Also important here was the extent of debt in the practice: income from clubs was more predictable than payment from individual poor patients.

A narrow band of the population – the upper and middle classes,

Table 5.4. *Fee Schedules and House Rentals, 1871 and 1901*

Patient class	Annual rental	% of houses 1871	% of houses 1901
III (i)	£10–25	22	44
III (ii)	£15–25	10	16
II	£25–50	9	10
I	£50–100	4	3

Source: The patient classes are taken from two recommended schedules of fees: *A Tariff of Medical Fees recommended by the Shropshire Ethical Branch of the BMA* (Shrewsbury, 1870 and 1874). The second edition moved the lower limit of patients for whom fees were recommended from those with a rental above £10 per year to those with one over £15. The Manchester schedule continued to use the £10 to £25 income band in 1879 (*Lancet*, 1879), i, pp. 621–2. The house rentals are taken from *Reports of H.M. Commissioners of Inland Revenue.*

together with the aristocracy of labour – was thus the source of the major part of the doctor's income: that from fees. The fees that doctors were recommended to charge to certain groups of patients are shown in Table 5.3. They should be understood to have operated as a lowest common denominator since more complex procedures might lead to a higher fee. (See Tables 3.1 and 9.1.) Fee schedules were mainly a feature of the last quarter of the nineteenth century, although there were earlier examples.

The first column of Table 5.3 shows fees as agreed in 1819 by Blackburn surgeons and apothecaries which were based on the earlier custom of charging mainly for medicine. Hitherto this had meant that up to four-fifths of the cost of medical attendance had been charged up to medicines supplied. (See Table 3.1.) This custom declined during the rest of the century as qualified doctors attempted to distance themselves from trade and from druggists. By the 1830s and 1840s there was collective professional concern about what was perceived as an anachronistic, unjust and impolitic method of charging for medicine rather than skill. In 1849 the *Lancet* remarked on the growing practice of charging for visits, time and skill rather than for physic. It considered a fee range of 2s 6d to 10s 6d fair recompense for visits alone.[56] Charging only for visits was certainly the norm at this time in areas with a more affluent clientele.[57] However, old habits died hard. In the 1860s there were still four methods of charging employed:

[56] *Lancet*, ii 1849, pp. 195–6.   [57] Granville, *Spas*, p. 242.

visits with medicine included; visits with medicine charged separately; visits alone with a prescription left to be taken to the chemist; and a charge for medicine alone.[58] Charging for medicine alone was falling into professional disrepute by this time. An FRCS put this well, 'What is the difference between a druggist and a medical man? I would have answered one charges for physic and the other for brains.'[59] There was, however, some resistance from patients to doctors charging for a visit as distinct from charging for a bottle of medicine. Similarly, there was a tendency to think that if the patient went to the doctor's home, rather than the doctor visiting the patient, there should not be a fee.[60] Professional self-interest eventually triumphed over patient concern in this instance, and charging just for medicine was said to be 'a thing of the past' by the 1870s.[61] By the end of the century practice advertisements indicated that only a minority even included medicine in the charge. These were usually rural practices which needed to dispense for patients living miles away from a chemist. It was also found more commonly in the north-west of England than in other areas.[62]

Fees were difficult to alter because they reflected local custom or might be inherited from one's predecessor in the practice. Practice advertisements for so-called 'death vacancies' indicated this clearly, since the fees of these elderly doctors frequently showed the pricing policies of the previous generation still in use. It was a nice point of judgement to calculate fees so that, without losing patients, they were as high as the market would bear. The Victorian philosophy, forcefully expressed by one GP, was that 'a doctor is often valued and appreciated according to his charges.'[63] Although the *BMJ* grumbled in 1878 that 'the payment of medical men has, in fact, not progressed with the general rise in modern expenditure, and the cost of living in modern society',[64] the contemporary decline in the general price level meant that recommended fees had to be reduced during the next decade.

Where practitioners located themselves in the medical market depended mainly on the practice location. Within the profession, however, an important influence on reputation was thought to be formal qualifications, and hence there were attempts to link fees to qualification in a systematic way. These were not as influential as the BMA tables based on patient rental/income which were widely

---

[58] *Lancet*, i, 1864, p. 537.   [59] *BMJ*, 9 February 1878.   [60] *Lancet*, i, pp. 709–10.
[61] J. F. Clarke, *Autobiographical Recollections* (1874), p. 98.
[62] *BMJ*, 24 August 1907.
[63] Letter from 'A Rural Practitioner', *BMJ*, 1878, (1), p. 250.
[64] Editorial, *BMJ*, 1878 (1), p. 57.

Table 5.5. *Distribution of minimum medical fees quoted by GPs in 1899
and 1909*

Fee	Visits 1899 %	Visits 1909 %	Home or surgery 1909 %
1/–	2	–	20
1/6	4	5	25
2/–	8	6	25
2/6	50	58	27
3/–	3	1	–
3/6	26	24	2
5/–	5	4	1
7/–	1	–	–
10/6	1	1	–
N	116	708	143

Source: Calculated from advertisements in *BMJ Advertiser* for 1899 and 1909.

adopted. One professional schedule of 1880 suggested, for example, that whereas fellows of the royal colleges might charge from one to five guineas for a consultation, mere members of the colleges should charge lower fees ranging from five shillings to a guinea for visits without medicine. Licentiates of various medical bodies should charge even smaller fees and, except for the lowliest, be discouraged from adopting open surgeries as their practice style.[65]

At the turn of the twentieth century doctors appear to have become more entrepreneurial in their pursuit of fees. In medical practice advertisements for 1877 fees were almost never included; they were more evident in 1899; and they were present in about a quarter of the advertisements in 1909. The frequency distributions of these fees repays analysis since they reveal the nature of medical practice.

The first two columns of Tables 5.5, 5.6, and 5.7 focus on the fees that I have calculated the doctor made when visiting patients in their own homes. They show the charges made exclusive of medicine. (Numbers of practices in these tables are lower than in Table 5.2 since not all practices included fee data in the advertisements that are the basis for these statistics.) Table 5.5 shows clearly the low minimum visiting fees that were charged at both dates, with two-thirds of fees at two

---

[65] W. E. Stevenson, *The Medical Act 1858* (1880), pp. 30–1. (The full table is reproduced in Peterson, *Medical Profession*, pp. 212–3.

Table 5.6. *Distribution of maximum medical fees quoted by GPs in 1899 and 1909*

Fee	Visits 1899 %	Visits 1909 %	Home or surgery 1909 %
1/– and 1/6	–	–	11
2/– and 2/6	3	4	56
3/– and 3/6	15	10	9
4/– and 4/6	–	2	–
5/– and 5/6	18	26	15
6/– and 6/6	1	1	–
7/– and 7/6	24	15	1
10/– and 10/6	24	32	6
15/–	1	1	–
21/– or more	13	9	2
N	98	592	115

Source: As for Table 5.5

shillings and sixpence or less, and more than nine-tenths at three shillings and sixpence or under. Fees may have been kept down in order to induce the low-income patient to visit the doctor's surgery instead of the free dispensary or the out-patient clinic. Table 5.6 shows that between 1899 and 1909 the maximum visiting fee was also modest with no more than 7s 0d or 7s 6d being charged by three-fifths of the practices.

Interestingly, Table 5.6 also indicates that the maximum had been raised between 1899 and 1909 in schedules of practices located towards the lower and middle parts of the market, where most patients would be. This is evident if we look at the lower part of the table, where more four- and five-shilling fees were being charged and fewer two- and three-shilling ones. The rationale was probably that of maintaining fees in real terms. An earlier strategy – to raise income absolutely – was evident in the supplementary suggestions in the Shropshire BMA tables where, in 1889, additional charges were recommended for night visiting, sleeping in the house by special request and for procedures such as the testing of urine.[66] Doctors may well have calculated that in this period of falling prices, the upward trend in the *real* wages of the general population increased demand for their services, since middle- and working-class patients had a

[66] *A Tariff of Medical Fees* (Shrewsbury, 1889).

Table 5.7. *Range of medical fees quoted by GPs in 1899 and 1909*

Fee	Visits 1899 %	Visits 1909 %	Home or surgery 1909 %
2/6 or less			
up to 3/6	19	13	75
up to 5/–	17	21	17
up to 7/6	10	8	1
to over 7/6	25	27	8
3/– or 3/6			
up to 7/6	14	13	–
to over 7/6	5	13	2
4/– or more			
up to 7/6	5	1	–
to over 7/6	5	4	–
N	100	592	115

Source: As for Table 5.5.

larger margin of income (once the cost of essential household items had been met) to spare for medical services. This may have offset some of the disadvantageous effects on doctors' incomes of an increased supply of doctors at that time.

Table 5.7 indicates a decline from 1899 to 1909 in the proportion of practices having their fee range from 2s 6d (or below) up to 7s 6d. This suggests an attempt to raise the range of visiting fees to combat the effects of a general price inflation upon real medical incomes. Nearly one in ten more practices were including seven shillings and sixpence or above in their fee schedules in 1909 than had done so a decade before. The final columns in Tables 5.5 to 5.7 also highlight another shift in medical practice in the opening of additional lock-up or branch surgeries, located away from the main surgery in the doctor's house. These predominantly urban lock-ups were an entrepreneurial device to extend practice by widening the market, and usually did so, by opening up premises in working-class districts to patients who paid their fees in cash.[67]

Table 5.8 indicates the charges that practitioners' committees laid down as suitable for panel doctors to charge the dependants of their

[67] Editor of the *Lancet* et al, *The Conduct of Medical Practice* (1927) p. 93.

Table 5.8. *Fee schedules for dependants of insured patients, 1913*

Practice location	Surgery attendance	Home visit
Brighton	2/6	2/6
Cheshire	2/6	3/6
Liverpool	2/0	2/6
London	2/0	2/0
Manchester	2/0	2/6
Middlesex	1/0	2/0
Newcastle	2/6	2/6
Plymouth	2/6	2/6
Sheffield	2/6	3/6

Source: BMJ 11 January to 24 May 1913.

national health insurance patients. Although the data are from 1913, and thus strictly speaking outside our period, they nevertheless throw light on the kind of charges likely to have been made by doctors to their poor patients in preceding years. It is clear that these were low, ranging from 1s 0d to 2s 6d for surgery attendance, and from 2s 0d to 3s 6d for home visits. As such they provide a useful corroboration of the representativeness of the data calculated from a different source in the final column of Tables 5.5 to 5.7. The lower surgery fees given in these tables indicate a wider range of practices, including those with cash and branch surgeries, that would not have been represented in the ranks of Local Medical Committees, and thus not have appeared in Table 5.8. Table 5.8 is also interesting in that it indicates that medical charges were similar from one region to the next, and thus that a national market had been created.

We thus found evidence of income-maximising fee strategies, a shrewd choice of practice location, improved rationality in use of time with the development of the surgery (since patient rather than doctor travelled), and a related increase in numbers of patients treated. This suggests how doctors tried to combat both an increase in their numbers and changes to their cost of living.

Debts, failures, bankruptcies

Dependency on fee income put a premium on prompt payment by patients and on efficient accounting by the doctor, but neither materialised very often. Patients' reluctance to pay was notorious among all classes. (See Plate 7.) Before 1911 debts were reckoned by the BMA at 6.5% of income, or 8% with the cost of an agent to do the collection.[68] In a minority of cases they were very much higher than this. A GP, practising in a large town at the beginning of the Victorian period, recorded how sending out his bills at Christmas mainly to tradespeople and artisans had produced by midsummer only £130 of the £800 owing, and his own estimation was that only a further £100 could be expected even after recourse to dunning or the law.[69] Half a century later another practitioner complained bitterly that he was losing 30 to 40 per cent of his notional income through bad debts.[70] Examples can also be found for the Edwardian period. A country practice making £350 a year gross income was advertised in 1909 with book debts of £250, of which only about £100 were seen as 'good and recoverable.'[71] Far worse was a Lancashire working- and middle-class practice – with a gross income of £600 annually – and book debts of £2000.[72] Presumably, these last two examples were not considered to be irredeemably debt-ridden practices, since otherwise this kind of detail on debt would hardly be mentioned in 'practice for sale' advertisements. How debts could swiftly accumulate was shown by the Teesdale practice of Dr George Pilkington, who got in only £207 out of bills for £544 in 1883–4.[73]

In order to practise and prosper doctors had to take vigorous action to bring in the money owing to them. The accepted custom was to bill once a year, usually at Christmas time.[74] There were ineffectual attempts in the profession to stimulate individual practitioners to put in their bills more quickly, and certainly no less frequently than twice yearly.[75] The *BMJ* thundered against 'that small portion of the public who ... are ... unfortunately to be found in every practice, who require their bills to be rendered five or six times, at intervals of six months, before they think fit to pay them.'[76] Undoubtedly, notions of professional gentility inhibited doctors from harassing their middle-class patients too frequently. In any case, practitioners had a fair idea of what kind of debt would have to be written off as 'bad debt'. William English recorded in his ledger beside an account for £230 in 1833, and a promissory note for that amount, 'It will never be paid.'[77]

[68] *BMJ Advertiser*, 5 January 1924, p. 4.   [69] *Medical Gazette*, 30 June 1838.
[70] *BMJ*, 2 April 1892.
[71] *BMJ Advertiser*, 12 June 1909.   [72] *BMJ Advertiser*, 1 May 1909.
[73] G. Stout, 'A Ledger initialled)G P', *Cleveland and Teesdale Local History Society*, 48 (1985), p. 18.
[74] *BMJ*, 20 February 1892.   [75] de Styrap, *Practitioner*, p. 202.
[76] *BMJ*, editorial, 9 February 1878.
[77] English, *Whitby Medical Family*, p. 45.

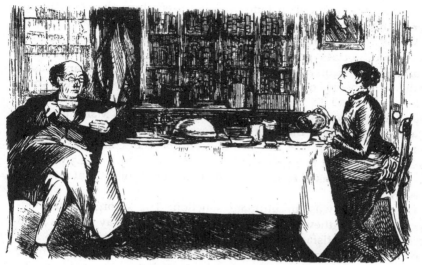

MEDICAL REMUNERATION.

Doctor. " UM ! MOST INSOLENT !" (*To his Wife.*) " LISTEN TO THIS, MY DEAR." (*Reads Letter aloud.*) " ' SIR,—I ENCLOSE A P. O. ORDER FOR THIRTEEN SHILLINGS AND SIXPENCE, HOPING IT WILL DO YOU AS LITTLE GOOD AS YOUR TWO VERY SMALL BOTTLES OF " PHYSIC " DID ME.' "

Plate 7 'Medical Remuneration' (*Punch*, 1878)

In contrast, there was 'good debt'; this might be reclaimable with some exertion. In some cases payment by instalment might be the only feasible solution to salvage a large account accumulated over several years by a less-than-affluent patient.[78] In other cases the doctor drove a hard bargain and renewed treatment only after payment by a patient of an earlier account. Dr Callender, a Northumberland country GP, adopted a more dignified course. He always sent his bills out, 'I know quite well they won't be able to pay me in full, some not even by instalments, but I want them to know what they owe for what they have had.'[79] There were other alternatives. Payment in kind, especially in rural areas, was often acceptable to the practitioner, although whether this was a recognition of economic necessity or a balance of convenience is not clear. In the late eighteenth century the Yorkshire surgeon, William Elmhirst, would accept payment accord-ing to the occupation of his patient and received variously a sheep, manure, cloth, coals and candles.[80] This predominantly rural tradition

[78] For example, Sheffield City Archives, Em 888, Elmhirst ledger, entry for Edward Hammond, 1774: Somerset RO DD/SAS/TN 28, Accounts of James Billett, surgeon and oculist, entries for Mrs Pyne, 1830–34.
[79] Cox, *Doctors*, p. 35. Callender practised in the 1890s at Haydon Bridge.
[80] Sigsworth and Brady, *William Elmhirst*, p. iv.

Making a medical living

of occasional payment in kind was followed through the Victorian period and into the twentieth century.[81]

Whilst repeated billing was the preferred strategy against recalcitrant middle-class non-payers there was an alternative for their working-class equivalents. Collectors were employed in urban areas to gather threepenny or sixpenny instalments, with a 12 per cent commission charged to the doctor. In some regions of the country – especially the north-west – this was very prevalent. In Manchester, for example, about half the bills in ordinary practice were put into the hands of the collector.[82] The income from the debt collector was seen as a valuable asset to a practice: 'collectors book brings in £5 weekly'; or 'transfer of debts of £300, which are being paid collector at rate of £5 weekly'.[83]

Legal action was an ultimate sanction. The Georgian surgeon-apothecary, Matthew Flinders, wrote of the 'never pay villains', and recorded his satisfaction that summonses not only brought him recompense but encouraged others to pay.[84] A more competitive medical market in the late nineteenth century led to more widespread legal action. When faced with very large and recalcitrant debtors who could pay if pressurised, recourse might be made to a professional protection society. Joining a society such as the British Medical Protection Society had the inestimable advantage of allowing professional dignity to be retained whilst attempting to make good outstanding claims. The society would chase up the debt, at first through writing letters and then with legal action, if the doctor so desired. More rarely, there was resort to legal action by practitioners on their own initiative.[85] Most practitioners saw this as a last resort. But for one doctor it was the norm:

If bills are neglected year after year I threaten proceedings, and if this is unavailing, I issue a summons. I never get my claims opposed, and it is frequently paid into court. I do not find this summary method to injure my practice; on the contrary, I am saved the trouble of attending those who do not mean to pay.[86]

[81] C. Wood, *Paradise Lost*, (1990) p. 113 and personal communication from Dr A. W. Maiden, who practised in Saxilby, Lincolnshire from 1935.
[82] *BMJ*, 24 August 1907.
[83] For example, practice advertisements, *BMJ Advertiser*, 11 November 1899.
[84] Lincs. RO, Flinders I, fo. 23, entry June 1777.
[85] For example, *Lancet*, 12 June 1875, and 25 December 1875; *BMJ*, 1878, i, p. 470 and 1892, i, p. 795.
[86] *BMJ*, 30 March 1878.

It is interesting to note that – after allowing fees to a Debenham surgeon – a judge in a Suffolk case in 1885 commented that he did not know a class of men worse paid than doctors.[87]

In these circumstances it is hardly surprising to find a surgeon recommending to his colleagues that cash payments were preferable to bills in running a practice.[88] Arguably, one significant cause of the move towards the cash practice at the end of the nineteenth century was this professional awareness of patients' propensity to debt. Between the 1870s and the 1900s there was a discernible shift towards cash practices, with the emergence of the 'sixpenny doctor' and the branch practice in larger urban areas. A cash orientation was seen as advantageous in selling such a practice: 'patients ... nearly always pay the fees at the time', or 'cash receipts average over £720 p.a. (of which two-thirds is from ready-money payments)'[89] Cash was always demanded from 'birds of passage';[90] non-ratepayers who might do a 'moonlight flit' when debts became pressing.

Patients' debts were one cause of practice failure, as the case of George Pilkington in the 1880s has indicated. Yet there were usually other factors involved; Pilkington seems to have assumed that all visits would merit payment. His rate of visiting was very high, averaging over nine domiciliary visits or surgery consultations per patient, compared with interwar rates of only half this amount.[91] There were equally high rates in a later abortive attempt to establish a practice in Stockton on Tees five miles away, when nine-tenths of contacts with patients were time-consuming visits to homes. And in setting up in Stockton he chose a place that was already well provided with doctors. Predictably, Pilkington ended life as a *locum*.[92] The need for insufficient medical income to be supplemented by familial help was not uncommon; Henry Peart who began a Midlands practice in 1830 also needed this kind of assistance, as did William Cook. Cook's wife, Harriet, had always to supplement medical earnings with her own successful journalistic and literary endeavours, whilst there was a substantial inheritance, and continual family subventions including an unpaid loan of £1200 for buying into a partnership. Cook first attempted practice in Tunbridge Wells in the 1850s where, unsuccessful in obtaining either sufficient patients or election to public office, his annual income was only £174 after three years' work. Deciding that a

---

[87] *Lancet* 4 April 1885.   [88] *BMJ* 31 December 1881.
[89] *BMJ Advertiser*, 5 and 26 June 1909.
[90] *BMJ*, 31 December 1881, letter from a provincial surgeon.
[91] Digby and Bosanquet, 'Doctors and Patients', p. 87.
[92] Stout, 'A Ledger', pp. 17–9.

double qualification would help make any future practice more viable he obtained an Edinburgh MD, became a partner in a St John's Wood practice, and in his third year here had earnings of £490. Considering that his fortunes could be improved still further he moved to a Hampstead partnership in 1863; two years later his gross practice income came to £576, of which £140 came from poor-law duties, and an equivalent sum from his office as public vaccinator. However, expenses continuously exceeded medical income.[93]

Whilst liberal family support enabled some to survive, contemporary advertisements of practice nuclei for sale indicated that many others were less fortunate. These advertisements cast a revealing light on the downside of the very competitive medical market of late Victorian and Edwardian England. Practice nuclei were generally advertised privately, and were more a catalogue of disappointed aspirations than a springboard to future prosperity. Most were self-revelatory, as for example, 'For disposal – surgery, only been open 3 months. At present doing little but good opening for a man who can afford to wait a little time. It is situated in a thickly populated working-class suburb of Manchester.'[94] Only the really credulous would have replied to such an advertisement. Sometimes the same message was conveyed less explicitly as in, 'presents a splendid opening for a young Irish or Scotchman [sic] with £100 cash', since the frugality and hard work of these practitioners was well-known.[95] A lack of certified books was conspicuous in these stereotypical 'splendid openings for a man not afraid of hard work' and figures of takings were few and far between. A handful did give income: 'recently established nucleus ... income for last 12 months over £100'; 'established 12 months, cash takings £159'; 'first years cash £200, second, £300, and capable of much more'; or 'four year's standing – last year's cash receipts £250'.[96] These were probably the better nuclei since there was some attempt to supplement hyperbole with quantification. But given that these figures were gross ones, so that practice expenses of 16 per cent would need to be deducted, and the remaining income taxed, the amount left to live on would not have sustained even threadbare gentility. In these circumstances even a good Edwardian practice nucleus – making £300 a year – would have yielded a net weekly income of only four pounds and eleven shillings.

[93] I. Loudon, 'Cash Book', p. 254; W. D. Foster, 'The Finances of a Victorian General Practitioner', *Proceedings of the Royal Society of Medicine*, 66 (1973), pp. 12–16. I am grateful to Magaret Pelling for drawing my attention to this article.
[94] *BMJ Advertiser*, 2 December 1909.   [95] *BMJ Advertiser*, 11 November 1909.
[96] *BMJ Advertiser*, 3 April, 24 April, 17 July, 7 August, and 11 December, 1909.

Success in practice was thus not easy to achieve. An earlier survey by the Medical School of St Bartholomew's Hospital of their recent graduates discovered in 1869 that for a variety of reasons, not all of them economic, many of these élite entrants had failed to make what was considered a fair living from their profession. Twelve per cent had had only limited success in practice, six per cent had failed entirely, and ten per cent had left the medical profession.[97] Beyond the low living standards of practice nuclei there were a number of alternatives within the medical sphere. Among the more respectable were those which traded off greater security against a low income: acting as an assistant or locum in another practice, or taking a salaried medical appointment. Other disappointed doctors emigrated. Australian evidence indicated that old problems might recur in the new land, although prospects might be better. For example, John FitzSimmons wrote from New South Wales in 1847 to his family in London:

My pay is 7/6 per day and am paying out of this £6 p[er] month and from New Colonial regulations we are obliged to find our own quarters, coal candle etc ... I pay £26 per annum for a house. I am allowed a male servant from the Gover[nmen]t but pays the female £12 p[er] year so you can judge my dear brother how I am situated and from my present rank I must appear respectable, the uniform being in itself expensive.[98]

And emigration could even prove disastrous as with the huge mortality amongst doctors who went to the Swan River, Western Australia.[99] For the less bold spirits who stayed at home, some might drift downwards into 'quackery' rather than regular practice. Understandably there were few written testimonies about this. One such, at the beginning of the nineteenth century, when the profession was notoriously overcrowded, was John Clark. He was a young Scottish surgeon who, having failed to make a living at Dunkeld under the Duke of Atholl's patronage, came to London as 'assistant with succession' to a Soho practitioner. Here he developed patent medicines such as 'Dr Clark's Cough Mixture' and – beset with worries about unpaid accounts – could only dream of future success.[100]

Economic uncertainties might be exacerbated by ill health, a particular professional hazard. Many Victorian medical practitioners suffered from mental depression, for example, and the suicide rate was

---

[97] J. Paget, 'What becomes of Medical Students?', *St Bartholomew's Hospital Reports*, 5 (1869), p. 238.

[98] Letter to Lawrence FitzSimmons, London, 22 July 1847. I am indebted to David Fitzpatrick for this letter.

[99] P. Joske, 'A Strange Fatality', *The Push from the Bush, A Bulletin of Social History*, 13 (1982), pp. 49–68. Eric Richards kindly drew my attention to this.

[100] Scottish RO, GD 80/932, Letters of John Clark, 1793–1804.

also high.[101] The impact of sickness or death upon the families of practitioners resulted in the creation of charitable societies to help them, such as the West Riding Medical Charitable Society, or the Society for the Relief of Widows and Orphans of Medical Men. Concern over the uncertainties of their professional lives led later to the creation of the Medical Sickness Annuity and Life Assurance Society in 1885. The perils of the country doctor in being thrown from horse or trap meant that 'in a minute [he] finds himself in much greater need of medical aid than most of those who send him urgent summonses.'[102] The *BMJ* discussed 'how many promising careers, especially among men engaged in general practice have been wrecked owing to some inability to tide over a temporary incapacity resulting from some acute illness.'[103]

Some practitioners found themselves beyond economic aid; the ultimate economic failure was that of bankruptcy. Small numbers of English doctors of medicine, surgeons or physicians became bankrupt during the period 1886–1914 when official statistics of occupational groups were made available in Board of Trade *Returns*, and their liabilities were low. A comparison can be made with a professional group that was not dissimilar in numbers to see whether the medical practice was particularly risky.[104] In absolute terms doctors suffered only half as many bankruptcies as solicitors whilst their liabilites were on average only one-eighth as great.[105] The small number of professional men reflected the fact that they dealt in services rather than commodities. In thus investing in their own human capital failure showed rather more in the wreckage of private lives than in public humiliation in the courts.

A comparative dimension

'At this time the proportion of briefless barristers is greater than ever, as well as the number of clergymen eager to be curates. And at this time, not only the bar and the established church are crowded with

[101] J. Oppenheim, 'Shattered Nerves.' Doctors, Patients, and Depression in Victorian England (Oxford, 1991), p. 155; O. Anderson, *Suicide in Victorian and Edwardian England* (Oxford, 1987), pp. 94–5.

[102] *BMJ*, January 1894.   [103] *BMJ*, 8 March 1884.

[104] Numbers of physicians and surgeons rose from 15,091 in 1881 to 24,533 by 1911, whereas barristers and solicitors increased from 17,386 to 21,380 in the same period (H. J. Perkin, 'Middle-Class Education and Employment in the 19th Century: a Critical Note', *Economic History Review*, second series, 14 (1961–2)).

[105] PP, 1899, LXXXVIII; 1904, LXXXVII; 1909, LXXXIX; 1919, X. I am most grateful to Mark Lester for generously supplying me with this data.

hungry competitors, but also every dissenting church, the attorney's branch of law, and all the branches of the medical and surgical professions ... two-thirds at the very least, of professional men, may be reckoned among the uneasy class.'[106] This comment of 1833 is interesting in the light of a recent controversy over professional incomes during the nineteenth century. Incomes in this period have hitherto been seen as broadly stable but a hypothesis was formulated suggesting that there was increasing income inequality, starting after the French Wars and peaking in the 1860s before a period of levelling off until 1914.[107] The key statistics underpinning this argument for widening inequality concerned the alleged gains made by professional groups in the first half century. That this data was 'hopelessly flawed' was comprehensively shown by two critics.[108] The controversy also highlighted the lack of data on incomes from *private* practice in law and medicine, as compared to that available for a few government officials.

The comparative length of working life, the spread of income within each profession, differences between specialist and general incomes, the extent of local variablity of income between rural and urban locations and/or, small or large centres of population, or the non-economic rewards of each profession would all be germane to a full discussion of this important question. Within a brief analysis we must perforce confine ourselves to a more generalised picture.

What then can be said about the relative rewards of the professions? The material rewards of ordinary clergymen were even worse than those of doctors. Professional handbooks suggested that 'without private means a clergyman will have a hard time of it.'[109] The legal profession was the reference group to which envious comparisons were frequently made by doctors. Lawyers were seen as being better placed in the market place since they were not circumscribed by society's assumptions about professional altruism towards the poor, nor confronted by powerful combinations of price-fixing clients. And lawyers had a more rational pricing system in which work was charged according to its difficulty and the degree of expertise,

---

[106] E. G. Wakefield, *England and America: a Comparison of the Social and Political State of Both Nations* (1833), quoted in M. F. Lloyd Prichard ed., *The Collected Works of Edward Gibbon Wakefield* (Glasgow, 1968), pp. 360–1.

[107] J. G. Williamson, 'The Structure of Pay in Britain, 1710–1911', *Research in Economic History*, 7 (1982).

[108] C. H. Feinstein, 'The Rise and Fall of the Williamson Curve', *Journal of Economic History*, XLVIII (1988), pp. 711–13; R. V. Jackson, 'The Structure of Pay in Nineteenth-Century Britain', *Economic History Review* second series, XL, (1987), pp. 564–7.

[109] F. Davenant, *What shall my son be* (1870), p. 18.

whereas the bulk of ordinary medical practice was charged by its quantity (i.e. the number of visits made). Class-differentiated medical treatment made only a crude attempt to adjust for this. The calculations of the early social statisticians were revealing in discussing the income of lawyers and clergy but not that of doctors. However, Colquhoun in 1815 suggested that the average income of all members of the medical profession was £200 a year, whereas that of all members of the legal profession was £300.[110] A more detailed later view of the relative rewards of the three traditional professions – law, medicine and the church – can be obtained from probates published for a single year, 1858. This is shown in Figure 5.1. The median for medical estates was lower than that for law or the church, falling in the one to two thousand pound range rather than the two to three thousand one.

More precise figures have been calculated by Routh from income tax returns for 1913–14 which gave average male earnings in these three professions.[111] However, when looking at GPs' incomes, it must be remembered that they had by this time received a very significant boost from the payments made by panel patients under the National Insurance Act of 1911. Routh's figures therefore gave a much more sanguine picture of medical incomes than had been the case for Victorian and Edwardian medical practice. Barristers earned £478, solicitors £568, GPs £395, and clergy £206. Barristers' earnings were thus one-fifth higher and solicitors' earnings two-fifths higher than those of the GP. The weighted average for *all* professions (including dentists, army officers, engineers and chemists) was only £328, so GPs were doing better than all but lawyers. However, it has been estimated that the majority of the GP's income of £395 came from panel patients.[112] Indeed, the panel payment of nine shillings per patient was double that found by the Plender Report to be the equivalent remuneration received by doctors in pre-insurance practice.[113] In turn this indicates that GPs' income had been much less buoyant earlier.

English GPs were no worse off than their medical counterparts abroad, since the overriding impression internationally is of low material rewards and much competition. There are two very real difficulties in attempting such a comparison: first, detailed work on incomes elsewhere is missing in most cases; secondly, variations in the structure of the medical profession and in the fluid relationships

[110] P. Colquhoun, *A Treatise on the Wealth, Power and Resources of the British Empire* (second edn, 1815), p. 124.
[111] Routh, *Occupation and Pay*, pp. 63, 120–1.
[112] Digby and Bosanquet, 'Doctors and Patients' p. 80.
[113] *Report on Medical Attendance and Remuneration*, PP, 1912–13, pp. 681–3, 699–701.

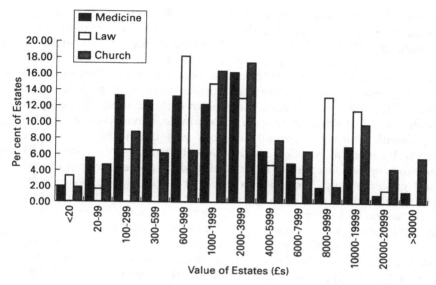

Figure 5.1   Probates of professional men, 1858

between regular and irregular practitioners makes any comparison problematic. There was, however, usually a distinction between élite and ordinary practitioners, and this discussion focuses on the latter. It must be emphasised that what follows can only be taken as an approximation.

Medical incomes in Scotland were notorious for their meagreness, and for the hard work that was needed to win them. Sir Walter Scott's verdict was an apposite one: 'There is no creature in Scotland that works harder or is more poorly requited than the country doctor, unless perhaps it may be his horse.'[114] At present we lack systematic evidence on medical incomes in Scotland, and the ensuing examples are taken from a small sample of medical account books and correspondence. Fees charged by ordinary practitioners appear to have been not dissimilar to those in England at the time. George Scrimzeour of Thornhill Pelmont charged half a crown in the 1800s, whilst W. C. Johnstone, a surgeon in St Andrews, billed his patients between one shilling and two shillings and sixpence during the 1840s.[115] Neither, however, was conspicuous by his professional acumen since each

[114] W. Scott, *The Surgeon's Daughter* (Waverley Novels, vol. XLVIII, Edinburgh, 1833), p. 185.
[115] Scottish RO CS 96 CS 236/Misc 9/1 nos. 90–1: and CS 237/F9/13 nos. 4347–8.

ended up in the bankruptcy courts. As in England there was very laggard payment of medical bills in all classes. Alexander Hamilton, a Haddington surgeon, made repeated and increasingly plaintive representations to have a bill for 'five pounds ten pence farthing' paid him by a gentry family.[116] In these circumstances, some practitioners found it impossible to make a living from practice alone and had to follow a dual occupation, as had been common in earlier periods, not only in Scotland but in England as well. For example, David Wishart, a late-eighteenth century Thornhill surgeon, was unable to keep afloat solely by medical practice and had also to run a general store. His accounts were a fascinating mixture of medical procedures performed and groceries sold: bread at sixpence, or sugar at two pence half-penny, alternated with drawing a tooth, or bleeding, each at sixpence. At times he had payment in from only one in four of his patients so that it is unsurprising eventually to find him a bankrupt.[117]

The Scottish medical profession recognised that medical incomes were lower than in England.[118] Income from medical appointments was a lesser supplement than in England: income from poor-law appointments, for example, did not routinely have extra charges for midwifery and vaccination as in England; and the annual salaries for medical officers and sanitary inspectors in Scottish burghs could be as low as one, two or three pounds.[119] In both countries there were attempts to exercise some collective professional muscle to standardise fees through recommended fee schedules. Table 5.9 shows three schedules from different parts of Scotland. It is of particular interest here in suggesting the higher levels of fees that Scottish doctors hoped to win from patients of a given income group, compared to those in England. For example, the Lothian schedule of 1868 aimed to charge the poorest group of patients what the BMA Shrewsbury table two years later contemplated exacting from its wealthiest ones! (See Table 5.9, col (iii) and Table 5.3 col (iv).) Given the actual fees in practitioners' account books quoted above, non-élite doctors appear to have charged much less than was recommended in fee schedules.

Practice in Europe did not produce larger average incomes for the ordinary practitioner than that in England or Scotland. Doctors in

---

[116] Scottish RO, GD 110/976/1–2. Hamilton graduated from Edinburgh in 1816.

[117] Scottish RO CS 96/1301–2, account books of David Wishart. S. W. F. Holloway points out that distinctions between medicines and drugs and food and drink were not so clear cut in the past (*Royal Pharmaceutical Society*, p. 53).

[118] For example, *Edinburgh Medical Journal*, April 1867, p. 953.

[119] *Edinburgh Medical Journal*, April 1867, p. 953; *Fourth Annual Report of Local Government Board of Scotland*, p. 318–9. Brenda White very helpfully drew my attention to this source.

Table 5.9. *Scottish fee schedules: ordinary visits, 1818–1868*

Patient income	Inverness 1818 (i)	Glasgow 1853 (ii)	Lothian 1868 (iii)
<£25	2/6	2/–	2/6–5/–
£25–£50	NA	2/6	2/6–5/–
£50–£100	NA	2/6	3/6–7/6
>£100	10/6	5/–21/–	5/–10/–

Note:
I am indebted to Dr Jacqueline Jenkinson for drawing my attention to these sources.
Sources:
(i) *Rules Adopted by the Medical Society of the North for the Regulation of their Fees* (Inverness, 1818).
(ii) *Glasgow S. Medical Society Code of Ethics Adopted in 1853* (1870).
(iii) *Edinburgh Medical Journal* (1868–9), p. 191.

Vienna had low remuneration, and in Berlin there had to be a frequent turnover of patients to ensure survival.[120] In late-eighteenth- and early-nineteenth-century France, there was tremendous diversity in the range of regular practitioners, yet patients were mainly confined to the bourgeoisie, better-off peasants and artisans, and treatment was usually for emergencies or terminal illness. Elite physicians made some use of sliding fee schedules to allow for the different economic circumstances of their patients but even so, found some resistance to paying for advice rather than medicine. Surgeons might practise profitably in the towns, but to survive financially in the countryside they usually needed another trade as well. Whatever the medical or social status of practitioners one-fifth of their fees might have to be written off, whilst even those accounts that were paid could be tendered in kind. Large incomes from practice were rare and complaints of an overcrowded profession frequent.[121]

Practice in lands with an expanding frontier was hard. That in early- and mid-nineteenth century USA was very competitive; 'chances of success were small' and numbers of aspiring practitioners in 'almost every location outnumbered the supply of fee-paying families.'[122] By

[120] Shryock, *Modern Medicine*, p. 266; P. Weindling, 'Medical Practice', p. 409.
[121] Ramsey, *Popular Medicine*, pp. 54, 57–8, 63, 69, 111–13, 118–19. This discussion excludes the post-Revolution salaried medical officers.
[122] C. E. Rosenberg, 'The Shape of Traditional Practice, 1800–1875' in G. Rosen, ed., *The Structure of American Medical Practice 1875–1941* (Philadelphia, 1983).

the end of the nineteenth century three-quarters of medical students failed to make a living as doctors.[123] Patients' reluctance to pay their doctor for services rendered was resented by the doctor. 'There are many persons in every community who would rather part with their eye-teeth than a five dollar bill', wrote Dr Samuel Gross.[124] And medical practitioners in early-twentieth-century Australia faced an equally hard struggle to achieve solvency, since there was only a limited supply of affluent patients who could pay on a fee-for-service basis, leaving doctors dependent, as in England, on equally hard-won income from friendly societies.[125] Interestingly, the fee schedules adopted in Victoria indicated higher fees from the 1840s to 1880s than were attempted in Britain and, understandably, higher mileage fees also.[126] In South Africa too, there was much late-nineteenth-century professional concern at what was seen as an over-supply of medical practitioners in Cape Province. The Medical Council received complaints that country medical men were keeping coffee shops, running stores, or acting as postmen, whilst wives ran bakeries, or taught dancing or the piano to make ends meet. However, even this was seen as preferable to still more doctors migrating to the towns and increasing professional competition there, with anxieties that this would lead to medical pauperisation and degradation.[127]

Practice before the 1911 National Insurance Act

This chapter has argued that there was a very competitive medical market. GPs had to be entrepreneurial in their attitudes to their patients and to commercial opportunities in society. Evidence of intense competition among practitioners for available practice opportunities was particularly obvious by the 1900s. A Bristol doctor commented in 1907 that many of the openings advertised for practices were 'illusory', and that 'the country is overstocked with doctors to an extent that no one but the unfortunates themselves has any idea: hence the sixpenny surgery.'[128] A sixpenny doctor suggested that the opprobrium attached to such men was misplaced. 'The disgrace attaches not to the man who accepts a small fee, but to those who

---

123 Shryock, *Modern Medicine*, p. 266.
124 G. Rosen and B. C. Rosen, eds., *400 Years of a Doctor's Life*, p. 181.
125 Gillespie, *The Price of Health*, chapter 1.
126 D. Dyason, 'The Medical Profession in Colonial Victoria, 1834–1901' in R. Macleod and M. Lewis, *Disease, Medicine and Empire* (1988), pp. 205, 215.
127 P. W. Laidler and M. Gelfand, *South Africa. Its Medical History, 1652–1898* (Cape Town, 1971), p. 503.
128 *BMJ*, 1907 (11), p. 1860, letter from 'Bristolian'.

thrust them down to that level.'[129] And a practitioner ruefully considered the trials and profits of practice:

For myself I can honestly say that the thought of my fee comes always second to the thought of my patient; but of an evening, after a twelve hours' day of physical and mental fatigue, it is somewhat hard to think that all that work and anxiety does not mean a good balance at the bank and a safe provision for the old age whose advent we are doing our utmost to hasten.[130]

To some extent such feelings were a subjective reaction to expectations of what medical incomes should be. Anxieties became acute whenever there were inflationary pressures or when other groups were seen to be raising their incomes – as in the 1860s and 1900s. The impression gained from the editorials of the *BMJ* and the *Lancet* for the late nineteenth and early twentieth centuries was of a beleaguered GP. Within the profession he was beset on the one side by wealthy consultants, and on the other by the sixpenny doctors – each group appropriating practice which GPs saw as rightfully theirs. Outside the profession there was perceived to be an equally competitive encounter, in which GPs felt themselves to be squeezed between charitable bodies indiscriminately giving medical charity, and penny-pinching clubs with organised patient power.[131] It was only national health insurance payments after 1911 that rescued a typical GP from economic struggle.[132] They made possible the middle-class professional lifestyle which had previously only been an aspiration; one or two cars, the parlour maid to open the front door, private schooling for the children, and the regular afternoon on the golf-course. This kind of affluent lifestyle had hitherto been much more conspicuous amongst physicians.

---

[129] *BMJ*, 1907, (11), p. 480, letter from 'Fair Play'.   [130] *BMJ*, 1903 (11), p. 1095.
[131] See for example the evidence given by GPs to the *SC on Metropolitan Hospitals*, PP 1890, XVI, QQ 1598–9, 3606–8, 4478, 3272–3.
[132] Digby and Bosanquet, 'Doctors and Patients', pp. 74–94.

6

Physicians

Physicians viewed themselves as a medical and social élite. They possessed a university degree in medicine, which gave them intellectual and theoretical knowledge of medicine.[1] Physic was concerned with treating through medical means the internal ailments and diseases of patients, so that physicians were perceived as practising medicine with their minds rather than their hands and, in making a diagnosis, emphasis was placed on the verbal and visual rather than the manual. During the late eighteenth century physicians were relatively plentiful in London, but in the provinces they were greatly outnumbered by other types of practitioners. However, in national terms, the disparity had lessened from one in seven to one in five by the mid-nineteenth century.[2] This numerical difference is largely explained by the fact that physicians in private practice practised with élite patients whilst surgeon-apothecaries and GPs treated a greater socio-economic range. The patients whom the physician treated belonged to the aristocracy, the gentry and the upper and middle classes; these groups comprised, at most, one in ten of the population. Since physicians were approximately about one in six amongst medical practitioners, élite patients had an unusually favourable doctor-patient ratio since they also employed surgeons and apothecaries.[3]

---

[1] Not all were as competent as their MD might suggest, however, since MDs could be purchased at Aberdeen or St Andrew's, whilst, at the beginning of the period, some might practise without any formal medical qualification as a 'physician'.

[2] In 1783 there were 3623 surgeon-apothecaries, surgeons, and apothecaries and 511 physicians (Lane, 'Medical Practitioners', pp. 353–71); The *Census* of 1851 enumerated 2328 physicians and 15,163 surgeon-apothecaries; that of 1861, 2385 physicians and 12,030 surgeon-apothecaries. Unfortunately, after 1861 the census aggregated numbers of physicians with surgeons and later also with general practitioners.

[3] In this calculation I have assumed that a minimum income of £100 per annum was a necessary precondition for employing a physician in the eighteenth century and only five to seven per cent of the English population fell into this category (P. Lindert and

The physician's Victorian practice also tended to become increasingly specialist in nature: proportionately more physicians were consultants, as those with hospital appointments often came to be called. Given this situation, many practised in London, in county or hospital towns, and in spas. Considerable problems were experienced in starting such a practice, whilst maintaining it was dependent almost as much on social attributes as on medical skills. Thus, the chances of achieving prosperity were slim. This chapter analyses the dynamics of this process.

Building a practice

Holding an honorary office in an infirmary or hospital provided an important key to expanding a physician's practice, although it was less vital to the physician than it was to the surgeon. Typically, the physician took longer to achieve an economic livelihood than did the GP. Typically this was through attaining a post as assistant physican in a hospital, before receiving the final professional accolade of a full consultancy post as a general physician. During the eighteenth century it wasn't particularly difficult for a London physician to achieve a hospital appointment, whereas it was later transformed into a mark of recognition.[4] In 1847, fewer than half of provincial physicians had positions at hospitals or dispensaries, although the proportion was higher in London, with three out of five. However, only one in twenty (of all medical men) made it to *senior* posts in London hospitals in 1878.[5] Hospital positions were much sought after since it gave the opportunity both for specialist work and for a high social profile in the community; not least through contact with the members of the local élite who were on the governing bodies of these institutions.[6] Private practice then might follow, either in the families that made up county society or in those constituting the urban middle classes. Once this had been achieved, Georgian physicians – though

J. G. Williamson, 'Revising England's Social Tables, 1688–1812', *Explorations in Economic History* (October 1982), pp. 385–408 and (January 1983), pp. 94–109). In the Victorian era one in ten upper- and middle-class families had an annual income of £100 or more. This was also the lowest income level for paying income tax (H. Perkin, *The Origins of English Society, 1780–1880* (1969), p. 420 and J. C. Stamp, *British Incomes and Property* (1916), p. 432). This figure of ten per cent was an upper limit, and it is plausible to think of the Victorian figure as little more than that of the eighteenth century.

[4] W. F. Bynum, 'Physicians, hospitals and career structures in eighteenth century London' in Bynum and Porter, *William Hunter*, pp. 115, 121.

[5] Loudon, *Medical Care*, p. 221; Peterson, *Medical Profession*, p. 137.

[6] Waddington, *Medical Profession*, p. 31.

not their Victorian successors - might resign their hospital appointments.[7]

For provincial physicians medical practice was of a more general
nature than for London consultant physicians, although patients were
equally select. Their practice focused on the upper social strata, except
that in their role of hospital consultant they would also come into
contact with some poorer patients. It was important, therefore, for
them to be socially visible and thus use a carriage to drive to their
patients. A polished social demeanour, with the ability to make good
general conversation, were important ingredients in that vital professional attribute – a good bedside manner. The norms of gentility
were seen as being crucial to a successful career, and it was suggested
that 'The character of a physician ought to be that of a gentleman.'[8]
Medical students (who stereotypically were thought to live profligate
lives) were lectured on their need to devote some of their time to
general cultivation of the mind in order that they could converse and
'be fitted to associate with' gentlemen.[9]

What of the young physician? Starting out in practice as a physician
was more problematical than for the surgeon-apothecary or the GP,
since a select clientele meant that work was less widespread. Handbooks for entrants to the profession dwelt on the necessity of private
means to finance young physicians through a longer, more specialist
apprenticeship, and to tide them over the longer period needed to
build up a practice.[10] For the mid-Victorian period, Peterson has
suggested that, typically, a position of Fellow of the Royal College of
Physicians was attained at the age of 33, the post of assistant physician
at 34, whilst that of full physician was not reached until 40 years of
age.[11] Even for such established practitioners private income was
helpful to bridge the unevenness of income, since the physician suffered – perhaps even more than his professional brethren – from
non-payment or belated payment of bills.

Some examples from the 1820s illustrate the divergent fortunes of
those attempting to develop practices as physicians. This is a good
period to study the phenomenon since, in contrast to the golden years
of the eighteenth century, professional competition was intense. John
Simpson articulated the feelings of an aspiring physician, 'As a young

[7] Bynum, 'Physicians, Hospitals', p. 118.
[8] T. Withers, *A Treatise on the Errors and Defects of Medical Education* (York, 1794). Withers
   was Physician to the York County Hospital.
[9] Brodie, *Discourse on Conduct of Medical Students*, p. 19.
[10] Thompson, *Profession*, p. 167.
[11] Peterson, *Medical Profession*, p. 137.

physician I cannot have practice to keep me fully employed. I read a great deal.'[12] He was writing in 1825, a time when young practitioners were finding it difficult to get started in an overcrowded profession. Simpson was starting up in Bradford, which he conceded was a 'bad situation for a medical man.'[13] But even in London – potentially a much better location – a young physician without connections found the going equally difficult. Samuel Warren wrote with some journalistic embellishment of his early struggles when, 'I had numbered twelve months almost without feeling a pulse or receiving a fee.'[14] Warren – like many others – regretted the 'vanity which led me to rely so implicitly on my talents for success. Had I but been content with the humble sphere of GP' he thought he would more easily have obtained what he termed 'a respectable livelihood.'[15] Warren stated that he got a lucky break through a street accident that led to practice in a titled household and thence to further introductions. More usual for a physician was career advancement through the patronage of a senior colleague.[16] For example, in his early years the physician-accoucheur, Charles Locock, benefited from the help of Dr Gooch. He rejoiced that:

I have been busy lately more with Dr Gooch's patients than my own, consequently have had to do more with Ladyships and Right Honourables – than with cobblers' wives and bakers' daughters – These serve as famous introductions to families, and Gooch has often sent me, where there has been little or no occasion for it, merely as a medium for getting me known.[17]

For the physician such personal connection was allegedly more important than a hospital appointment, but connection operated powerfully in the punishing elections to such offices and, once gained, hospital appointments then facilitated further connections. With these circular and reinforcing processes a distinction between connection and office appears to be more apparent than real. Birth and family

---

12 Wilmott, *Dr John Simpson*, p. 11. John Simpson (born 1793) came of a medical family, and only practised for a short time, when a timely inheritance allowed him to become a county gentleman.
13 Wilmott, *Journal*, p. 30. See also the comment by H. Marland that in the West Riding Wakefield had more physicians relative to population than Bradford (or Leeds) because of its middle- and upper-class clientele (*Medicine and Society*, p. 261).
14 Samuel Warren, *Passages from the Diary of a Late Physician* (2 vols., Paris, 1839) vol. I, p. 2. Warren only practised for a short time between 1821–7 before becoming a medical journalist.
15 Warren, *Passages*, p. 8.
16 See J. Keevil, *Hamey the Stranger* (1952) for an account of the uncertainties of patronage in an early-seventeenth-century career progression.
17 R. C. Maulitz, 'Metropolitan Medicine and the Man-Midwife: the Early Life and Letters of Charles Locock', *MH*, 26 (1982), p. 34.

have traditionally been seen as more important factors for the physician's professional success than for the more mundane work of the surgeon-apothecary or GP. Valuable analyses of the élite who became Fellows of the Royal College of Physicians has indicated that this social card has been over-emphasised. In origin, few had aristocratic connections, whilst those from a professional backgound came from the middle ranks and, tellingly in this context, were not the first-born, but the younger sons.[18] This is not to deny that once a physician had a fashionable practice, hobnobbing with the great brought further valuable professional rewards. The professional life of Sir Henry Halford centred during the early nineteenth century on a wide consultancy practice with a genteel and aristocratic clientele.[19] He eventually attracted the patronage of the King and was perceived subsequently by his colleagues as more of a courtier than a doctor. Arguably, this was a specialist application of a highly developed, professional bedside manner to an august social context.[20]

Another means of assisting professional advancement was publication; enhanced public visibility meant that practice might thereby be fostered. Physicians – having time on their hands in their early professional days – were more prone than surgeons or GPs to publish; in mid-century one in five provincial physicians, and one in two London physicians, put their thoughts in print.[21] Robert Lee was one such author; a physician specialising in gynaecology and obstetrics, who was Physician to the British Lying-In Hospital before becoming Professor of Midwifery at St George's Hospital, and in 1841 a Fellow of the Royal College of Physicians. He published extensively first on his teaching and then his research.[22] Despite this he devoted an anxious passage in his diary in 1843 to analysing whether he was keeping a due balance between his practice and his research, and this preoccupation was still troubling him seven years later, when he concluded that further publication would extend his practice.[23]

Whilst it is easy to isolate general factors that contributed to professional success it is harder to pin down why some careers failed to

[18] Peterson, *Medical Profession*, pp. 147, 204–5.
[19] Leics. RO, DG 24/941 and 943, Diaries of Henry Halford.
[20] Clarke, *Autobiographical Recollections*, p. 113.
[21] I. Loudon, 'Two Thousand Medical Men in 1847', *Bulletin of the Society for Social History of Medicine*, 1983, p. 7. These figures are based on a sample of 2000 randomly selected entries in the London and Provincial Medical Directories for 1847.
[22] His books during the 1840s included *The Anatomy of the Nerves of the Uterus* (1841), *Clinical Midwifery* (1842), *Lectures on the Theory and Practice of Midwifery* (1844), *Memoirs on the Ganglia and Nerves of the Uterus* (1849) and *Pathological Researches on the Diseases of the Uterus* (1840–9).
[23] Wellcome MS 3218, Diary of Robert Lee (1793–1872).

take off. In Lee's case a difficult personality, with a degree of intolerance and combativeness, appears to have made for professional awkwardnesses, whilst ensuing bitterness at a lack of professional recognition by his peers no doubt exacerbated the situation.[24] Others at this time failed to make a successful practice until late in life, despite apparently having all the means to do so. Edmund Lyon, Physician to the Royal Manchester Infirmary was a case in point. Born of a clerical family, and with an Edinburgh medical degree, he was elected in 1817 – at the early age of 27 – Physician to the infirmary by a very large majority. On his retirement he was said by the board to have given 'unremitting, exemplary and zealous services' for almost a quarter of a century. It might have been expected that contact with members of the board, plus the status of his office, would have brought in much lucrative practice. So too might his other office as Honorary Physician to Henshaw's Blind Asylum, especially when enhanced by public visiblity gained from his publications, which included *A Sketch of the Medical Topography and Statistics of Manchester*. Yet his biographer commented that Lyon did not manage to make a successful practice until late in life.[25] One might speculate that the shyness which made him a reluctant teacher was part of a wider and professionally more crippling social diffidence.[26] As with Lee it was social rather than medical talents that were apparently deficient.

An important element in creating a practice was establishing good professional contacts with colleagues. This was all the more important in an era when the prosperous patient might turn to more than one practitioner. Jane Walls described how in 1788, during her brother's 'dreadful illness', his family turned in desperation to several physicians:

It's two months since he had Dr Kilvington's advice of Ripon, he kept him for weeks in a terrible state, mistook his case. He grew worse. We brought him to York for the advice of a Dr Hunter who mistook his case. Also, Mr and Mrs Weddell sent to Dr Fothergill in London for his advice. The first medicine he took from his prescription gave him ease.[27]

How this sequence of practitioners occurred was important for professional goodwill; hence the contemporary handbooks on etiquette and ethics. Etiquette prescribed that doctors should not advertise for

[24] See diary entries for summer 1845 and the *DNB* comment on the profession not giving him due recognition.
[25] S. Crompton, *Memoir of Edmund Lyon, M.D.* (Manchester, 1881).
[26] Manchester RO Papers of E. Lyon, M134/1/2/8.
[27] Wilts. RO uncatalogued Ailesbury Papers, letter from Jane Walls to the Lord Bruce, 1788. Dr John Fothergill (1735–80) was a prominent Quaker and a highly successful

patients or poach another's patients. But the initiative lay with the patient who might have a shrewd idea of the relative professional competence of individuals. Claver Morris's diary included the entry:

I went to Sherborne and saw Mr Shirley who was very ill of a jaundice, and his physician Dr Bull not discerning rightly his disease, prescribing very languid medicine for what he thought it to be, he [Mr Shirley] desired my assistance, and I prescribed.[28]

Rancorous relationships between colleagues might develop over consultations even in this 'golden age of physic', when competition in the medical market was less intense than in the ensuing period. In a series of pamphlets three practitioners in Bury St Edmunds exposed their hostilities to the world in 1764: the physician, Dr Sharpin, and his surgical colleague, Mr Steward, accused a Dr Norwood of unprofessional conduct in taking over the treatment of their patient. Norwood was an extra-licentiate of the the College of Physicians, and the author of *An Essay on the Treatment of Cancerous Tumours*, so that it is possible that he succeeded his colleagues because, being better-known, the patient preferred to trust his fate to him. This was certainly not an isolated example of professional enmity. Thirty-five years later in the same county of Suffolk, a practitioner in Halesworth, a Dr Langslow (who earlier had been the Physician to the Lying-In Charity of London), sued his rival, a Mr Dalton. This was in order to recover medical fees due to him from his treatment of a Master Day, who was a schoolboy in whose treatment Dalton had succeeded Langslow. Dr Langslow complained of the jealous assertions of his medical colleagues, which he thought had damaged his practice by discouraging patients from seeking his help. The volatility displayed by the protagonists in these unseemly intra-professional disputes gave a revealing insight into the precarious nature of Georgian practitioners' professional livelihoods, not least in their own perceptions.[29]

Maintaining a practice

For the physician maintaining a practice was not only dependent on clinical skills and diagnostic acumen but also on relationships with

London physician. Dr Alexander Hunter (1729–1809) was a founder, and later Physician to the York Asylum.

[28] Diary entry, 17 March 1720 in E. Hobhouse, ed., *The Diary of a West Country Physician* (1934), p. 78.

[29] Dr Sharpin and Mr Steward, *An Appeal to the Public in General and to the Gentlemen of the Faculty in Particular With Regard to their Medical and Chirurgical Treatment of Mr John Ralling* (Bury, 1764): Dr William Norford, *A Letter to Dr Sharpin in Answer* (Bury, 1764); Dr R. Langslow, *The Case of Master Day of Yoxford* (Bungay, 1800).

individual patients. This contrasted with the social dynamics of a surgeon-apothecary's practice, where there was a larger 'throughput' of patients at modest fees. The contact of physicians with their patients is well documented; characteristically this was friendly rather than intimate in nature although this varied according to their relative social status.[30] For the gentry friendships with the medical fraternity typically formed part of the outer rather than inner circle, as they did for the Verney family during the eighteenth century.[31] Physicians clearly valued their contacts with leading families, not least because it was their best advertisement, and a source of further practice through personal recommendation. Crucially, such social connection helped distance them from trade. They were therefore prepared to work hard at maintaining a friendly as well as a professional relationship. Dr Thomson of Worcester dispatched fresh salmon as a gift to his patient at Ferry Hall in Ludlow in 1776, and Dr Edward Beck of Ipswich sent some garden cuttings to Sir W. F. Middleton in 1858.[32] Some patients reciprocated in traditional style: the Ailesbury family customarily sent half a buck to the family physician during the late eighteenth and early nineteenth century.[33] Yet the social distance between the élite patient as patron and the physician, was not entirely bridged by such gifts; a certain note of ingratiation was evident in the tone that physicians adopted so that the physician signed letters very formally, 'your lordship's most obedient and humble servant' or 'yours gratefully and obediently'. Doctor and patient were on more even terms in the special circumstances of the spa. Dr Arbuthnot, for instance, referred to his patients at Tunbridge Wells in 1731 who, 'filled my belly with good dinners at noon, and emptied my pockets at night at quadrille.'[34]

Lay patronage contributed to the overlapping nature of practices within a diffuse medical market. The patient's choice of medical practitioner was eclectic and wide-ranging and resulted in a competitive professional life for the physician. This gives a useful insight into the social dynamics of keeping up a friendly relationship with local fami-

---

[30] See *A Seventeenth Century Doctor and his Patients, John Symcotts, 1592(?) – 1662* (Bedfordshire Record Society, xxxi, 1951) for the friendly correspondence of Symcotts with Mr Power of Ramsey.

[31] Margaret Maria Lady Verney, *Verney Letters of the Eighteenth Century* (2 vols. 1930).

[32] RCSL, uncatalogued letters of William Thomson. Letter to Mr Walker, 24 March 1776; East Suffolk RO, HA 93/9/419, letters of Dr Edward Beck, 1858.

[33] Wilts. RO uncatalogued papers of the Ailesbury family; venison was sent to Dr Adair in the 1760s, Dr Warren in the 1780s and Dr Phipps in 1813.

[34] Letter to Lady Suffolk, 6 July 1731, quoted in G. A. Aitken, *The Life and Works of John Arbuthnot*, second edn (New York), pp. 134–5.

lies lest they prefer a competitor. The patronage of the old Roman Catholic gentry family of the Blundells is particularly instructive during the early eighteenth century. In these years the Blundells employed some 25 orthodox practitioners, as well as midwives and two fringe practitioners. Ten physicians were used, three regularly, whilst a further seven were consulted occasionally for more serious illnesses. The regular physician, Dr William Lancaster, was a local man from Ormskirk six miles distant, who shared the family's Catholic persuasion.[35] Others were consulted on an occasional basis for more serious afflictions: they were brought in from Liverpool (slightly more distant), Wigan (some 15 miles away), Chester (nearly 30 miles) and even – on the occasion of terminal illness – from Whitchurch in the neighbouring county of Salop, which was more than 40 miles distant. Interestingly, the Blundells sometimes travelled to consult their doctors, although it was more usual for them to be visited.[36] For Nicholas, medical practitioners, and more especially his physicians, seem to have became as much friends as professional advisers. A congenial personality was an essential element in a 'bedside manner' and a generally convivial disposition was advantageous in employment; the physicians, William Lancaster, and the father and son, Frances and Thomas Worthington, were in this category. That the Blundells were not exceptional in the way they deployed local physicians is shown by the Purefoy family from the 1720s to the 1750s. The Purefoys' home at Shalstone was at the conjunction of several counties so that it was natural for them to recruit widely, as well as employing a spa physician; their physicians thus included Dr Kimberley of Northampton, Dr Pitts of Oxford and Dr Rayner of Bath.[37]

By the mid-nineteenth century improved communication meant that even country-based families could regularly call on London practitioners, if they could afford to do so. There was a marked difference between the use made of local physicians and other practitioners by the Blundells or the Purefoys, and the much greater reliance later placed on the metropolitan physician. A good example of this was Charles Darwin during his sojourn at Downe in Kent from 1842 to his death in 1881.[38] In part, this pattern of medical consultation may also have been influenced by the nature of Darwin's ill-health, with par-

---

[35] The evidence for this statement is indirect, in that the diary states that a priest lodged with the doctor's brother, a Liverpool grocer.
[36] *Great Diurnall*, entries 19 August 1709, 4 December 1724, 16 January 1725.
[37] G. Eland, ed., *Purefoy Letters* (2 vols., 1935), pp. 328, 341.
[38] My analysis of the pattern of consulation is based on the valuable data given in R. Colp, *To Be An Invalid. The Illness of Charles Darwin* (Chicago, 1977).

ticularly poor spells during 1839–42, 1848–9, 1863–4 and 1865. This, it may be inferred, would have resulted in a search for alternative specialists since once one consultant physician with a favoured regime had been tried and found wanting, another was selected. Only Darwin's own father, Dr Robert Waring Darwin, retained the long-term confidence of his patient. During this entire period Darwin consulted physicians, with but two exceptions: first, Mr James Startin, a London skin specialist, who treated his eczema in 1863 and 1865; and secondly, a local surgeon, Charles Allfrey, who was called in during Darwin's terminal illness. But for the most part élite London physicians treated him, including three who advised him on diet: Frederick Headland, whose regimen delighted his patient in 1860 because it included wine; Bence Jones who recommended his well-known 'starvation' diet in 1863–4; and Andrew Clark who prescribed a strict diet with physic during the 1870s. Other top London physicans were also called in to advise on Darwin's flatulence and sickness including: the very fashionable Henry Holland in 1848; William Jenner in 1863 (who thought chalk would do the trick); William Brinton in 1863–4 (who prescribed mineral acids); as well as John Chapman in 1865 (who recommended applications of ice to the spine). However, on several occasions between 1849 and 1863 Darwin was prepared to travel in order to gain the benefit of the water cure; he was treated by two Malvern physicians, James Gully and James Ayerst, as well as by their colleagues Edward Lane at Moor Park, and Edmund Smith at Ilkley. For his final cardiac troubles he was advised by three physicians: Andrew Clark, Norman Moore, and F. C. McNalty.[39] Interestingly, Darwin who was skilled in the etiquette of the medical profession, took pains in 1881 when consulting alternative practitioners to his regular attendant, Dr Clark, to have Dr Moore and Mr Allfrey 'in nominal consultation' with Dr Clark.[40]

[39] Robert Waring Darwin 1766–1848 had an extensive practice around Shrewsbury; James Startin (1806–72) was noted for the complexity of his prescriptions for skin diseases; Charles Allfrey (1839–1912) practised at St Mary Cray; Henry Bence Jones, FRS (1813–73); Sir Andrew Clark (1826–93); Frederick Headland (1830–75) was Physician to Charing Cross Hospital and an expert on the action of medicines; Sir Henry Holland (1788–1873) had a very extensive fashionable practice; William Jenner (1815–98), was Physician in Ordinary to Queen Victoria; William Brinton (1823–67), was Physician to St Thomas's Hospital and had several publications on diseases of the stomach; John Chapman (1821–94) was the author of *Functional Diseases of the Stomach* (1864); James Manby Gully was probably the best known hydrotherapist and the author of *The Water Cure in Chronic Disease* (1847); McNalty practised in the Lake District, and was consulted when Darwin was on holiday in Patterdale; Moore (1847–1922) was then a rising young London physician.
[40] Cope, *Invalid*, p. 94.

In dealing with affluent patients much of the therapeutic inter-vention was thus concerned with chronic ailments in which the physi-cian might undertake a long-term management of the disorder. The character of the medical encounter is important in appreciating the dynamics of the physician's practice in its economic dimension. Fortu-nately, in the pre-railway era, the correspondence between physician and patient was relatively abundant because so much medical treatment was prescribed by letter rather than by face-to-face contact. In part this arose from the mobility of the upper classes with their town and country houses, journeys to spas, and frequent visits to family or friends. Correspondence was also produced by the uneven distribution of physicians who tended to congregate in populous towns, and thus not be available for any but acute or life-threatening illness in the more distant parts of the rural hinterland. Since four-fifths of the illnesses and ailments for which the physician was consul-ted probably were not acute but chronic in nature, diagnosis and treatment was often through letter rather than interview. That this was the case is of inestimable value to the historian, although it may have been of less value to the patient.

A letter to Mrs Christian from Dr Willam Brownrigg (who practised in Whitehaven for 30 years from 1757) gives a clear insight into the type of relationship that a country physician might wish to develop with a patient. That the letter of April 1741 is an unpolished draft is helpful, since it shows the practitioner struggling to put his own professional objectives into a form that was socially acceptable to the patient:

Although it is not expected of a physician to give his opinion of the nature [of the] disease and [the] reasons for which he does [i.e. acts], yet something [like this is] absolutely necessary if he expects a compliance, and [it is] always satisfactory if he can explain himself [so] as to be understood and his method of proceeding appears rational, nor do I think it is revealing my art to explain so much to every one who is capable of understanding it, as for your accurate description of your case I find and conclude you are. As I am therefore desirous of doing everything which may contribute [in] any way to your satisfaction I hope it will not be thought too troublesome if I endeavour to give you a short view of my sentiments of the nature of the disorder in as intelligible a manner as the nature of the subject will admit of. The first observation I shall make is that you have an exceeding soft and lax habit of body.[41]

Brownrigg thus indicated that he was aware that he needed to get his patient's compliance if he was to succeed in imposing a regimen, and with shrewd psychology took the patient into his confidence as to his

[41] Carlisle Library, E104, W. Brownrigg's Casebook, 1737–41.

proposed treatment of her illness. This was particularly necessary in an age when lay knowledge of, and interest in, disease was not much – if at all – inferior to that of the Faculty. By assuming and acknowledging the patient's intelligence and self-knowledge, Brownrigg delicately paid Mrs Christian a compliment which he might also hope would win her trust in his diagnostic acumen. This professional strategy is interesting in relation to a later professional handbook for physicians in which John Gregory advised a physician to use 'judgement and discretion'. Gregory acknowledged that whilst 'The government of a physician over his patients should undoubtedly be great ... an absolute government very few patients will submit to.' He thus counselled the physician to prescribe a regimen that was realistically 'the best that will be observed'.[42]

The geographical distance between physician and patient made Gregory's advice problematic because the doctor needed to acquire precise details of the illness. This meant that epistolary social pleasantries of a genteel character had to be commingled with physical details of an intimate kind. The letter in 1776 from Dr William Thomson, Physician to the Worcester Infirmary, to Mr Walker of Ferry Hall is a nice example of this genre:

I am just now favoured with your letter, and will, with great pleasure, pay every attention to the circumstances you mention relating to your health. But before I prescribe for you, I must beg leave to enquire a little about this frequent making of water in a morning after drinking your chocolate. You must tell me what colour the water is, and whether it remains clear after being made, or turns muddy and afterwards drops a sediment. I also wish to know what water you make through the day and night, both as to the frequency of making it, and the quantity you make at a time. Mention also the quantity made at a time in the morning, when you have such frequent calls, and whether you make it with perfect ease, or if it gives you pain while you make it or after it is over. When you have informed me of these particulars, I shall be able to say whether you ought to take anything for the complaint or not, and (if anything be necessary) what is most likely to do you service.[43]

In some social contexts, notably venereal disease, patients were reluctant frankly to divulge sufficient information to their doctors. William Cullen wrote sternly that, 'Dr Monro and I ... are of the opinion that it [the illness] has continued longer from a mistaken notion ... which prevents him from reporting freely and fairly ... without which it is impossible for a physician to conduct any obstinate disease to a final cure.'[44] The earlier aphorism by Dr Cheyne seems apposite here: 'Fine

[42] J. Gregory, *On the Duties and Qualifications of a Physician* (second edn, 1820), p. 21.
[43] RCSL, Uncatalogued letters of W. Thomson, letter of 20 March 1776.
[44] RCPE, Cullen correspondence, 30/2, fo. 78, Mr Mees case, 24 August 1769.

folk use their physicians as they do their laundresses [and] send their linen to be cleaned in order only to be dirtied again.'[45]

In these circumstances the general tone of physicians' letters to their Georgian patients was deferential but not obsequious; they were concerned to show that the doctor belonged to the same genteel world, yet was grateful for the patronage bestowed. This subtle blend was particularly well illustrated in letters which gently reprimanded the patient and must, therefore, have caused considerable anxiety to the physician in achieving the right tone of solicitous concern. Take, for example, that written in 1741 by Dr Hardinge to his patient Sir William Robinson of Newby Hall, Yorkshire:

> I will not be very impertinent as a physician, but think I have full right as a true friend to you to put you in mind of the great negligence which I have lately observed in you. For God's sake show a little more wisdom, and do not treat your health as a trifle; it is certainly in your power to enjoy a tolerable share of it, and therefore you must expect a little scolding when you take too little care of it.[46]

Sir William suffered from asthma which – with gout, dyspepsia, rheumatism, and varied nervous/hypochondriacal disorders – appears to have been among the most common chronic afflictions of the affluent. In some cases the long-term nature of these diseases tended to transform the status of the physician from that of professional expert to family doctor and friend. However, this did not preclude the patient from consulting other members of the Faculty. Sir William contacted no less than four physicians over his sufferings, a large but not exceptional number among those with chronic ailments.[47] Dr Hardinge accepted with good grace Sir William's use of a Hull physician (Dr Flemyng), and corresponded amicably with the Bath physician (Dr Hartley) whom his patient saw during a visit to the spa. But Hardinge showed irritation at advice being given Sir William by a Dr Wintringham, as can be inferred by his denial that he was conducting a 'paper war' against the latter.[48]

The letters of Dr Hardinge to Sir William exemplify much of the nature of Georgian medicine, with their revealing sequence of long-distance history-taking, diagnosis, and therapeutics. As this was based

---

45 C. F. Mullett, *The Letters of Dr George Cheyne to Samuel Richardson (1733–1743)* (University of Missouri Press, 1943), p. 3.
46 Leeds Archives, Newby Hall Papers, letter dated 23 September 1741.
47 Identification of these practitioners is problematical but it is likely that three of the individuals concerned were: Caleb Harding, MD, FRS, a royal physician practising in Mansfield, London and Derby: Clifton Wintringham, MD of York; and Malcolm Fleming, with an MD from Rheims, who practised in Hull and York.
48 Leeds Archives, Newby Hall Papers, letter dated 29 October 1742.

on symptomatology, the chief source of information about the disease was the patient, so that the physician was very willing to listen to the patient's own account of his or her illness. Knowledge of the sufferer's past history of illness, of the family, and of heredity, were of enormous importance in diagnosis. A preceding chapter argued that before the development of pathological anatomy created an understanding of the specific nature of diseases, the physician's 'medical gaze' was not focused locally; concern lay with general indicators of the patient's physical state within a broad humoral interpretation of the body. And, because the physician was less concerned with precise physical measurements at this time, it was frequently as useful to read a patient's account, as it was to listen. Equally, it was thought to be just as acceptable to diagnose without the need for a physical examination. It is in this context of medical practice that we should place Dr Hardinge's letter to his patient, 'In such cases as yours I will be directed by nothing but your own experiences, and would form my proceedings and hints for further trials from such things as you are able to inform me of.'[49] Unfortunately, Sir William's letters to his doctors have not survived, but we know from extant letters sent by sufferers to a consultant such as William Cullen, that great detail was sent to the doctor.[50] No doubt this lengthy process of revelation and self-interpretation – coupled with the confidence that the physician valued such testimony – had considerable therapeutic value for the patient. Typically, such outpouring covered much of the individual's history of ailments, complaints of his or her pains, together with a view of self-perceived abnormalities in the body, or the mind. This had the inestimable value of giving an experienced practitioner good insight into the personality of the correspondent, and hence the opportunity of making a better diagnosis. The replies by the consultant showed that psychological as well as linguistic skills were of considerable professional importance.

In diagnosis, the physician used mainly non-technical language so that such understanding of the illness as was possible was shared between patient and practitioner. Thus, Hardinge explained to Sir William that:

I take your asthma to proceed from the making of a chyle by successive indigestions, as your lungs cannot well deal with it; I take it that the very labour of the [asthmatic] fit does grind and comminute [i.e. pulverise] that birdlime, if I may call it, which occasions it, and that when it is so comminuted, the fit is regularly over.[51]

---

[49] Leeds Archives, Newby Hall Papers, letter dated 29 October 1742.
[50] RCPE, Cullen Correspondence, 31/1–17, (1755–90).
[51] Newby Hall Papers, letter dated 1 November 1740.

In prescribing suitable treatment for the patient, a Georgian physician was able to practise holistic medicine, based on insight into 'the whole person'. Medical theories of the day retained classical medicine's belief in the interaction of body and mind,[52] so that the physician was well equipped to give due weight to the psychosomatic factor in a patient's illness. It was perhaps predictable in this context that Sir William's employment of four physicians should have led to disagreements in diagnosis and treatment, with varying importance having been given to the nervous and the physical origin of his asthma. While Hardinge saw it in physical terms (in which overeating produced chyle), Hartley and Flemyng saw it as 'chiefly nervous' but aggravated by over-eating.[53] And while Hartley and Flemyng advocated a more vigorous set of medicines (including the eating of soap for flatulence) and a regimen of cold bathing for Sir William, his longstanding doctor and friend, Hardinge, thought gentler methods were apposite for the patient's tender constitution and weak lungs. All were persuaded, however, of the need to take into account in their diagnoses singularities of physique and personality and to actively involve patients in the understanding and management of their condition.

Only gradually was the physician able and willing to supplement careful observation of patients' appearance, and the account by them of their symptoms, with new manual techniques, first using percussion and then auscultation in diagnosing chest disorders. The adoption of newer mechanical aids to diagnosis was slowed by the traditional perception of the physician – as a remote intellectual rather than a close-contact, manual operator – since adoption of these new methods would have meant physical contact with patients. Social considerations might also impede contact with patients. In the case of George III by Sir George Baker in 1788, for example, only the pulse was counted, and inspection of the tongue and excreta was neglected, whilst case notes were kept only as an *aide memoire*.[54] By the 1830s guides were published to help medical students (and their elders) conduct a systematic physical examination using the latest technological aids. By mid-century it seems probable that physical examinations were more generally acceptable socially, although more so with male than female patients. And, as the misrepresentations implicit in some patients' accounts of their illness were then more readily appre-

[52] L. J. Rather, *Mind and Body in Eighteenth Century Medicine* (1965), pp. 1–2, 9, 16–7; Rather, 'Six Things Non-Natural', p. 337.

[53] Newby Hall Papers, Dr Hardinge to Dr Hartley 10 September 1745, Dr Fleming to Sir William 13 October 1747.

[54] I. MacAlpine and R. Hunter, *George III and the Mad-Business* (1969), pp. 22–3.

ciated, along with an acknowledgement of the deficiencies in using external symptoms as a guide to diagnosis, there was perhaps a greater readiness to use the growing range of medical technology to improve diagnostic accuracy. From the middle of the nineteenth century to the end of the century it became technically possible to use a thermometer to take the temperatures of patients, and a sphygmomanometer to measure their blood pressure.[55] Unfortunately, there is little evidence to show the extent of the take-up of these advances in private practice. One might speculate that their adoption was slow since not only did they run counter to the intellectual tradition of physic but, particularly for older practitioners might also have impinged on their self-image as skilled healers who intuitively used the art of empirical experience unlike scientists who relied on machine-made measurement. In some instances, physicians seem to have preferred to adopt a less scientific approach since this ensured better communication with the patient and the family. For example, Dr Vaughan (later Sir Henry Halford) refused to sign the post-mortem report on the Duchess of Devonshire in 1806, because he considered that the language used in the report by Everard Home was too technical for the family to understand.[56]

Achieving prosperity

There were two principal kinds of relationships between physician and patient – medical and business; historians have tended to neglect the latter. Whereas for the surgeon-apothecary or GP there may be surviving ledgers, the standard documentation for the business side of a physician's life is usually an isolated few items in the family papers of erstwhile patients. From these illustrative pieces of evidence it appears that the standard physician's fee of one guinea (for a consultation given at his own home) was raised for night visits or prolonged daytime visits. For example, a mid-nineteenth-century Suffolk physician charged a double fee for sitting up all night with his patient, and did the same for an all-day visit.[57] Much larger fees resulted either when the physician had a considerable clinical and/or social reputation, or if the patient was perceived to be wealthy or titled. For instance, Dr Addington at the height of his profession charged £100

[55] S. J. Reiser, *Medicine and the Reign of Technology* (Cambridge, 1990), pp. 21–3, 29, 31, 38, 105, 115.
[56] Leics. RO Harland MSS, DG24/812/25–31, 1 April 1806.
[57] E. Suffolk RO, HA 61, 436/26, Accounts of Dr Beck for attendance on Sir P. Broke, c. 1858.

for his services during the fatal illness of Harriet Brudenell, the daughter of the Earl of Cardigan in 1767. In contrast, his colleague, Dr James (well-known for his invention of 'James' Powders') felt able only to demand a more modest £23 in the same case.[58] Authoritative estimates in the 1860s were that physicians charged one guinea for a visit or one to two guineas for a consultation.[59] In the late seventies fees of one guinea for a consultation, followed by a further guinea for writing a letter to the patient's GP, was the standard rate.[60] One contemporary estimate was higher in suggesting that the standard physician's fee was then three guineas. This was probably too high because three guineas was still being quoted as the standard fee for a Harley Street consultation as late as the 1930s.[61]

The issue was further complicated because in some cases the physician travelled to the country seat of the patient. For a long period physicians did not price their time appropriately when making visits in the countryside. (Historically, this was a parallel problem to that experienced by the profession in charging for their expertise rather than for their medicines.) Claver Morris, for example, practising in early-eighteenth-century Wells, rarely charged more than a guinea for such a local visit and only charged a maximum of twelve guineas for unusually distant visits to neighbouring counties.[62] Others were more realistic; in 1775 charges made by physicians during the last illness of Theresa Parker of Saltram House, were £250 by Dr Glass for eight visits and £150 by Dr Caldwell for 'a few' visits.[63] Adequate payment to recompense the physician for travel away from home and for loss of income whilst away was a matter of continued professional anxiety. Twenty-one years later Dr Erasmus Darwin replied to his Bristol colleague, Thomas Beddoes, who had asked for advice on this subject:

> I went to Margate, about three years ago, which is 200 miles from Derby, and was 6 days and had a present of £100. I have twice been to London and had about 10 guineas a day given me and what was supposed to be travelling expenses. When a physician goes far from home he loses the custom of families: as they will not wait for his return, as when he goes but one day's journey. And those families apply to another. Your staying so long from home must have been attended with much loss. I think you should have 10

---

[58] J. Wake, *The Brudenells of Deane* (second edition, 1954), p. 276. It is, of course, impossible to estimate how much time each spent with the child.

[59] Farr's introduction, *Census, 1861*, p. 243; *Lancet* 18 June 1864.

[60] *BMJ*, 19 January 1878.

[61] Rivington, *Medical Profession*, p. 52; PEP *Report on the British Health Services* (1937), p. 160.

[62] Holmes, *Augustan England*, p. 224.

[63] R. Fletcher, *The Parkers at Saltram* (1970), p. 122.

guineas a day, and a sum for what should be conceived as to be chaise expenses.[64]

The attractions of good fees in spas and watering places during the late eighteenth and early nineteenth centuries made it worthwhile for physicians to migrate from London during the summer season to Tunbridge Wells, Buxton, Scarborough or Brighton.[65] With the advent of rail travel in the 1840s journeys became much quicker and the geographical range of practices widened for everyday – rather than just for seasonal – consultancy.[66] Physicians also began to price their time with greater economic rationality, charging either one guinea per mile for visits to the country, or two-thirds of a guinea for each mile travelled by rail. A professional manual of 1870 suggested that distant visits might incur charges of up to 100 guineas.[67]

Physicians tended, as we have seen earlier, to congregate in county and hospital towns and in the capital, since these were the locations of affluent patients. Wilkes referred to his Wolverhampton colleague, Dr John Collins, who had removed to London, 'thinking this way of life too great slavery.'[68] Spas were the physicians' other professional honey pot. Table 6.1 indicates that there the ratios of physicians to other regular practitioners were far higher than the national average, where ratios varied between 1:10 in the late eighteenth century to 1:5 in the mid-nineteenth century. Figures of doctors are taken from local *Directories* so that only a general order of magnitude is indicated. Nevertheless, this is very striking. In the period between the 1740s and the 1870s ratios of physicians to other doctors varied in Bath between 1:1.4 and 1:3, whilst during the early nineteenth century those in Tunbridge Wells were of the order of 1:2.3, and in Cheltenham between 1:1.5 and 1:4.[69]

Not that physicians got it all their own way with affluent patients,

[64] D. King-Hele, *Letters of Erasmus Darwin* (Cambridge, 1981), pp. 297–8.
[65] *Clifford's Guide of Tunbridge Wells* (fourth edn, 1818), pp. 27, 170; *Medical Register*, 1783, pp. 112, 123; *New Buxton Guide* (Buxton, 1837), p. 13.
[66] Granville, *Spas*, I, p. ix.
[67] *Census*, 1861, p. 243; Rivington, *Medical Profession*, p. 52; F. Davenport, *What Shall My Son Be* (1870), p. 54.
[68] Wellcome MS 5006, fo. 25, entry for May 1739.
[69] Figures for Bath were obtained in local directories for 1773, 1778, 1784, 1792, 1800, 1805, 1809, 1812, 1819, 1822, 1826, 1830, 1833, 1842, 1846, 1848, 1849, 1850, 1852, 1860–1, 1872–3, as well as *Universal Magazine* (1747); and W. Baylies, *Practical Reflections on the uses and abuses of the Bath Waters* (1757). For Tunbridge Wells, figures were obtained from *Clifford's Guide to Tunbridge Wells* (1828) and (1834), and from *Visitors Guide to Tunbridge Wells* (1830). For Cheltenham figures were gleaned from E. Humphries and E. C. Willoughby, *At Cheltenham Spa* (1928), p. 86; *Griffiths New Historical Description of Cheltenham* (Cheltenham, 1826), p. 47; and Granville, *Spas*, II, pp. 307–8.

Table 6.1. *Ratios of physicians to other regular practitioners in Bath,*
Tunbridge Wells and Cheltenham, 1740–1870

	Bath	Tunbridge	Cheltenham
1740	1:3	–	–
1750	1:2	–	–
1760	–	–	–
1770	1:2.5	–	–
1780	1:3	–	1:4
1790	1:2.5	–	–
1800	1:1.7	–	1:2
1810	1:1.2	–	–
1820	1:2.2	1:2.3	1:1.5
1830	1:2.3	1:2.3	1:2
1840	1:1.7	–	–
1850	1:1.7	1:2.3	–
1860	1:1.6	–	–
1870	1:1.4	–	–

Note: Other regular practitioners include surgeons, surgeon-apothecaries,
and apothecaries.
Sources: See footnote 69.

either in spas or in the metropolis, since other practitioners also
wished to acquire prosperity. A surgeon wrote from Bath in 1791:

It is not my intention to confine my practice to those cases which fall
especially under the province of the surgeon, having been persuaded to
extend it to cases which are more strictly the object of medicine, but I shall not
keep or dispense medicines. All the surgeons of this place, and most of them
in London are occasionally employed in cases that do not entirely belong to
the practice of surgery.[70]

Nationally, there was an uneven distribution of physicians, with striking regional disparities. The concentration of physicians in the southern half of England was even more pronounced than that for the
profession as a whole. Table 6.2 indicates that in 1851 the south-east
and south-west of England were twice as well provided as were the
areas with the fewest physicians, whilst London – with the most
physicians – was four times as well endowed.

Top London physicians could attain substantial wealth. Particularly
in the earlier part of the period, many were very effective self-

---

[70] Wilts. RO, Uncatalogued Ailesbury Papers, letter of 20 November 1791 from Garlick
to the Lord Bruce. Garlick appeared in the 1780 and 1783 *Medical Register* as practising
in Marlborough.

Table 6.2. *Ratios of physicians to regional population in 1851*

Region	Numbers of physicians	Population per physician
London	552	4279
S.E. Counties	229	7110
S. Midlands	80	15,429
E. Counties	63	17,682
S. W. Counties	213	8466
W. Midlands	176	12,118
N. Midlands	67	18,127
N. W. Counties	153	16,279
Yorkshire	102	17,539
N. Counties	82	11,818

Source: Census, 1851.

publicists and made a point of being visible in fashionable society. John Radcliffe, who died in 1714, made a legendary fortune which included a capital gift of £45,000 to the University of Oxford. His successor, Richard Mead, made £5–6000 annually for fifteen years and at his most successful earned over £7000 (despite the fact that his individual charges were modest). John Fothergill, with an exceptionally successful London practice from the 1740s to the 1770s was variously estimated to have earned £5000 to £11,000 annually, while J. C. Lettsom (who took over his practice) made up to £12,000 a year. Richard Warren, a favourite physician in London society at the turn of the nineteenth century bequeathed £150,000 on his death.[71] He shared the best medical business of London with Matthew Baillie. Baillie himself earned £10,000 a year during the early nineteenth century, whilst William Chambers made 7–9000 guineas in the early Victorian age.[72]

Sir Henry Halford's peak earnings reached £12,000. The figures for his annual income are given in Table 6.3 and illustrate clearly the typically low earnings of the young physician, followed by the riches to be acquired once fashionable status was attained. His annual income rose from £220 in 1792 to £9850 in 1809, and £12,000 by 1824. In real terms the increase over the period as a whole is very impressive since the price level in 1792 and 1823 was almost identical. However,

[71] W. Munk, *The Life of Henry Halford* (1895), p. 42.
[72] Holmes, *Augustan England*, p. 221–3: R. Porter, *English Society in the Eighteenth Century* (1982), p. 92; Waddington, *Medical Profession*, p. 32; J. J. Abraham, *Lettsom* (1933), p. 208.

Table 6.3. *Henry Halford's annual income, 1792–1824*

Year	Annual income £
1792	220
1793	164
1794	327
1795	401
1796	399
1797	511
1798	905
1799	1403
1800	2153
1801	3214
1802	5081
1803	5947
1804	7632
1805	7727
1806	7909
1807	9434
1808	8902
1809	9850
1824	12,000

Source: W. Munk, *The Life of Henry Halford* (1895), p. 39.

very rapid war-time inflation in the earlier part of the period (when cost of living indices rose from 122 in 1792 to 212 in 1809), meant that the early growth in nominal income, although impressive, was less spectacular than a first glance would indicate.[73] Halford was the son of a provincial physician, James Vaughan – a Physician to the Leicester Infirmary – who settled in London in 1792. Elected Physician to the Middlesex Hospital the following year, and becoming a Fellow of the College of Physicians the year after that, it still took another four to five years before a good income was attained. A good marriage, succession to the Halford estate in 1809 (when he changed his name), and attendance on four monarchs – George III, George IV, William IV and Victoria, confirmed his pre-eminence and ensured a fortune.

Many of the largest Georgian medical incomes were based on royal patronage, since both reputation and pocket book benefited. There was a standard daily consultancy fee of 30 guineas for a royal physi-

[73] The Schumpeter-Gilboy price index has been utilised here and indicates that the consumer's cost of living index then fell to £128 by 1823. (B. R. Mitchell, *Abstract of British Historical Statistics* (Cambridge, 1962) p. 469.)

cian, whilst retainer fees of several hundred pounds per annum were also customary. Bynum's study suggests that a total of 480 doctors held a royal appointment at the English court for the period between 1688 and 1837. Medical bills for the last eight years of George III's reign amounted to a colossal £271,691.[74] The most successful of royal doctors was acknowledged to be Halford, since he was called in to attend no less than seven royal deathbeds. For prolonged attentions to King George IV, he received £2000, whilst his charges during the King's terminal illness amounted to £4800.[75] With such rewards, only the very successful would turn down a royal appointment as did William Heberden Senior, who actually refused George III's offer of the post of physician to Queen Charlotte in 1761 because of his extensive private practice.[76] This did not impede him, however, from attending a consultation on George III in 1788.

Including as it did the possibility of court attendance, and the better chance of hospital appointments, teaching and prosperous patients, income from metropolitan practice was undoubtedly greater than a provincial one. For example, Dr James Hope's income rose steeply in the late-Georgian and early-Victorian eras. Without connections, and as a young physician in London he earned only £200 pounds in his first year of practice in 1828, yet by 1840 (when he was House Physician at St George's Hospital) he earned £4000 per annum. The exact nature of the difference – in fees charged and income gained – between metropolis and provincial practice is difficult to evaluate. A successful physician in early-eighteenth-century Wells, Claver Morris, had medical earnings which rose from £100 to £300 in the period from 1707 to 1723. Morris had a sliding scale of fees for consultations at his home which ranged from two shillings and sixpence for the poor, five shillings for artisans and tradesmen to half a guinea for more substantial citizens, and one guinea for the gentry or clergy. Geoffrey Holmes's view is that a provincial physician would have needed to be doing very well indeed to make £500 in Augustan England.[77] Yet incomes of £400 a year were estimated for *young* Norfolk physicians before the end of the century.[78] Although fees were larger in metropolitan areas, the premium that the London physician could

[74] W. F.Bynum, 'Medicine and the English Court, 1688–1837', in V. Nutton, ed., *Medicine at the Courts of Europe, 1500–1837* (1990), pp. 280, 282–3.
[75] Leics. RO, Halford MSS, DG 24 859/3.
[76] MacAlpine and Hunter, *George III*, p. 23.
[77] Holmes, *Augustan England*, p. 224–5. Claver Morris (1659–1726) was an extra licentiate of the College of Physicians.
[78] K. Garlick and A. Macintyre, eds., *The Diary of Joseph Farington* (1978), vol. 4, p. 1244. I am grateful to Colin Pedley for this reference.

command over his provincial colleagues was stated variously. In the early eighteenth century a lay view – that of Lady Fermanagh – was that London fees were five times greater than in the provinces,[79] and that would appear to be of the right order of magnitude if a comparison is made with well-known London physicians.[80] However, Thomson's survey of the profession in 1857 indicated a smaller, yet still substantial differentiation, with estimates of provincial physicians earning from £500 to £1500, and successful (but not top) London colleagues earning from £800 to £3000.[81] London certainly had more affluent patients than the provinces whilst its physicians were typically better qualified. In 1880 a suggested table of fees, based on qualification, recommended from one to five guineas for the payment of a consultant who was a Fellow of the Royal College of Physicians.[82]

The tendency of physicians to congregate in capital cities – whether London or Edinburgh – meant that they frequently extended their practice through consultation. Consultation amongst several colleagues in a difficult case might be a means to extended practice in the longer term. Georgian illustrations of consultations among large groups of physicians reveal that some contemporaries suspected that this was a means of fee-grubbing. Such a consultation certainly doubled the standard guinea fee for a Georgian physician.[83] The grasping image of the profession led to some attempts at damage-limitation, as with this example of eloquent pleading, where contrasts drawn with an ideal type of physician unwittingly undercut the case:

The art of physic fairly and honestly practised I honour as the first of professions, [and] ... I think a real physician the most liberal of characters on earth; by which I do not mean every doctor that goes about taking guineas, but him who will neither flatter the great not deceive the ignorant, and who would prefer the satisfaction of making one invalid a healthy man, to the wealth of a Radcliffe or the vogue of a Ward.[84]

Correspondence was an important aspect of the consultative art. It was also seen as a satisfactory resolution of a Georgian provincial physician's dilemma. Through this means more expert advice could be

---

[79] Margaret Maria Lady Verney, *Verney Letters of the Eighteenth Century from the MSS at Claydon House* (2 vols. London, 1930), vol. II, p. 84.

[80] Holmes indicates an order of magnitude of four times rather than five, but suggests that the London practitioner, Richard Mead, had modest charges (*Augustan England*, p. 224).

[81] Thomson, *Choice of Profession*, p. 169.

[82] W. E. Stevenson, *The Medical Act (1858) Amendment Bill and Medical Reform: A Paper Read Before the Abernethian Society at St Bartholomew's Hospital* (1880), pp. 30–1.

[83] C. D. Leake, ed., *Percival's Medical Ethics* (Baltimore, 1927), p. 102.

[84] J. Ruhrah, ed., *William Cadogan. His Essay on Gout* (New York, 1925), p. 17.

obtained in a non-life-threatening illness without the need to bring in
local competitors who, if they impressed the family or patient, might
well displace the regular attendant. Brownrigg's case book indicated
the importance in difficult cases for a provincial physician of consultation by letter with distant colleagues, since he consulted Monro in
Edinburgh and Mead in London.[85] However, the physician with the
greatest Georgian consultation practice was the Edinburgh-based
practitioner, William Cullen, who had a standard fee of one guinea for
a written opinion, but who was adamant that 'nobody ... shall suffer
from my want of advice.'[86] He asked his patients to pay what they
could afford:

You put a question to me about my fee which I am never willing to answer for
the most part submitting my own opinion to that of others in this matter but if
I must speak to you I shall tell you that my fee is according to the circumstances of the person and the trouble I have from the case.[87]

Indeed, Cullen seems to have waived his fees entirely in the most
deserving cases, since we find a Mr John Rogers writing to him that 'I
am the more ashamed to put you to the present trouble since you
have generously given your advice without any fee or reward.'[88]

Billing a patient was one thing but obtaining payment was quite
another. Patients themselves might be cynical about what they saw as
the obtrusive fee-grubbing of their physician. Richard Wilkes was
notorious for this, and his death came in characteristic fashion, according to one of his patients. 'He was at Wolverhampton the day he died
and took several fees, and the week before he rode 50 miles; so the
love of money held him to the end.'[89] No doubt the physician felt
equally sour about the meanness of patients. There are a number of
apocryphal stories of an eminent physician being paid half a guinea,
stooping down and pretending to look for something on the floor. On
being asked what was the object of the search, the reply was that, 'I
was only looking for the *other* half guinea.'[90] A physician's initial
outlook might be one of benevolence but this could be soured by
contact with economically-minded patients. William Cadogan
observed pithily that 'a man should be a skilful and honest physician
(unless he be sent for too late and dismissed too soon, which is

[85] Carlisle Library, E 104, William Brownrigg's Casebook, 1737–42.
[86] Risse, 'Doctor William Cullen', pp. 343–4.
[87] RCPE, Cullen MS 31/1, Letter dated 17 March 1774.
[88] Cullen MSS 31/1, Letter dated 28 March 1774.
[89] Quoted in R. and D. Porter, *Patient's Progress*, p. 68.
[90] Most stories focus on the surgeon, Abernethy (e.g. F. Davenant, *What shall my son be* (1870), p. 54), but others give different characters.

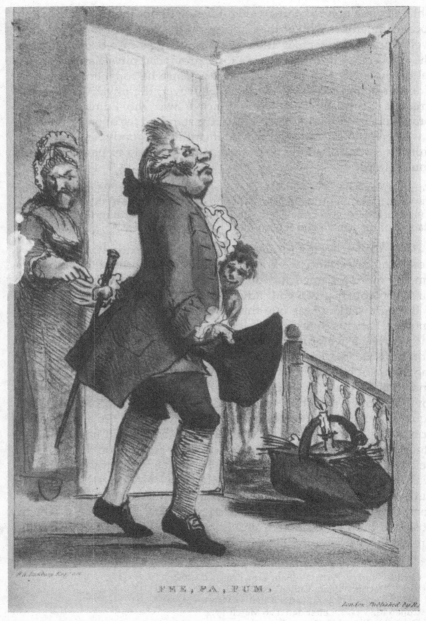

Plate 8   A Discreet Payment for a Housecall, by H. W. Bunby (1750–1811)

generally the case).' The ability to ensure an efficient conduct of the business side of the relationship with a patient without marring the socio-medical relationship was a difficult yet essential art. (See Plate 8.) Non-payment of fees was a particularly serious professional hazard since, by their own professional rules, physicians were unable to recover their fees at law.[91] The problems this caused with more affluent patients as a result of bills that have survived in family and estate papers can frequently be seen. Occasionally, it seemed to have been assumed by the more prestigious patient that the gain to reputation alone was more than adequate remuneration for the doctor. Dr David Dundas, for instance, complained that he got nothing for his attendance on King George III in 1788. He concluded philosophically, however, that it 'was undoubtedly of good use to me in my profession and made me known.'[92]

Where genteel rather than royal patients were concerned, remuneration was less a game of chance but the swings and roundabouts of fortune still operated. A grateful patient might well round up the bill that the physician had charged: in mid-nineteenth century Suffolk, for instance, Sir P. Broke paid £100 to Dr Beck instead of the £92 that had been indicated on the bill.[93] Gentry families were notoriously slow in meeting their obligations. The papers of the Carew family of Crowscombe Court in Somerset from the mid-eighteenth to the mid-nineteenth century show that typically the family's physicians had to wait for two or three years for payment of quite large cumulated bills.[94] However, some had to wait for their patient's eventual death and the settlement of the estate by trustees before their endeavours were recompensed, as did Dr Ling for his patient, G. H. Carew in 1842. Nor was this predicament confined to England; for example, Dr William Sinclair of Thurso waited more than a decade for his bills to be paid during the mid-eighteenth century.[95] Of course not every physician depended on medical fees for income and lifestyle. Advantageous marriages, for example, might make all the difference between a genteel and a struggling standard of living. Claver Morris in the early eighteenth century made three good marriages: the first to a wealthy woman, the second to a propertied widow, whilst his third wife brought him capital of £300.[96]

Precisely because of the restricted group of patients and the limited

[91] Davenant, *My son*, p. 54.   [92] Scottish RO GD 35/236/13.
[93] E. Suffolk RO, HA 61 : 436/26, bill c. 1858.
[94] Somerset RO, DD/TB 13/7–8; DD/TB Box 14 20; DD/TB 15/30.
[95] Scottish RO GD 136/1085/1 and 2, bills of 1741–53 in Sinclair of Freswick papers.
[96] Hobhouse, *Country Physician*, pp. 12–4.

kinds of treatment offered, choosing to become a physician involved even greater risks of failure than did that of the GP. The stereotypical life of the *successful* physician was pleasant and well-remunerated; the nature of its rewards were social as well as economic. It corresponded most closely to the historical stereotype of the doctor in the 'good old days': an intimate knowledge of patient and family; plenty of time for careful diagnosis and treatment; and a pleasant social relationship with patients. The medical nature of these encounters is analysed in the following chapter.

PART III

Patients and doctors

7

Medicalisation and affluent patients

This chapter focuses on two privileged groups – affluent patients and physicians – and their economic and medical relationship to each other. From the late seventeenth century there was a growth in numbers and incomes of the 'middling' sort of people; mainly those with mercantile, professional and business occupations. In London, for example, they formed one-fifth to one quarter of all households. This development meant that a physician's services could now be applied beyond a narrow élite group to a much wider section of English society.[1] The urban renaissance of the eighteenth century fostered sociability between urban middling groups and country gentry which involved the drawing into the town of visitors from a wide geographical area. A luxury or leisure economy in the town, of which medicine was one element, expanded the medical market.[2] Also helpful in increasing practice were the mercantilist views of the age since these could be skilfully applied to suggest that a need for health in the future could – under a physician's guidance – be assisted by careful attention to lifestyle in the present. As the heroic interventions of traditional physic became less fashionable, and the moderate measures of regimen correspondingly more attractive, so the physician's role increasingly focused on advice, support and psychological reassurance. The widespread eighteenth-century interest in the mind – whether sane or insane – was shown in the conspicuous and explicit psychologising of Georgian correspondence between physician and patient.[3] Whether this was deployed instrumentally is difficult to

---

[1] Earle, *The Making of the Middle Class*, pp. 13, 80–1.
[2] Borsay, *Urban Renaissance*, pp. 271, 282, 316–7; A. McInnes, 'The Emergence of a Leisure Town: Shrewsbury, 1660–1760', *Past and Present*, 120 (1988), pp. 61, 83–4.
[3] Earlier, during the late sixteenth and early seventeenth centuries the Stratford physician, John Hall, had shown intuitive understanding of patients, as did the

judge, but it had the inestimable advantage for the medical man of deepening the dependence of the sufferer on the physician, and thus in reducing the odds of this being only a short-term relationship. Changing cultural relations between leisure and health meant that a gamble for health under professional direction could be easily assimilated into the Georgian predilection for gambolling for pleasure at the spa. This medicalisation of 'taking the waters' might replace or supplement lay attempts to reach a cure. An expanding range of spas and treatments enabled the physician to offer even more specialist advice on their selection and utility than had his predecessors, through suggesting that water, like medicine, needed to be taken with discrimination and under expert guidance. Of Bath in 1766 it was aptly said that 'today, many persons of rank and condition/Were boil'd by command of an able physician.'[4]

Regimen

Extending the medical market within élite and middling groups was a subtle task. Traditional lay wisdom on the value of exercise and good diet was very similar to the professional position on regimen, with its stress on healthy living. The Lancashire merchant, William Stout (1665–1752), had his own salubrious routine; this was apparently uninfluenced by any contemporary medical debates on regimen, yet was remarkably similar in character. The habits of a lifetime were to: rise with the sun and walk for two miles; do a day's business; spend an hour or so in his garden in the evening; to eat the 'simple product of our own country'; and, even when invalided after an accident, to take no physic.[5] Habits of life rather than the doctor's physic, were perceived to be the key to health. This lay sagacity was encapsulated in Dryden's lines:

> Better to hunt in fields, for health unbought,
> Than fee the doctor for a nauseous draught,
> The wise, for cure, on exercise depend;
> God never made his work, for man to mend.[6]

mid-seventeenth-century Bedfordshire physician, John Symcotts, but it was the clerical practitioner, Richard Napier, who had been notable for his distinctive psychological healing. (H. Josephs, *John Hall, Man and Physician* (1976), p. 24; M. MacDonald, *Mystical Bedlam* (Cambridge, 1981); *A Seventeenth Century Doctor and his Patient, John Symcotts* (Bedfordshire Record Society, xxxi, 1951).
4 *The New Bath Guide* (second edn, 1766), pp. 15–16.
5 J. D. Marshall, *The Autobiography of William Stout of Lancaster 1665–1752* (Chetham Society, third series xiv, Manchester, 1867), pp. 219, 226–7, 237–8.
6 'To John Driden of Chesterton', lines 192–6.

It was thus desirable to limit physic and recourse to a doctor, and instead to manage one's own health, through a regimen of exercise, moderate diet, and a judicious blend of business and pleasure. Dr Johnson later personified a more widespread reaction against physic in which the lateness of his conversion to regimen was matched by the enthusiasm with which he publicised its virtues. He advised a friend in 1783 that 'It does not appear from your doctor's prescription that he sees to the bottom of your distemper. What he gives you strikes at no cause ... I do not think you have so much to hope from physic as from regimen.'[7]

In an age when medicine produced uncertain results, and frequently caused discomfort or distress to the patient, alternatives to physic were likely to be at a premium as physicians acknowledged. John Locke, physician and philosopher, recognised this in suggesting to a patient that 'Half your cure depends on the doctor's prescriptions and the other half is in your own mind. Cheerfulness will have a great[er] efficacy towards your recovery than anything the apothecaries shops can afford.'[8] In constituting themselves as experts not just on physic but on psychotherapy, physicians might seek to intervene widely in everyday life. Physicians were aware that management could not be delegated entirely to sufferers since paying patients must be retained. Swift's ironic lines, 'The best doctors in the world are Doctor Diet, Doctor Quiet, and Doctor Merryman'[9], were given an extended meaning. Instead of being alternatives to medical care the Georgian doctor used such traditional prescriptions for a growing social sector of the population. Therapeutic interventions were facilitated by a mercantilist view of health as a commodity whose stock – like gold – could be augmented by careful management and hoarding. A Lake District physician wrote to a patient in 1742 that he would 'prescribe such methods as are most proper to be prescribed in order to preserve your future health.'[10]

Relationships between physicians and their patients suggested an evolving partnership that had sufficient flexibility to accommodate a moving frontier; varied professional inputs were complemented by fluctuating patient dependency. This was desirable since frequently the physician was physically distant, yet still wanted long-term

---

[7] G. Birkbeck Hill, ed. *Letters of Samuel Johnson* (2 vols. 1892), II, p. 355.
[8] K. Dewhurst, *John Locke, Physician and Philosopher* (1963), pp. 296–7, advice to Mrs Clarke, 8 March 1694.
[9] Swift, 'Dialogue 2'.
[10] Carlisle Public Library, E104, William Brownrigg's Case Book (1737–41), entry on J. Christian, 4 August 1742.

involvement. Thus a consultant wrote in a letter to a sufferer from spasmodic asthma, that 'Mr Russell has now had so much experience of his disease that he is already acquainted with the most part of the management that is necessary.'[11] The crucial words were 'with the most part' since these ensured that continued advice was necessary. And, in light-hearted mood, Dr Hardinge wrote to Sir William Robinson in 1743 that 'it gives me great pleasure to hear, that you pretend to be above all waters and all doctors.'[12] From the physician's perspective, confidence that such a stance was a pretence was grounded in experience of the chronic sufferer's dependency on medical aid. From the viewpoint of the patient such confidence does not appear misplaced. Between 1741 and 1746 the elderly John Wyndham kept a medical diary, containing daily entries about his chronic bladder complaint. These show that although he was ready to alter the amount and frequency of his medication, and also to listen to his friends' accounts of their doctors' advice, he retained overall confidence in his own physician, Dr Hele, and the advice he gave him.[13]

North of the border, Sir John Clerk exhibited a similar pattern of long-term dependency. This is shown by correspondence with doctors between 1706 and 1751, together with Sir John's memoranda on health, his health diary and a journal kept by his son during his father's serious illness in 1718. He was a chronic sufferer, not only from gout, and gravel, but from the usual kinds of aches and twinges, imagined or real, experienced by a hypochondriac, including back pain, coldness on his thigh, and a rough palate. The advice on regimen of his physicians, Drs Burnet and Rule, was framed with a shrewd insight into the psychology of their patient, and the need to encourage him. '[We] think you have no reason to fear any hazard. Howsoever, to show how ready we are to be serviceable to you in our art, we have thought upon the following advice.'[14] Sir John's regular purging in Spring and Autumn was under the superintendence of his physicians. And his later regimen of rising early, regular mealtimes, avoidance of liquor, and some cold bathing had been laid down in 1710 by Dr Baynard. He advised that 'Nothing conduces more to health than a regular way of living.'[15] In his diary, Sir John reflected on the health consequences of his actions; the benefit of cold bathing

[11] RCPE, Cullen Correspondence, 31/1, letter from Dr Cullen, 12 July 1770.
[12] Leeds Archives, Newby Hall Papers, letter dated 11 June 1743.
[13] Somerset RO, DD/WY box 1, Medical Diary of John Wyndham (1674–1750), of Norrington, Wiltshire.
[14] Scottish RO GD18/2131, Clerk papers, queries to Drs Burnet and Rule, 1696, and their reply.
[15] Scottish RO GD18/2133.

and the harmfulness of hearty eating. 'Ill this night', he recorded and then reflected that he 'ate too much at dinner of boiled ham, soup, pudding, milk' for a poor digestion.[16] An attack of gout he found 'very uneasy and dispiriting', the more so since it 'kept me from rest in the night time' and 'resisted fasting, purging, vomiting, bathing, and all usual external topics.'[17] Significantly, a swift recourse to the Faculty resulted from a serious attack of acute illness in 1718, when a tumour led to the involvement of six surgeons and two physicians. Convalescence was also superintended by a physician, Dr Eizat, who modified Sir John's regimen to take account of his greater bodily weakness. He counselled moderation, 'for tho' you have got good by these things formerly, you cannot expect the same now when you are weaker.'[18] Despite his reliance on doctors, the patient retained an independent tenor of mind in his dealings with them. He was critical of his practitioners during his serious illness in 1718. And minor decisions on health were taken independently, including vomits during a digestive illness in 1722, and choices on taking spa water. Like so many other sufferers he had his favourite cures, which he exchanged with other sufferers.[19] Physicians themselves recognised that in an era of private patronage a degree of patient autonomy was inevitable. 'From these plain principles you may easily deduce rules for management in like case', counselled one of Sir John's physicians.[20]

In dealing with long-standing complaints Georgian physicians sought to understand the psychology of the sufferer to an even greater extent than their predecessors. The relationship of mind and body was seen as of crucial importance, and a considerable number of nervous and hypochondriacal disorders in their affluent patients underlined the utility of physicians concerning themselves with this. In a discussion on regimen, John Gregory in his *Elements of the Practice of Physic* of 1744 stated that 'The mind should be kept in as tranquil a state as possible.'[21] Such advice figured prominently in the medical correspondence of the day. In laying down a regimen for his nervy patient, John Christian Esq. in 1742, Dr Brownrigg stated that a 'cheerful and easy disposition of mind will also greatly contribute towards preserving your health.'[22] Conventional Georgian wisdom was that such cheerfulness was often to be gained from exercise, which acted as

[16] Scottish RO GD18/2137, 2139.   [17] Scottish RO GD18/2135.
[18] Scottish RO GD18/2137.
[19] Scottish RO GD18/2138.   [20] Scottish RO GD18/2143.
[21] Second edn, 1744, p. 17.
[22] Carlisle Public Library, E104, Brownrigg's case book, letter of 4 August 1742.

tonic to both body and mind. This emphasis on exercise as a central element in regimen was innovatory. In 1775 William Thomson, the Physician to the Worcester Infirmary, when consulted by his Ludlow colleague, the surgeon Edward Cole, advised that the patient, a Mr Walker, should 'rely greatly on his horse, whom he will find the best doctor among us.'[23] Individuals reacted variously to this ambiguous relationship between doctor (or horse) and patient, medicine and management, or physic and regimen. However, a clergyman wrote enthusiastically to the *Gentleman's Magazine* in 1738 commending Dr Cheyne's temperate rules for living, 'the doctor's system is pretty near that sort of medicine which nature calls for.'[24]

Cheyne's notable *Essay on Regimen* of 1740 marked the climax of a twenty-year medical campaign to moderate the high living of the early Georgian age.[25] His methods had already been tried out on his patients, but without winning a wider fashionable acceptance. 'If I could cure my patients with burgundy and ham pie I might be cried up to the skies', he wrote ruefully.[26] Undeterred, the polemically-inclined Cheyne wrote his *Essay* in order 'to instruct all sober and serious persons, how to preserve, or regain their health.' His 'philosophic medicine' was addressed to the whole person in its recommendation of exercise, low-living and a low diet. 'Riding is the best of all exercises to get health, and to promote the digestions . . . but walking is best to preserve health', he considered.[27] His contemporaries, Arbuthnot and Mead, placed diet in a central position in regimen, but Cheyne carried his enthusiasm for the subject to the point of framing a dietetic gospel.[28] He placed particularly strong faith in his low diet of milk and seeds, which would 'mend' the juices of the body, and cool and sweeten the circulating fluids. This was of strategic importance in restoring health because of his humoral conception of the body as a 'hydraulic machine' of pipes and tubes through which flowed the vital fluids.[29]

[23] 'Of the regimen of life' in *The Medical Works of Richard Mead M.D.* (Dublin, 1767), pp. 435–7. Richard Mead (1673–1754), was a member of the College of Physicians, a royal physician, and Physician to St Thomas' Hospital. RCSL, correspondence of William Thomson, letter of 14 June 1775; *Eighteenth Century Medics*, p. 123.

[24] *Gentleman's Magazine*, VIII (1738), p. 362.

[25] L. S. King, 'George Cheyne, Mirror of Eighteenth Century Medicine', *BHM*, 48 (1974), 517; *Cheyne's Observations concerning the Gout* had been published in 1720, and his *Essay on Health and Long Life* had appeared in 1724.

[26] C. F. Mullett, ed. *The Letters of Dr George Cheyne to the Countess of Huntingdon* (San Marino, 1940), p. 41. Letter dated 3 August 1734.

[27] Cheyne, *Regimen*, pp. i, xvi; 'Medical aphorism 25' in *Regimen*, p. lxv.

[28] J. Arbuthnot, *An Essay Concerning the Nature of Aliments* (1731); Mead, *Works*, pp.435–7.

[29] Cheyne, *Regimen* pp. i, ii, xxviii.

Cheyne's long correspondence during the 1730s and early 1740s with two of his patients – Selina, Countess of Huntingdon and the novelist, Samuel Richardson – although carefully attuned to their different social status, were remarkably similar in their emphasis on regimen, rather than occasional physic, as the way to alleviate their complaints.[30] The former was urged to stand by 'the simplicity of the dietetical gospel', consisting mainly of vegetables and milk, to drink the Bristol water, to take exercise, and also a regular vomit and a mild purge. The doctor congratulated her that this had been successful in that it had 'sweetened your blood, [and] opened the obstructions in the glands.'[31] Richardson was reassured that 'all chronical cases require time, patience and perseverance in a proper method', and that Cheyne's rules would direct him 'in the most proper method to lengthen your useful life.'[32] This correspondence exemplified very well the mixture of exhortation, advice, reassurance, modified prescription and congratulation 'on your state of rejuvenescence',[33] that marked the dealings of the eighteenth-century physician and patient. Richardson's close application to business had led to continuous psychological and physical problems which Cheyne treated by a combination of traditional physic – medicines and seasonal vomits and bleeding taken at the equinoxes – and of regimen. The patient was advised to adopt a temperate diet (preferably vegetable), and to take exercise (either by walking or on an indoor parlour-horse).[34] He should also drink mineral waters, take cold baths, and spend three or four weeks at a spa. Cheyne contrasted the power of medicine and regimen; the former 'will but relieve, not cure you, and for but a short time', whereas with regimen 'you are cured for ever'. There was also the significant advantage of regimen over medicine that 'you run no risk, nor ever can by it make symptoms worse than they are at present.'[35] Equally, one might infer that the risks of the physician in alienating the patient were also lessened.

---

[30] The correspondence with Selina, Countess of Huntingdon (1707–91), took place throughout the 1730s, and that with Samuel Richardson – novelist and also printer of Cheyne's books – from 1733 to 1743.

[31] *Letters to the Countess*, pp. 58–9, letters of 25 February and 20 August 1737.

[32] Mullett, *Letters to Richardson*, pp. 48–9, letter of 13 May 1739.

[33] *Letters to Samuel Richardson*, p. 78, letter of 30 December 1741.

[34] 'The chamber-horse ... has all the good and beneficial effects of a hard trotting horse except the fresh air ... the board ought to be as long as the room will permit ... and the chair you sit on with a cushion on the board as a bottom to it with a two armed hoop and with a foot-stool.' Letter 20 April 1740, quoted in *Letters to Richardson*, pp. 59–60. There is an unusual example of a Chippendale exercising chair without arms in Stanway House, Oxfordshire.

[35] *Letters to Samuel Richardson*, p. 76, letter of 12 December 1741.

'The scorbutic, gouty, consumptive, or nervous valetudinarian' had been the principal object of Cheyne's concern. Amongst these, the gouty were an important category of sufferer to whom contemporary doctors directed their advice on regimen since it was a disease they attributed to high living. William Cadogan's *A Dissertation on the Gout and all Chronic Diseases Jointly Considered* of 1771, covered much the same intellectual territory as had Cheyne's Essay. Indeed, Dr Johnson concluded that 'Tis only Dr Cheyne's book told in a new way.'[36] Cadogan's prescriptive advice was given with a more brutal clarity, however, and his ideas on the role of physic, in relation to nature, were much more restrictive, referring to 'idle acts and tricks of medication and quackery; never once lifting their eyes to Nature.'[37] Chronic diseases such as rheumatism, stone, colic, jaundice, palsy and gout were to be remedied by 'activity, temperance, and peace of mind.' This involved an entire recasting of lifestyle. 'It is the constant course of life we lead, what we do, or neglect to do, habitually every day, that if right establishes our health, if wrong, makes us invalids for life.' Characteristically, Cadogan posed the sufferer's dilemmas starkly: it was not from 'natural defects' of the constitution but from 'abuses' of it, through 'indolence, intemperance, or vexation', that chronic illness came. Gout arose from 'the daily accumulations of indigestion', in which the body threw off 'bad humours' to the extremities.[38]

It was therefore worse than useless for the gouty to send for the doctor, take medicine, and briefly adopt a temperate regimen.[39] Such blunt advice was doubtless of great benefit to those sufferers sufficiently disciplined to heed it, but taken by itself it was of dubious economic value to the medical profession. At a stroke Cadogan had removed four-fifths of its patients! Contemporaries were not slow to draw the moral, and in the satiric *The Doctor Dissected or Willy Cadogan in the Kitchen* all 'disciples of Galen' were advised to 'shut up your shops.' Instead:

> Physicians, I beg of all rank, and degrees
> You'll learn the new method of getting your fees:
> Politeness discard, and adopt in its stead.
> The manner now practic'd of being well bred:
> Tell your patients their folly deprives them of health,
> And prefer honest bluntness to fame and to wealth.[40]

[36] J.Boswell, *Journal of a Tour to the Hebrides* (New York, 1936), pp. 168–9.
[37] J. Ruhrah, ed. *William Cadogan. His Essay on Gout* (New York, 1925), pp. 13–4.
[38] *Cadogan's Essay on Gout*, pp. 33, 34, 31, 85.   [39] *Cadogan's Essay on Gout*, p. 5.
[40] Reprinted at the end of Ruhrah, *Cadogan*. On opposition to Cadogan see J. Rendle-Short, 'William Cadogan, Eighteenth Century Physician', *MH*, 4 (1960), 301–5.

Being an entrepreneurial profession, however, medics exploited this situation so that rather than being disadvantaged by it, positive benefits accrued. Instead of regimen replacing physic, it became complementary to it. This meant that in cases of chronic ailments – where the line between sickness and health was blurred – the doctor's advice could be proffered not only on occasions when physic was appropriate, but on a more permanent basis through providing rules for health, continual psychological encouragement to the patient in pursuing them, and modifications of the regimen as these became expedient. Such a process was facilitated by the friendly relationships that were carefully built up between physician and affluent patient.

Cheyne's *Essay of Health and Long Life* was criticised in 1724 in *A Letter to George Cheyne Shewing The Danger Of Laying Down General Rules* for ignoring the fact that no disease affected two persons alike, and hence that regimen needed to be adapted to the *individual* sufferer. A rather different criticism of the use made of regimen by eighteenth-century doctors came later from the leading London physician, William Heberden, who argued on the basis of forty years' practice that 'many physicians appear to be too strict and particular in the rules of diet and regimen' they lay down.[41] Cullen similarly continually emphasised the importance of regimen and 'good management' but without prescriptive extremes.[42] He understood that physicians had to work with patients towards a common objective; it was better to gain the foothills of partially-regained health successfully than totally fail to scale the mountains of complete fitness. Hence he overturned accepted wisdom in allowing patients accustomed to drinking alcohol to continue to do so.[43] Cullen gave authority and currency to the idea that the alleviation or management of chronic conditions lay principally in regimen. And his shrewd insight into the place of disease within an overall lifestyle gave a central place to the sufferer's personality.[44]

Whether advice by physicians was accepted depended on the individual personalities of their patients. Sufferers might despair of the imperceptibly slow effects made by regimen on their disorder. Mrs Waters, for instance, an infirm gentlewoman suffering from long-term

---

[41] W. Heberden, *Commentaries on the History and Cure of Diseases* (New York, 1962), p. 1.
[42] RCPE, Cullen Correspondence, 30/2, letter concerning Mr Somervel, July 1769. See also G. B. Risse, 'Doctor William Cullen, Physician, Edinburgh: A Consultation Practice in the Eighteenth Century', *BHM*. 48 (1974), pp. 339–40, 346–8.
[43] King-Hele, *Erasmus Darwin*, p. 132; *Works of Alexander Monro*, pp. 635–6.
[44] See for example, RCPE, Cullen Correspondence, 30/2, letter concerning Captain Johnson of 18 July 1769, that on Mrs Watson of 7 June 1769, and that about Benjamin Gavin of 31 May 1769, which illustrate Cullen's psychological insight.

ill health, became tired of 'constant riding in the country air' and 'a proper diet.' In 1739 she 'importuned' her doctor 'to prescribe further' and, seemingly rather against his better judgement, her physician obliged her by applying a blister and giving her a strong purge.[45] And the hypochondriacal poet, William Shenstone, who was always, as he wrote in 1743, 'in hopes of gleaning up a little health', was prepared to try out a prescribed regimen, but was disappointed by its results. 'I ride every day almost to fatigue; which only tends to make my want of sleep more sensible.' Despite this he persevered and wrote that 'tomorrow morning I set out for Cheltenham, to make trial of the waters there.'[46]

Taking the waters

Taking the waters had been practised since the classical period when it was thought that immersion in spa water brought the humours into harmony. Bath had been popular in Roman times, and bathing was revived in the sixteenth century, but it was not until the following century that drinking mineral waters became fashionable there. In this early modern period doctors emphasised the need for medical advice and condemned the 'independent' bather.[47] A proliferation of advice books from the late sixteenth century suggested that both doctors and their patients took the therapeutic claims of spas seriously. These trends were to intensify in the period under consideration here. Taking the waters might not only involve a prolonged stay by members of the social élite at a fashionable spa or resort, but also included drinking mineral waters at home. Drinking the spa in this manner might come from the laity's own initiative, but was increasingly prescribed by doctors as a purge.[48] Another alternative to travelling to famous spas lay in patronage of local ones. For instance, although Harrogate was the Victorian queen among northern spas by the early Victorian period, there were seven others in Yorkshire advertising their water as 'like Harrogate'.[49]

Given that there was often a spa nearby, it is interesting to speculate

45 Carlisle Public Library, Brownrigg's case book, Mrs Water's case, May to August 1739.
46 M. Williams, ed., *The Letters of William Shenstone* (Oxford, 1931), pp. 67, 69, 79.
47 For example, Bath City Reference Library, MS 1495, directions to Sir Alexander Fraser, 1675.
48 For example, this was part of the prescription by Sir Hans Sloane for Lady Fermanagh in 1722 for colic (*Verney Letters*, II, p. 93); and of Erasmus Darwin for Thomas Wedgewood in 1793 for eye disorders thought to arise from intestinal worms (King-Hele, *Darwin*, p. 233).
49 Granville, *Spas*, I, pp. 105–7, 132–5, 202–9, 211–7, 229.

why sufferers chose to subject themselves to the acute discomforts of long-distance travel in order to visit the major spas. In some cases it is possible to see a progression from local to national spas: at the end of the eighteenth and beginning of the nineteenth centuries members of the Gray family of York used Hovingham – a nearby but undeveloped local spa – for convalescence, Scarborough for more serious illnesses, and Bath (where they had relatives) only when these had failed.[50] In contrast, others immediately travelled to a spa some distance away having been influenced by medical recommendation, fashion, royal or noble patronage, spa facilities and amenities, or therapeutic claims. Also relevant in sufferers' choice of spa, given the expense of spa living, was the presence of relatives or friends nearby. And geographical convenience together with coach facilities was important: those living in northern England or Scotland tended to patronise Scarborough or Buxton; Londoners were inclined to go to Tunbridge, Brighton, or Bath (the latter having better coach services to the capital than Cheltenham); while those living in the south or west typically went to Bristol, Cheltenham, Leamington or Bath.

Bath always attracted many sufferers and patients since it was the most well-established spa. In the era of Beau Nash Bath had led the way in emphasising the social as much as the medical nature of its attractions, so creating the sparkling psychology of the Georgian spa where a gamble for health matched that for pleasure. In the 1720s Defoe foreshadowed many moralistic commentators with his view that 'bathing is made more a sport and diversion than a physical prescription for health.'[51] In contrast to his view of this 'close city', Defoe liked the open Derbyshire countryside around Buxton, the inland spa reputed second only to Bath.[52] It was not until the 1780s that the social infrastructure of a fashionable spa was created at Buxton with the Grand Crescent, assembly room, card and billiard rooms, shops and hotels. And, by the late eighteenth century, Tunbridge had also become fashionable, being patronised by royalty and literary luminaries. The fluctuating esteem in which resorts were held was nowhere better exemplified than in Cheltenham: fashionable in the 1740s; much less popular during the next thirty years because of smallpox outbreaks; restored to favour after George III's visit in 1788; and climbing to unprecedented heights of social brilliance in the Regency period. A new Cheltenham began to be laid out, architecturally harmonious, and with superb facilities for visitors. Contempo-

[50] E. Gray, *Papers and Diaries of a York Family, 1764–1839* (1927), pp. 23, 47–8, 52.
[51] D. Defoe, *A Tour Through the Whole Island of Great Britain* (2 vols., 1974), II, p. 34.
[52] Defoe, *Tour*, pp. 166–7.

rary with this was the rival development of nearby Leamington, where sumptuous hotels replaced humble inns, and attracted visiting dukes and duchesses. By this time Harrogate was occupying the niche provided earlier by Cheltenham. Buxton, its nearest rival in the north, had only 2000 visitors whereas estimates put the number of visitors to Harrogate at between seven and ten thousand annually. The opening of the Royal Pump Room in 1842 increased the attractions of the spa, so that eight years later some 12,000 people made the pilgimage to Harrogate each year, of whom nine out of ten drank water at the Pump Room.[53]

The focus of attraction for the seasonally health conscious gradually passed from the inland spa to the seaside resort. An early indication was Cowper's poem, 'Retirement', which described how those who had been 'content with Bristol, Bath and Tunbridge Wells' now 'fly to the coast' and all agree 'with one consent to rush into the sea.' The dual attractions of spa and sea at Scarborough, for example, by the 1720s and 1730s seemed more attractive to many northerners and Scots than the restricted amenities of Buxton.[54] During the late eighteenth century several other seaside resorts began to attract a growing number of summer visitors, including Weymouth (especially after George III's visit in 1783) and Brighton (under the patronage of the Prince of Wales). Such resorts, with their reliance on a diffused benefit to be derived from unorganised leisure beside the seaside, eventually reduced the social attractiveness of more regimented spa life to all but the valetudinarian. Certain spas – notably Bath and Harrogate – survived in that role to the end of our period, offering increasingly specialist medical facilities to the invalid, the convalescent and the sick. Others – such as Cheltenham, Tunbridge and Leamington – attracted permanent residents because of the social amenities that had earlier served to recruit seasonal visitors.

Speedier and more comfortable rail travel widened choice, and contributed to spas developing a more defined therapeutic image for their waters. Influencing the sufferer's choice of spa was the hope of cure: optimism was an enduring quality, as indeed it had to be in the context of traditional medicine, so that expectations of the benefit to be received from a spa were correspondingly high. Elizabeth Verney wrote from Bath in 1736 that 'Parson Chaloner is here ... he looks

---

53 A Hunter, *A Treatise on the Mineral Waters of Harrogate* (1830), p. 9; W. Grainge, *The History and Topography of Harrogate and Knaresborough* (1871), p. 154; Granville, *Spas*, I, pp. 61–2; E. Lee, *The Watering Places of England* (1914), p. 63.
54 Defoe, *Tour*, II, p. 247; *Gentleman's Magazine*, II (1732), p. 741.

sadly but he has a great opinion that these waters will do him good.'[55] Faith in their healing power – the *placebo* effect – may have been as important as any scientific efficacy the waters possessed. Confidence in the waters' powers was essential given the self-discipline that the adoption of a health-restoring routine imposed. A Buxton visitor described a day beginning at seven:

Our plan of living is now so fixt that you may know where to find us any hour of the day. We rise at 7, drink water till nine, breakfast, pray at 10, jumble and trot from eleven till one, drink water, put on a clean shirt, dine at past 2, write, read, work and play upon the guitar all the evening, sup at 8, bathe at 10 and then to bed.[56]

Not surprisingly she exclaimed in a later letter, 'what machines we are.'[57] Yet a visitor to Tunbridge Wells in 1749 suggested that such a timetable was worthwhile, 'I really find myself so well here that I shall be afraid to leave off the waters for fear of losing the joy of health'.[58]

The large numbers of spa visitors suggest a continued belief in the value of taking the waters. Few enjoyed sufficiently good health to scorn the opportunity to improve it; hence for many the enjoyment of fashionable activities also involved therapeutic pursuits. And spa organisation facilitated this by unifying the two activities; the pump room was both the place to be seen socially, and to drink the mineral waters. A perceptive analysis of how – in a business-like pursuit of health – therapeutic dedication was related to pleasurable diversions, was given by a female visitor to Tunbridge in 1749:

Having been a long time out of health ... I have been a fortnight in a most flourishing state of health, which to acquire and maintain has cost me time and pains; drinking waters, riding on horseback, airing in a post-chaise, continued dissipation, and uninterrupted idleness.[59]

Wisely, the medical profession recognised that social amenities 'help greatly in restoring the elasticity and buoyancy of spirits, which is, at one and the same time, the cause and effect of renovated health.[60] While certain individuals decided to go to a spa on their own initiative, others had been persuaded to go by their physician. Cobbett's view that those at spas had resorted there 'at the suggestion of silently laughing quacks'[61] had a substantial element of truth. Once at a spa

---

[55] *Verney Letters*, II, p. 143.
[56] Lady Newdigate-Newdegate, The *Cheverels of Cheverel Manor* (1898), p. 33.
[57] Newdigate-Newdegate, *Cheverels*, p. 47.
[58] Quoted in Melville, *Tunbridge Wells*, pp. 190–1.
[59] Mrs Elizabeth Montagu, quoted in Melville, *Tunbridge Wells*, pp. 190–1.
[60] Granville, *Spas*, I, p. 50.
[61] Ponsonby, *Diaries*, p. 284.

the invalid was soon the object of attention by the Faculty who, – having been in some cases alerted by the 'home' physician, visited new arrivals as soon as possible. Detailed instructions were then given on drinking the mineral waters, bathing, diet and exercise. For her rheumatic disorder in 1752 Lady Luxborough was told by Doctors Oliver and Price to take three glasses of the Bath water every day.[62] Prescriptions might also be given. Mrs Elizabeth Purefoy was given medicines in 1742 by Dr Rayner. She wrote that 'I hope they will perform a cure on my legs, and then I shall think my journey to Bath very fortunate.'[63] Under the tutelage of the medical profession, the spa came to be seen not so much as an independent means to a natural cure as a centre for medical direction and expertise. The significance of this growth in more specialist medical provision was that the patient came to outnumber the sufferer, invalids became more numerous than idlers, and the spa became a health, rather than a pleasure resort. There was a certain irony in this, since although valetudinarians had more regular need of the doctor and thus constituted a captive market, their numbers were more restricted.

The physician's role

'The physicians here are very numerous, but very good natured. To these charitable gentlemen, I owe, that I was cured in a week's time, of more distempers than ever I had in my life. They had almost killed me with their humanity ... In vain did I modestly decline their favours.'[64] In his ironic depiction of early-eighteenth-century Bath Steele noted the process of medicalisation. The growing popularity of watering places, which in the freedom they gave to sufferers to seek out their own remedies, might have challenged the position of the medical profession, could also serve to reinforce and extend the doctor's influence. The medical profession profited by, and also contributed to, the increasing vogue for taking the waters. They did this in a number of discrete but mutually reinforcing ways: as leading lights in the campaigns to increase the amenities of spas;[65] as practitioners who either settled in a spa town or migrated thence during the season to benefit from the more lucrative or specialist practice there; as doctors who – at least for a time – managed to free themselves of their more hopeless cases or troublesome patients by advocating a spell at a spa;

---

[62] Williams, *Lady Luxborough*, p. 14.   [63] *Purefoy Letters*, p. 331.
[64] *The Guardian*, 30 September 1714.
[65] R. S. Neale, *Bath, 1680–1850. A Social History* (1981), pp. 251, 256.

and as writers of 'spa books' extolling the benefits to be obtained from taking the waters, and giving detailed advice on how to do so.

The medical literature on the waters amounted to 414 publications between 1660 and 1800. Granville's classic account of English spas in 1841 highlighted the role of doctors in publishing these books, but the very proliferation of literature posed a challenge, since it meant that it was difficult for them to retain control over the water bibber. Overall, the role of chemists in analysing the waters seems likely to have complemented rather than challenged the role of doctors.[66] In extolling the virtues of their local spa, doctors attracted sufferers and patients, thus furthering the interests both of the spa and of the profession. Predictably, therefore, spa guides then incorporated the medical prescriptions on the correct mode of taking the waters. Thomas Benge Burr wrote on Tunbridge Wells in 1766 that:

We must not suppose that the water alone, without regular management and suitable assistance, is capable of curing these numerous disorders. No, as well may you expect to have a house built by throwing the materials into a heap, as to have a disease removed by an irregular and injudicious use of any mineral water whatsoever.[67]

'Injudicious' was by implication the use by lay sufferers without professional advice. Water was depicted as a dangerous commodity which was not to be trifled with since contra-indications were increasingly perceived by the medical gaze; a steadily increasing amount of detail was given as to restrictions and timetable. Seen through the eyes of doctors, taking the waters was not an optional pastime for sufferers but part of a prescribed medical routine for patients. Dr Scudamore laid down in 1828 the proper way to imbibe the waters of Tunbridge. Aperient medicines had to be taken before treatment by the waters. Then, 'being favourably prepared', the first dose of water should be taken between 7 am. and 8 am., the second at noon, and the third at 3 in the afternoon; the quantity of water being progressively increased from about a pint at first to 2 pints daily. At the same time there should be appropriate exercise, and 'attentive regard to diet,' with tea and coffee taken only in the evenings when there was no water in the stomach, and dinner no later than 4 or 5 pm. The Tunbridge waters were to be taken for at least three weeks but no

[66] C. Mullett, *Public Baths and Health in England from the Sixteenth to the Eighteenth Century* (Baltimore, 1946), p. 54; C. Hamlin, 'Chemistry, Medicines and the Legitimisation of the English Spa, 1740–1840' and D. Harley, 'A Sword in a Madman's Hand' in R. Porter, ed., *The Medical History of Water and Spas* (1990).
[67] *The History of Tunbridge Wells* (Tunbridge Wells, 1766), p. 87.

more than two months at a time, and visits to the spa were to be made between May and November.[68]

Those seeking relief for their ailments through taking the waters were not only drowned in prescriptive advice on how, but also where, to take them. Each spa claimed to alleviate an amazing variety of sicknesses but typically made its pitch for a defined spectrum of disease for which its water was said to be particularly efficacious. Thus Dr John Nott, for instance, extolled the Hotwell waters at Clifton in Bristol for their especial value for phthisis (i.e. TB), and for diabetes. However, he claimed that they also had more general healing virtues since they possessed 'antiseptic' qualities, resolved obstructions, dissolved coagulations and 'impacted humours', quickened a sluggish circulation, corrected acidities, and mitigated fever. This was skilful advertisement since it was likely to have a strong appeal to valetudinarians and sufferers from many chronic diseases. Indeed, the entrepreneurial character of much of this 'spa literature' is very striking. Resident spa doctors claimed that they alone understood the nature and efficacy of their spa. And within the local faculty – as Falconer noted in *An Essay on Bath Waters* in 1770 – rival doctors each had a financial interest in advancing their own view of the water.[69] There was a direct connection between persuasive medical promotion of a spa and the professional success of doctors who practised there. Practitioners were loud in their praise of the efficacy of local waters and vague in their warnings about the perils of more distant ones. Not that such Georgian 'puffing' was inherently insincere or fraudulent. Given the limitations of medical knowledge it was natural to construct correlations on the basis of individual cases, and to assume that since some sufferers from gout, for example, felt relief after a sojourn at Bath that its water had specific therapeutic value for this disease. However, this medical writing by 'regular' practitioners was not dissimilar to the promotion of specific remedies by 'quacks' that was widely condemned by the medical faculty.

The prolific writers of promotional literature on Georgian Bath suggested that its waters, when drunk or used for bathing, were helpful for gout, rheumatism, jaundice, paralytic afflictions, stiff joints,

---

68 Quoted in Clifford's *Descriptive Guide to Tunbridge Wells* (fourth edn, Tunbridge Wells, 1828), pp. 22–6.
69 J. Nott, *Of the Hotwell Waters near Bristol* (third edn, Bristol, 1793); N. G. Coley ' "Cures without care". Chymical physicians, and mineral waters in seventeenth-century English medicine', *MH*, 23 (1979), 200; N. G. Coley, 'Physicians and the chemical analysis of mineral waters in eighteenth-century England', *MH*, 26 (1982).

palsy, nervous disorders and obstructions, distempers of the stomach and intestines, and women's and children's cases. In the following century writers also claimed that they were particularly effective in cases of sciatica, dyspepsia, liver complaints, chlorosis, cutaneous eruptions, biliary afflictions, colic, and uterine diseases. By this time the pastime of 'taking the waters' had become medicalised as 'hydrology'. Dr Granville claimed substantial credit for this and suggested that before his survey of English spas in 1841 'English bibliography was deficient in modern scientific and practical works on mineral hydrology.'[70] This concern for scientific validation was particularly noticeable in Victorian writing on spas but from the late-seventeenth century analyses had been made by doctors using precipitation of the salts, and by the second half of the nineteenth century spectographic analysis by chemists greatly increased the precision of the results. In the *Lancet*'s survey of Bath in 1899 twelve mineral salts were recorded as being present in the water, with 165.927 grains of salts per gallon of water.[71] After listing complaints for which Bath water was 'of eminent service' (including metallic poisoning and a number of disorders of the nervous system), the report concluded that 'Bath possesses in a most satisfactory manner all the requirements of a valuable resort for the treatment of disease by hydro-therapeutic measures.'

In the growth of seaside resorts – notably that of Scarborough and Brighton – it is interesting to discern very similar developments to those in the inland spas. Scarborough was doubly blessed with both salt and spa water. Its fame sprang from Dr Wittie's *Scarborough Spa* of 1660, where the spa was commended for everything from wind to leprosy, and within a few years it was being visited by 'a multitude of scorbuticks, hypochondriacks and other valetudinarians.'[72] By the early eighteenth century Scarborough water sold in London for the same price as that of Bath, and fashionable metropolitan doctors such as Mead recommended their patients to come to the Yorkshire resort.[73] Later in development, but ultimately eclipsing the northern resort in popularity, was Brighton. Dr Richard Russell, who practised in Lewes nearby, published in 1753 his *Dissertation on the Use of Sea Water in Diseases of the Glands* which laid the basis for Brighton's popularity as a health resort. Russell suggested that the sea was 'designed to be a kind of common defence against the corruption and

---

[70] P. B. Granville, ed. *The Autobiography of A. B. Granville* (two vols., second edn,1874), II, pp. 337, 349.
[71] *Lancet*, 14 October 1899.   [72] W. Simpson, *Hydrologia Chymica* (1669).
[73] A. Rowntree, ed,. *The History of Scarborough* (1931), p. 260.

putrefaction of bodies.'[74] He was succeeded by other physicians who
promoted the salubrious qualities of Brighthelmston, as it was then
called; Dr Relhan who praised the air, and Awitser who commended
sea water as a drink and opened sea-water baths for all-year-round
bathing.[75] Granville gave an authoritative seal of approval to the
health-giving character of Victorian seaside resorts, 'Sea-bathing, judi-
ciously prescribed, and properly employed ... [is] next to the use of
mineral waters, one of the most powerful means a medical man can
wield for the restoration of his patients.'[76]

The categories of patients that physicians particularly recommended to visit the sea or a spa were the chronic sick (whose illness
was not responding to physic), those convalescing from an acute
illness, women worn down from over-frequent childbearing, and a
residual group of troublesome individuals – hypochondriacal or with
diffuse complaints that were difficult to diagnose or treat. Mr Richardson – a Harrogate practitioner of long experience – remarked in the
1840s that while his colleagues tended to be 'sceptical, and inclined to
laugh at his faith in the waters ... they will send me patients very
often to be treated and cured by the very waters they seem to des-
pise.'[77] For the doctor advising a trip to a spa the rationale may well
have been simply the very human desire to win a breathing space
from one of his more tedious clients, coupled with a professional salve
to the conscience that such treatment could do no harm and might
even do good. For the sufferer from chronic ailments sea air might
well be prescribed. Mary Brigham, at the opening of the nineteenth
century, had had 'spasmodic asthma' for two years 'without any relief
from medicines [and] it was at last recommended to her, to go to the
seaside, which she did, and since her residence there she has not had a
single attack, and is now getting quite well.'[78] Not that all the patients
sent were in a condition to benefit and it was said of Clifton that in
most instances it was a corpse that arrived there.'[79]

That these were good locations in which to practise seems to have
been an unchallenged assumption, since to the usual attraction of an

[74] Richard Russell, MD, FRS, practised as a physician in Lewes and Brighton (*Eighteenth Century Medics*, p. 518).
[75] *A Short History of Brighthelmston, with Remarks on its Air and Analysis of its Waters* (1761). Dr Anthony Relhan, MD, FCP (1715–76) practised in Brighton and London; *Thoughts on Brighthelmston Concerning Sea-Bathing and Drinking Sea-Water with some Directions for their Use* (1768).
[76] Granville, *Spas*, I, p. 184.   [77] Granville, *Spas*, p. 76.
[78] Wellcome MS 1145, S. Berry's Notebook (notes on patients at St Bartholomew's Hospital, 1829–36).
[79] Granville, *Spas*, p. 362.

affluent resident clintele in a gentrified town was added a large number of well-heeled visitors. Medics were 'invariably found to multiply in a city which possesses a mineral spring in great vogue.'[80] Certainly Bath acted like a magnet to practitioners as well as patients. And it is also likely that the number of the Faculty in Bath was inflated by doctors who thought the costs of pleasant semi-retirement could be offset by opportunities for occasional practice, as was the case with John Haygarth, who had previously practised in Chester. Local directories gave a somewhat imprecise impression of this growth in practitioners. By 1773 Bath already had 17 physicians, 10 surgeons, and 27 apothecaries, and numbers continued to grow thereafter. By 1800 there were 22 physicians, 14 surgeons, 9 surgeon-apothecaries and 15 apothecaries, and in 1852 there were 41 physicians and 51 surgeons.[81] Since the number of residents was also growing the doctor to resident population ratio remained on a plateau, but at a level in the mid-nineteenth century that was nearly twice as well provided as the national average.[82] Unfortunately, no accurate statistics of visitors exist to facilitate a more accurate estimate of the ratios of doctors to either resident or transient populations, and hence to reach a more realistic view of doctor-patient ratios. (See Table 6.1.)

Not all spas attracted doctors in such numbers. Tunbridge Wells had far fewer doctors; in 1766 it was 'a public misfortune that no regular physician has constantly resided in the place to register cases.'[83] Instead, a London physician would come down in the season, as did Dr Yeats between 1815 and 1828. Only in 1829 did Yeats find it worth his while to practise permanently; presumably because demand had then expanded sufficiently.[84] By this time patients had become available not only in the summer season (from May to November), but also on an all-year-round basis from the growing number of residents who found a spa an agreeable place to live. In recognition of this the number of practitioners in 1830 had risen to four physicians and nine surgeons.[85] This provided only half the ratio

---

[80] Granville, *Spas*, p. xxxix.

[81] R. Crutwell, *The Stranger's Assistant and Guide to Bath* (1773), pp. 60–2; *Robbins Bath Directory* (1800); *A Directory of Bath and its Environs* (Bath, 1852).

[82] Bath's population in 1801 was 32,200 and in 1851 it was 54,240 giving doctor to resident population ratios of 1:533 in 1801 and 1:589 in 1851. Nationally, in 1851, the ratio was 1:1028.

[83] Burr, *Tunbridge Wells*, p. 76.

[84] *Clifford's Guide to Tunbridge* (second and third edns, 1828 and 1834). David Grant Yeats (1773–1836), MD, FCP, FRS (Munk, pp. 137–8).

[85] *Visitors Guide to Tunbridge Wells* (Tunbridge Wells, 1830).

of doctors to resident population of Bath at this date.[86] The ratios in
Tunbridge were very similar to those of Cheltenham from the 1820s to
1840s when the town was at its most fashionable as a spa. Whereas at
the beginning of the century Cheltenham only had four or five
medics, in 1826 it had 11 physicians, and 20 surgeons, and by 1839 it
had 12 physicians, and 30 surgeons.[87]

The financial returns of a fashionable spa practice were usually
assumed to be considerable. It seems likely that the rewards were
exaggerated. For example, Dr Jephson, who was amongst the most
successful of the Cheltenham physicians in the early nineteenth
century, was said to make £20,000 a year by the 1840s. But the account
book of another very successful Cheltenham physician, Dr Boisragon,
gives more modest – though still considerable – annual earnings of
£3000 for the years 1830–2.[88] Since Boisragon had been established for
several decades by this time, it is unlikely that his practice would have
taken off during the 1830s to the extent necessary to validate Granville's larger figure, although the enhanced reputation acquired from
having been royal physician-extraordinary had no doubt inflated the
fees he could charge. For the less well established or fashionable
physician, fees were harder to come by, and increasingly competitive
conditions made fee grubbing imperative. (See Plate 9.) It was said
of Bath that whereas physicians had been accustomed to attend
the pump room and merely charge a fee to their patients on their first
and last visits, by the 1840s they no longer saw their patients in the
pump room but visited and charged more frequently.[89]

In the eighteenth and early nineteenth centuries visitors apparently
did not regard medical fees at spas as exorbitantly high. While diaries
and correspondence of this period contained numerous grumbles
about the high charges for lodgings, food and amusements, expenditure on doctors passed without adverse comment. How is such a
silence to be interpreted? Did it mean that – as much contemporary
doggerel suggests – the Faculty were expected to make rich pickings,

---

[86] At this date Bath had 6 apothecaries, 33 physicians and 58 surgeons (*Pigot's Directory
of Bath*, 1830) and a population in 1831 of 38,063, giving a ratio of practitioners to
resident population of 1:392. Tunbridge had a resident population in the *Census* of
1831 of 10,381 and thus a practitioner to resident population ratio of 1:796.

[87] In 1831 the *Census* stated that the town had 22,942 residents and in 1841 it had 31,411,
giving doctor to resident population ratios of 1:740 and 1:748, if these are related to
the figures for practitioners for 1826 and 1839, given in Griffiths *New Historical
Description of Cheltenham* (Cheltenham, 1826), p. 47, and Granville, *Northern Spas*,
p. 307.

[88] G. Hart, *A History of Cheltenham* (Leicester, 1965), p. 198; Granville, *Spas*, p. 245. Henry
Charles Boisragon, (b. 1780) was physician to George IV.

[89] Granville, *Spas*, p. 402.

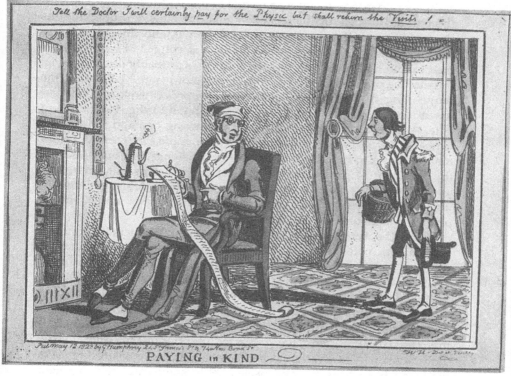

Plate 9   W. Heath, 'Paying in Kind' (1823)

in which case any comment was regarded as superfluous? This seems unlikely since the privacy of letters or journals would have encouraged uninhibited complaint, if such had been felt. Or was the recovery of health seen as an almost priceless commodity? In this case the precise level of fees – within certain broad customary limits – was more or less irrelevant and demand for medical care inelastic. This hypothesis has a certain persuasive attraction, especially for the Georgian period, when it is placed in the financial context of the very high levels of overall expenditure incurred in a visit of several weeks or even months to a health spa. Undercutting this argument for the early Victorian period, however, is evidence which indicates that visitors were patronising less expensive alternatives to the physician. At Cheltenham, for instance, it was noticeable by the 1840s that there were three surgeons who acted in the same way as physicians, in that they charged a fee for their attendance, but in their case only seven shillings rather than the guinea or two of the physician, and then sent the patients to pick up their medicine at a chemist's shop.[90] By this time there were seven such shops in the town, and this growth was another possible indication of patients resorting to less expensive medical alternatives. To some extent this was probably due to a social broadening of those who patronised the spa or resort; by this time the burgeoning of the middle classes and improvements in transport meant that visitors were less and less confined to the really affluent élite. As a result there was likely to be growing demand for medical care at a lower level of charges. But it is possible that these developments were also indicative of consumer resistance and that this took the form not of grumbling at medical expenditures but of seeking alternatives. This was part of a progressive and more general unwillingness to accept uncritically the pretensions of spas with their implicit promises of restored health.

Taking the waters was not always as pleasant or beneficial as sufferers had anticipated; like physic its nastiness did not always guarantee results. Some found the water undrinkable, as did Lady Tenterden in Cheltenham in 1829, although she had the consolation of finding bathing there beneficial.[91] Others recorded comments after bathing such as, 'I was much out of order after I came out and continued so for some hours.'[92] And bathing in the sea might prove equally disappointing. The barrister, John Baker, reflected ruefully in 1777, that 'I grow daily weaker. [Neither] the sea baths nor sea air has any effect to make me better but all are flat and useless.'[93] In some cases the comment reflected the personality of the sufferer rather more than the experience, as was the case with the hypochondriacal Baker. Relatives might also undercut the faith of the sufferer. One sceptical husband wrote of his wife's sojourn at Weymouth, 'all [are] expected to drown their nervous fears, and hysteric wanderings in the sea.'[94] Sufferers could become sceptics if they did not find spa water beneficial. In 1713 Swift declared that 'I have given away all my spa water', since he considered that it made his symptoms worse rather than better. Later, Dr Johnson – despite his patronage of Cheltenham – grumbled, 'There is nothing in all this boasted system ... medicated baths can be no better than warm water; their only effect can be that of tepid water.'[95] This

90 Granville, *Spas*, p. 242.
91 Leics. RO, Halford MSS, D6 24/871/5, Baron Tenterden to Sir Henry Halford, 6 September 1829.
92 *Great Diurnall*, III, p. 49.   93 Ponsonby, *Diaries*, p. 214.
94 Andrews, *Torrington Diaries*, I, p. 88, comment of J. Byng in August 1782.
95 Quoted in J. Walvin, *Besides the Seaside* (1978), p. 15.

scepticism was also shared by some contemporary doctors – amongst them Smollett. He wrote a treatise debunking Bath's waters which he thought 'can have little, or any effect on the animal economy.'[96] At this time, however, the faithful – both lay and medical – far outnumbered the unbelievers, but disbelief became a creeping disease which by the mid-nineteenth century had become more widespread. Expense, changing fashion, the disappointment of sufferers when their high hopes of cure had not been realised, together with a misunderstanding by practitioners of the relative part to be played by mineral water and medication were mutually reinforcing factors.[97]

In an unsuccessful attempt to counter Victorian lay and professional scepticism an increasing specialisation in spa water and facilities became available. In Wales there were flourishing spas at Llandridnod and Llangammarch, offering a mild climate and a choice of sulphur, saline or chalybeate waters. In the south of Scotland the well-established Hartwell waters, near Moffatt, continued to draw those wanting a cure for obstructions or cutaneous eruptions. Newer centres – at Bridge of Earn, Pitcaithly, Innerleithen, and most notably at Bridge of Allan – offered saline draughts for those with digestive problems. And in the 1890s the new northerly resort of Strathpeffer in Rothshire offered the dual attractions of the strongest sulphuretted water in Britain with the most varied, continental styles of balneology. In England there were Droitwich (with its salt water), and Woodhall Spa (with iodine mineral waters). Hydropathy, or the 'water cure', also became a popular alternative to balneology, the most flourishing centres being at Ben Rhydding and Malvern, where pure cold water was used internally and externally to regulate the body and tranquillise or stimulate the nervous system.[98] Water cures were seen as particularly suitable for the nervous ailments of the Victorian intelligentsia.[99]

In a more positivistic age doctors followed chemists in making an increasingly precise evaluation of spa waters through scientific analyses of the constituent mineral salts. There was also a greater specificity in the diseases that each spa claimed its waters were able to alleviate or cure. The patient was therefore able to benefit from the growing choice of specialist treatments in balneology. By the end of the Victorian period, for example, Bath had separate treatments for gentlemen,

---

96 *An Essay on the External Use of Water* quoted in L. Melville, *Bath under Beau Nash – and after* (1926), p. 122.
97 Granville, *Spas*, pp. xxxix, 302–3, 402, 419–20.
98 R. Price, 'Hydropathy in England 1840–1870', *MH*, 25 (1981), 269–80.
99 B. Smith, *A History of Malvern* (Leicester, 1964), pp. 195–6.

for ladies, and for children, including: deep baths (with the option of a
deep chair or reclining bath); mineral water and pine or sulphur
baths; electric mineral water or electric hot air baths; vapour baths –
either local or general; as well as a varied range of supplements and
alternatives including douches, sprays, and massage for all or part of
the body.[100] The contrast with a doctor's description of Georgian
bathing in the same town is illuminating, 'Diseased persons of all ages,
sexes and conditions, are promiscuously admitted into an open
bath.'[101] However, despite English spas' conscious imitation of the
more varied facilities of continental spas in the late nineteenth and
early twentieth centuries, English resorts were still seen as operating
at a disadvantage compared to European ones which were cheaper
yet offered a greater variety of mineral waters, more specialist bathing
facilities, and attractive social arrangements.[102] As a result, only one in
a thousand patients at British spas was a European compared to one
in every thirty at European watering places who was British.[103] In the
second half of the nineteenth century, the most fashionable continental resorts (Wiesbaden or Baden Baden) attracted from four to six times
as many visitors as the then most popular English resort – Harrogate.[104]

A Georgian sufferer setting out for Cheltenham confided that 'if I
get over this ill habit of body, depend upon it I will have a reverend
care of my health.'[105] And a Victorian visitor to Harrogate justified his
trip by stating that he was 'laying in an additional stock of health.'[106]
Such solicitude for health might have perpetuated the self-
management of health; a development that would have harmed the
financial interests of the medical profession. But an enhanced appreciation of the desirability of positive health – rather than merely absence
of disease – created expanded opportunities for a flexible profession to
intervene with more patients. It is, of course, problematical how
dependent such patients were, since they retained freedom over their
choice of physician.[107] Physicians were concerned with the everyday
maintenance of health for an increasing number of patients from
middling and genteel social groups as well as with the occasional

[100] *Bath as a Health Resort* (Bath, 1905), p. 46.
[101] Smollett, *An Essay on the External Use of Water* (1752).
[102] Wood, *Spa Treatment*, pp. 49–50; E. Lee, *The Watering Places of England Considered with Reference to their Medical Topography* (third edn, 1914), pp. 5–6.
[103] N. Wood, 'British Health Resorts for Foreign Invalids', *Contemporary Review*, C (1911), p.376.
[104] J. Macpherson, *The Baths and Wells of Europe* (1869, 1873, and 1888 editions).
[105] Williams, ed., *Letters of Shenstone*, p. 69.
[106] Granville, *Spas*, I, p. 49.   [107] Jewson, 'Medical Knowledge', *Sociology*, 8 (1974).

alleviation of disease. Affluence thus created opportunities for expanded Georgian and early Victorian medical practice. The following chapter suggests that poverty also increased practice for an entrepreneurial occupation.

Office, altruism and poor patients

This chapter is concerned with the lowest tier of patients – those who were unable to pay ordinary fees to a regular medical practitioner – and their treatment without direct payment by practitioners in an increasing range of statutory, voluntary and charitable bodies. Whereas the previous chapter was principally concerned with physicians this one focuses on surgeon-apothecaries and GPs. Although medical practitioners benefited by an increase in the number of offices (discussed earlier in Chapter 4), they continued to have to exercise medical altruism in the treatment of some impoverished patients. This chapter sets out to evaluate poor patients' quality of relationships with medical practitioners, and the degree of separation and differentiation between the facilities offered to the poor and those offered to other social groups in this expanding medical market.

The Old Poor Law

Generalising about the quality of medical services under the Old Poor Law is problematic because of the patchy survival and dispersed location of parochial archives. However, the overwhelming impression gained from surviving medical bills for treatment, and from contracts for the employment of parish surgeons, is of a considerable array of medical services before 1834. This implied that the medical profession were able to get payment for cases which earlier might have had to be treated without charge. Generally, good relationships between the parochial officers and members of the medical profession contrasted with those found after the Poor Law Amendment Act of 1834.

During the eighteenth and early nineteenth centuries there was a broad regional divide between the north and south of England, with northerners being much less prone to apply to the poor law and hence to receive parish medical services.[1] Southern parishes varied in their arrangements for the treatment of their poor; the majority seemed to have preferred to pay for medical and surgical treatment on the basis of services actually performed by the local surgeon-apothecary, although with an occasional supplementation by a physician on the one hand or an alternative practitioner (most commonly a bonesetter) on the other. A minority of parishes placed their medical arrangements on a more regular footing and drew up an annual contract, hoping thereby to provide more cost-effective treatment. There were some examples of contracts early in the eighteenth century in certain areas (in Essex, for example), but a more rapid general growth was evident from mid-century.[2] A clear view of the attitudes that motivated such treatment can be gained from these contracts. In March 1752 the rural inhabitants of Cannington in Somerset drew up a painstaking contract with Richard Clarke who, for five guineas:

Promises and undertakes to perform all chirurgical operations for all the poor of the said parish as well as those that actually receive relief from the said parish as also such person and persons as shall be thought objects of compassion by the principal inhabitants of the said parish (for the time being) and will also provide at his own expense all physic necessary to be administered in the operations aforesaid.[3]

A comparably sympathetic attitude towards the poor, as well as an inclusive specification of surgical treatment, was also found in urban areas at this time, as this example from Sheffield indicates. John Bourne and John Browne were to supply in 1756:

Good and sufficient drugs and medicines, meet and proper for the several sicknesses and disorders which such poor persons may respectively be afflicted with or labour under, and shall diligently attend and visit them, and do every thing in their power and skill for the recovery of such persons from their disorders and ailments and … do and perform according to the best of their skill and knowledge every act and operation in surgery or whatsoever which shall or may be needful or necessary to be done or performed.[4]

[1] *SC on Medical Relief*, PP 1844, IX, QQ 9698–9, 9700, 9703, evidence of Sir John Walsham, poor-law inspector.
[2] J. R. Smith concludes both that Essex contracts were found at the beginning of the century and that all but the very smallest or poorest parish had them before 1800. This interpretation suggests an earlier, and ultimately a more comprehensive, adoption than was usual elsewhere (*The Speckled Monster* (Essex Record Office, 1987), p. 54).
[3] Somerset RO, D/P/Can 13/2/2, Poor Book, 1732–63, Agreement of 30 March 1752.
[4] Sheffield City Archives, TC 166, Appointment of Surgeons to Sheffield Workhouse, 1756. John Browne was a midwife, apothecary and surgeon, and John Bourne a surgeon and man-midwife (*Eighteenth Century Medics*, pp. 66, 83).

Joan Lane has suggested that in Warwickshire poor-law contracts were an urban phenomenon, whereas rural parishes paid fees for country practitioners.[5] From a broader geographical perspective it is clear that some country parishes also had contracts, and that the proportion of both country and town parishes that resorted to them increased during the early nineteenth century. It is likely that the desire to achieve certainty and continuity in care were factors in leading to contracts, as had been the case in parishes having medical practitioners on a retainer basis since the sixteenth century.[6] Some parishes banded together to buy common medical services and Thomas cites ten parishes in Oxfordshire in 1824 that were included in one medical contract.[7] This reflected a trend towards more systematised poor-law administration, as with the so-called Speenhamland scales of outdoor relief. Also evident was a more competitive medical market since (particularly after 1815) an increased number of practitioners competed for available poor-law medical appointments. The parish could strike a harder bargain, either paying doctors less or demanding more services for the same contract payment.

Payments for the eighteenth-century parish doctor were as variable as the parishes they served. In his *State of the Poor* of 1797 F. M. Eden described thirty annual payments: four were under £10; ten from £10 to £19; six from £20 to £29; and ten over £30. For those willing to occupy a full-time residential post in a large workhouse the salaries were £60–£70. Eden's sample was not representative, however, being weighted heavily towards urban areas and so reflecting the more substantial payments made to the parish doctor who cared for large numbers of paupers.[8] In rural areas the usual range of eighteenth-century contract payments appears to have been five to ten guineas per annum, but in a few cases salaries were as high as 18 guineas.[9] Payments to parish doctors tended to increase, partly as a result of wartime price inflation from 1793 to 1815, and also because they became skilful at inserting a growing range of exclusions in their contracts as they gained a market advantage. Experience taught them that midwifery, inoculation or vaccination, treating accidents or performing the more difficult surgical procedures (usually fractures and dislocations) were very time consuming and might be charged for

[5] J. Lane, 'The Provincial Practitioner and His Services to the Poor, 1750–1800', *Bulletin of the Society for the Social History of Medicine*, 28 (1981).
[6] M. Pelling, 'Healing the Sick Poor: Social Policy and Disability in Norwich 1550–1640', *MH*, 29 (1985), pp. 122–3.
[7] E. G. Thomas, 'The Old Poor Law and Medicine', 5, *MH*, 24 (1980), p. 8.
[8] F. M. Eden, *The State of the Poor* (1797), vols. 2–3.
[9] Loudon, *Medical Care*, p.232.

separately.[10] Less common was the practice of charging extra for venereal cases.[11]

This contrasted with an earlier inclusiveness, which accorded with the ledger entries of the Somerset surgeon, Benjamin Pulsford, who was paid ten guineas annually as parish doctor, but made additional charges for unusually complicated surgery.[12] Parish overseers appear to have later adopted an exclusionary stance and became more stringent about the poor people for whose medical treatment they would pay. Increasingly they tended to state that it must be the *resident* poor of the parish and that, as the parish of Bradford on Tone specified in 1781, the surgeon was 'not to make any charge upon this parish for any poor person or persons whatsoever without a written order from an officer of this parish.'[13] Parish overseers sometimes refused to pay, as did Backwell in 1822, 'There being no order given for John Brown and there being a doubt whether he is a parishioner the vestry refuses to allow the charge for him.'[14] In the later context of a financial tightening of the parochial belt towards the end of the Old Poor Law era, it was unusual to find an entry such as that for Toddenham in Gloucestershire in 1826, where the vestry 'agreed to give Mr Hale £2.2s.0d in addition to his salary in consideration of the very sickly state of the parish during the past year.'[15] This seemed to partake more of earlier sentiments and relationships, thus illustrating the local variation which was an abiding characteristic of the Old Poor Law.

A concern that the poor should have skilled attention during sickness was evident in the kind of treatments they received. In parishes that had not drawn up a contract with a surgeon-apothecary, the custom at this time of charging for medical attendance, through the medicines given or the surgical procedures performed, provides a detailed record of the care given to the poor from the bills and vouchers attached to overseers' accounts. For making a journey where the pauper lived at a distance, the parish doctor charged his usual fees of 2s.6d (or 3s.6d at night), although the more established practitioners

[10] For example, Dorset RO, PE/SPV/OV/5, Agreements of Stour Provost Parish, 1787, 1804, and PE/POY/OV/1, Contract of Mr Fussell with Poyntington Parish, 1834; Gloucestershire RO, P 336, VE 2/1, Toddenham Select Vestry Book 1819–34, 24 April 1827, 22 March 1834; P 81, OV 7/2, Chipping Camden Agreements with Surgeons.

[11] Somerset RO, DD/FS/48, Benjamin Pulsford's Ledger, fo. 6, 23 April 1758, where the charges were ten shillings a case; Leicestershire RO, DE 2934/44, Watton in the Wolds Surgeon's Agreement 1817.

[12] Somerest RO, DD/FS/48, Benjamin Pulsford's Ledger, fo. 5, 11 November 1759.

[13] Somerset RO, D/P/Bra 13/2/2, Account Book of Overseers 1762–1788, 16 April 1781.

[14] Somerset RO D/P/Back 13/2/6, Overseers' Vouchers.   [15] Glos. RO, P336 VE 2/1.

occasionally charged 5 shillings. Then there were charges for medicines supplied with a very considerable range prescribed, including: powders, boluses and lozenges; draughts, juleps, mixtures and elixirs; embrocations, liniments, salves and ointments; as well as drops, cordials, electuaries and linctuses. Plasters, poultices and dressings were applied; blistering, purging, bleeding or leeching often took place; and difficult cases of childbirth were attended. Less commonly, limited surgery was attempted: dislocated bones were put back in place; hydroceles tapped; ulcers and fistulas treated; abcesses drained; fractures reduced and set; and, more rarely, amputations performed. Charges for these more complicated surgical procedures ranged from half a guinea to two guineas, although in total the charges for an entire course of treatment might occasionally be far more. In Backwell, Somerset, for instance, John Hipsley was paid £11.16s.0d for curing the wounds of Betty Weaver and attending her from December 1751 to March 1752.[16]

Occasionally, parishes resorted to payment by results, thus underlining the ambiguous relationship between medicine and trade, as well as continuing a practice that had been much commoner earlier. This rarely involved the parish surgeon, but in Great Bentley, Essex, the parish surgeon was promised five pounds if he made a perfect cure of a widow's broken leg.[17] In Gissing, Norfolk in 1740 William Crow (elswhere referred to in the parish records as 'Dr' Crow), undertook 'to make a perfect cure' of the leg of a poor boy, and if he made 'him or his leg perfectly sound' he was to receive thirty shillings from the parish overseer, and another twenty shillings for maintaining him in his house whilst the cure was effected. If no cure was made then only the initial down payment of ten shillings was to be paid.[18] (See Plate 10.) Another example concerned an apothecary in Camerton who took only half payment because his patient, a badly-burned collier, had died.[19] That such instance of payment by results was largely confined now to the poor law (and also the fringe) sectors of medicine by this time suggests the growing power of practitioners in the medical market, since earlier in the sixteenth and seventeenth centuries the custom had been more widespread.

Infectious diseases, amongst which the most recognisable was smallpox, were widely feared so that parish authorities made arangements to meet the challenge as best they could. From the 1760s

---

[16] Somerset RO, D/P/Back 13/2/6, Overseers' Vouchers.
[17] Thomas, 'The Old Poor Law', *MH*, 24 (1980), pp. 2, 5. Unfortunately no date is given.
[18] Norfolk RO, PD 50/49, Overseers' Accounts.
[19] Cited in W. Brockbank, 'Country Practice in Days Gone By', *MH*, 6 (1962).

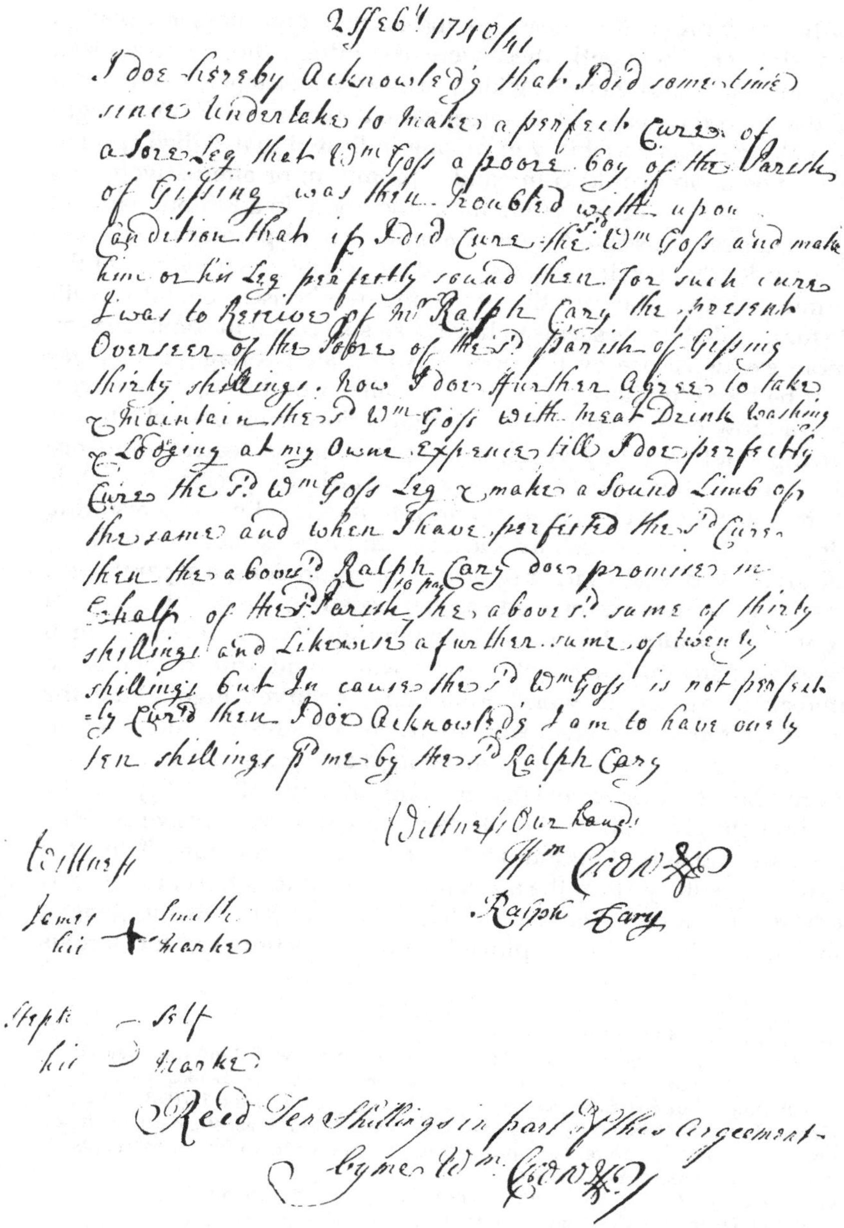

2 Feb. 1740/41

I doe hereby acknowledge that I did some time since undertake to make a perfect cure of a sore leg that Wm Goss a poore boy of the parish of Gissing was then troubled with upon condition that if I did cure the sd Wm Goss and make him or his leg perfectly sound then for such cure I was to receive of Mr Ralph Cary the present Overseer of the Poore of the sd Parish of Gissing thirty shillings. Now I doe further agree to take & maintein the sd Wm Goss with meat drink washing & lodging at my owne expences till I doe perfectly cure the sd Wm Goss leg & make a sound limb of the same and when I have perfected the sd Cure then the abovesd Ralph Cary does promise in behalf of the sd Parish the abovesd same of thirty shillings and likewise a further same of twenty shillings but in cause the sd Wm Goss is not perfectly cured then I doe acknowledge I am to have onely ten shillings pd me by the sd Ralph Cary

(Witness Our hands)
Wm Crow
Ralph Cary

Witness
James [+] Smith
his mark

Steph [—] Self
his mark

Recd Ten Shillings in part of this agreement by me Wm Crow

Plate 10   Payment by results under the Old Poor Law in Gissing, Norfolk (1740/1

parishes took preventive measures and arranged for mass inoculation of parishioners. Frequently these were of children who, being without prior infection and hence lacking acquired resistance, were most vulnerable to the disease.[20] Charges varied enormously.[21] One might speculate that this variability in pricing indicated that skilled specialists in inoculation could command a premium, or alternatively that parishes obtained cut-rates for a mass operation. In addition, parishes organised pest houses to be either temporarily or permanently available in order that smallpox cases could be isolated from the rest of the community. An earlier practice of making pest houses generally available for all inhabitants seems to have been succeeded in some areas by a more exclusive use by the poor.[22] An isolated cottage or cottages might be hired temporarily during a smallpox outbreak, as the overseers of Stow on the Wold did during a serious outbreak which was 'proving fatal in many cases, and spreading its fearful influence around us.'[23] Alternatively, a cottage could be built specifically for this in 'a remote part' of the parish, 'to prevent its spreading' and resulting in 'many inconveniences', as had been the case earlier in Chipping Sodbury.[24] And, in the larger poor-law incorporations, a separate pest house was sometimes erected, as happened in Bristol, the Isle of Wight, Shipmeadow, Melton and Smallburgh. But these were a small minority of institutions so that there was a widespread fear of an outbreak of disease in workhouses. Eden's survey highlighted the dangers: references were made to recent or present outbreaks of smallpox, measles, and malignant, spotted and putrid fevers.[25]

Both the comprehensive nature and the overall quality of the medical help given under the Old Poor Law were impressive as other historians, notably Loudon and Lane, have concluded.[26] In the eighteenth century, as in the sixteenth and seventeenth centuries, this medical assistance differed little from that available to the general population. The parish employed regular practitioners for serious

20 Thomas, 'The Old Poor Law', p. 10.
21 In 1810 fourpence was charged in Badgeworth, Somerset, whilst in Broomfield in the same county in the late 1760s, and also in West Stour in Dorset in 1804, payments of five shillings were recorded (Somerset RO, D/P Badg P3/2/5; and D/P/Broo 13/2/3; Dorset RO, PE/WSR/Ov 3). Thomas cites five shillings as standard in Essex, Oxfordshire and Berkshire, but Smith records a tremendous variety of payments.
22 Smith, *Speckled Monster*, pp. 149–53.
23 Glos. RO, P 317/VE 2/1, Stow on the Wold Vestry Book, 23 January 1833.
24 Glos. RO, D 2071 B6, Chipping Sodbury Erection of Pest House, 1757.
25 E. Suffolk RO, ADA 9/AH5/1/1, Agreement for Building a Pest House at Shipmeadow; Norfolk RO Minutes of Smallburgh Incorporation; Eden, *Poor*, pp. 576, 663, 679.
26 Loudon, 'Provincial Medical Practice', p. 27:, Lane, 'Provincial Practitioner', pp. 10–11.

cases of sickness, and the records of their treatment of these showed few significant differences from those given to their other paying patients. Plate 11 suggests that the range and cost of parish treatment was not of a second class nature. To some extent this indicated the non-stigmatised condition of the pauper under the Old, as distinct from the New, Poor Law. It may also hint at the limitations of contemporary medical treatment. The ledgers of the Somerset surgeon, Benjamin Pulsford, are interesting in indicating the overseers' confidence in the doctor's judgement that quite extensive treatment of paupers was necessary, and their subsequent approval of appropriate levels of compensation.[27] There were fewer complaints about practitioners' standards of medical care under the Old, than under the New, Poor Law. And, although it is difficult to make a comparison, in my judgement there was a substantive deterioration in the quality of medical care after 1834. Thus, the larger number of complaints after 1834 was not just a matter of more highly developed bureaucratic procedures for the New Poor Law which made abuses easier for contemporaries to detect.[28]

In addition to the regular male medical practitioner, parishes also employed others in the care of the poor, and it is interesting to find that surgeonesses were found in parish employment.[29] The custom of paying a midwife for deliveries was widespread, as was payment to a village woman to assist her. The former might be a professional midwife, licensed by the bishop at the beginning of our period, or merely a respectable village woman; the latter was often a pauper. Such pauper women were also employed to nurse accident cases, or more serious cases of sickness and chronic disease. Unqualified practitioners (sometimes known as 'wise women'), were used to perform standard, simple procedures such as dressing wounds. In West Yorkshire it has been estimated that a quarter of all pauper medical complaints were attended by fringe personnel.[30]

Apart from this varied care of the outdoor poor there was some limited indoor provision for the more seriously ill. In a few large towns, such as Liverpool, there might be recourse to the sick wards or infirmaries of workhouses.[31] In addition, individual or incorporated parochial authorities took out a subscription, typically of five guineas,

---

[27] Somerset RO, DD/FS/48 Benjamin Pulsford's Ledger, fos. 5–6, entries for 1758–9.
[28] See Thomas, 'Old Poor Law', p. 8 who cites complaints by the poor in Woodford in 1779–80 which were found to be well-founded.
[29] A. L. Wyman, 'The Surgeoness: the Female Practitioner of Surgery, 1400–1800' *MH*, 28 (1984), p. 37.
[30] Marland, *Medicine and Society*, p. 61.   [31] Eden, *Poor*, p. 330.

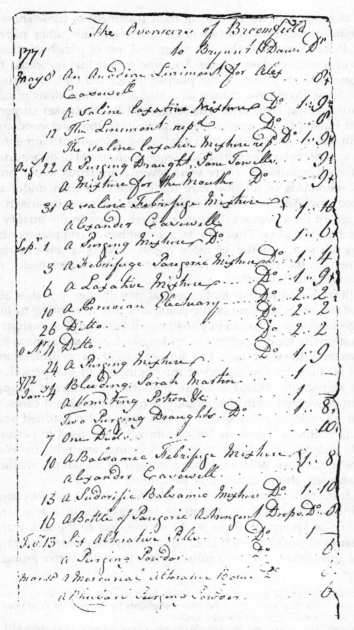

Plate 11 Treatment by the poor-law doctor, from the overseers' accounts of Broomfield, Somerset (1771)

to the local voluntary hospital or infirmary, and so were able to send more intractable cases – such as cancers or serious leg ulcers – for treatment.[32] Mary Fissell has emphasised how – until the late eighteenth century, when the infirmary became medicalised – the poor law and the voluntary hospital could be used flexibly and interchangeably by the poor.[33]

Early voluntary hospitals

Numbers of English voluntary hospitals had grown from one in 1720 to thirty-three by 1800.[34] It is with this period and with provincial infirmaries that this section is concerned. Founded for a variety of motives, they were intended for the poor. Society had an interest in the recovery of members of the labouring classes: the Salisbury Infirmary intended to provide for 'the laborious poor, the most useful part of society, the riches and strength of our nation ... [whose] condition is of the deepest sickness added to poverty.'[35] Although in general there is little direct connection between industrialisation and the rise of the hospital, in particular cases there was a relationship, as in Huddersfield, where the infirmary was to provide cheap medical care to those suffering industrial accidents.[36] Unusually, in the case of the Edinburgh Infirmary, the presence of servants' wards meant that the affluent might pursue their own self-interest in that their subscription to voluntary hospitals ensured that sick domestics would have treatment outside their households.[37] The founding statements of voluntary hospitals had a paternalistic theme offset by a counterpoint of social calculation. The apparently disinterested humanitarian and philanthropic motivation was, however, eloquently expressed, in terms that would 'paper over the cracks, between plebeians and patricians.'[38] In 1783 the Leeds Infirmary outlined its objectives in these terms:

Of all the passions benevolence is the most amiable ... the relief of the distressed must be acknowledged to be an indispensable duty ... It will be readily granted, that sickness and infirmity are likely to be sooner removed,

---

[32] Eden, *Poor*, pp. 301, 347, 547 634.
[33] M. Fissell, ']The Sick and Drooping Poor in Eighteenth century Bristol and its Regions', *SHM*, 2 (1989), p. 36.
[34] J. Woodward, *To Do the Sick No Harm*, pp. 147–8.
[35] Wilts. RO, J8/110/1, Auditors Report on the State of the Salisbury Infirmary, 1766–7.
[36] Marland, *Medicine and Society* , p. 130.
[37] G. B. Risse, *Hospital Life in Enlightenment Scotland* (1986), pp. 98–101.
[38] R. Porter, 'The Gift Relation: Philanthropy and Provincial Hospitals in Eighteenth-Century England', in Granshaw and Porter, eds, *The Hospital in History* (1989), p. 153.

when they are under the regular direction of the physician and surgeon ...
The experience of this truth first suggested the idea of a GENERAL
INFIRMARY, where the objects of distress might enjoy proper diet, medicines,
and cleanliness, and it be under the certain inspection of persons of acknowledged merit in the medical profession.[39]

This rhetoric of charity, with all its moral and religious resonance, was
used as a powerful inducement in hospital annual reports, and was
designed to reinforce the self-esteem of participants and thereby
induce citizens (or parishes) to give funds to the institution. The
annual charity sermon was perhaps the clearest exemplar of this
process at work, since collections taken after it were a regular part of
the institution's funding. In both reports and sermons it was therefore
necessary to idealise the institution's care. For example, in the
infirmary wards 'everything about them was comfortably clean and
decent', with officers 'attentive' to needs, and 'the most experienced in
their respective professions, with unwearied care and assiduity, with
the utmost tenderness and humanity, administering their advice and
assistance.'[40] The cultural conceptualisation of the poor is interesting
in showing who were seen as the deserving poor that merited assistance; the standard criterion for in-patient care was inability to pay
either for medicines or subsistence. Beyond this there was variability,
not only in the long list of exclusions but also in the type of poor
person infirmaries particularly wanted to assist. Salisbury targeted the
rural poor; Bath the day labourers and other poor persons meeting
with accidents; whilst Birmingham wished to help those unsettled
poor suffering from disease or accident, who had only recently found
work in local manufactures.[41]

Rules for hospital patients showed a disjunction between original
ideals and practical realities. They also illustrated the moralising function that the infirmary was intended to perform. For example:

Another good effect proposed by this institution, and that of the highest
importance, is the reformation of the manners of many dissolute people, who
may be admitted into the infirmary: this may reasonably be expected from the
endeavours of the clergy who will give their attendance, whose advice and
instructions will be rendered more effectual by those serious reflections,
which sickness and death naturally give.[42]

---

[39] *Reports of the General Infirmary at Leeds, 1782–3.*
[40] Wilts. RO, J8/110/1, Auditor's Report on the Salisbury Infirmary, 1768–9.
[41] Wilts. RO, Auditors Reports on Salisbury Infirmary; Wellcome Institute, London, MS
1094, Rules and Orders of the Casualty Hospital, Bath, 1788–1817; *An Account of the
Proceedings for the Establishment of the General Hospital* (Birmingham, 1766), p. 1.
[42] Quoted in E. M. Mumford, *Chester Royal Infirmary, 1756–1956* (1956).

It is important to appreciate that hospital care was conceived almost as much a moral or spiritual opportunity as a clinical one. The influential, contemporary *Reports* of the Society for Bettering the Condition and Increasing the Comforts of the Poor were interesting in this context in showing the intellectual climate of opinion in which infirmary rules were later developed and those of houses of recovery and dispensaries first formulated. These reports clearly and repeatedly promoted the connections between sickness and idleness, or between disease, death and the partaking of spiritous liquors or tea. Equally, there was an emphasis on the desirability of sobriety, industry, cleanliness, and morality in promoting health.[43] Prohibitions for infirmary in-patients thus included: indulging in spiritous liquors or drinking tea; smoking or chewing tobacco; playing at cards or dice; swearing or using abusive or indecent language; engaging in rude or indecent behaviour; and going into the wards of the opposite sex.[44] The practice of Bible reading and prayers in the wards was intended to elevate patients' behaviour. Such decorum was particularly important during periodic visits by governors or official visitors. And, when convalescent, patients were expected to resume the customary role of the poor and to labour in the wards at cleaning, washing, ironing or nursing in obedience to the instructions of the apothecary and matron.[45] The difficulty experienced in getting patients to conform to these models of virtue was suggested by the Devon and Exeter Infirmary, which stated its intention of making its patients sign that they would obey the rules, and charged them five shillings a week (for the provisions they had consumed) if they did not conform.[46] All institutions reserved the right to discharge patients for irregular behaviour. Manchester Infirmary grumbled in the 1760s that there was 'a growing irregularity amongst these poor people' once they had been discharged, in that they failed to 'notify their cure or return their thanks.' Even worse was the fact that some had apparently made 'complaints in town of ... pretended ill-treatment', and warning was given that in such instances there would be no readmittance.[47]

[43] For example, *Reports of the Society for Bettering the Condition and Increasing the Comforts of the Poor*, vol. 1, pp. x-xii; vol. 2, p. 231; appendix IV, p. 21; vol. 3, appendix V, pp. 39–40; Vol. IV, appendix 2, p. 24.
[44] This is based on an analysis of the infirmary rules of Bath, Birmingham, Bristol, Chester, Devon and Exeter, Leeds, Leicester, Norfolk and Norwich, Salisbury and York.
[45] See for example, *The Statutes and Rules for the Government of the General Hospital near Birmingham* (Birmingham, 1779), patients rule XVI; *Leeds General Infirmary Rules and Orders* (Leeds, 1782), rule 85.
[46] Devon RO, HS1 Statutes and Rules of the Devon and Exeter Hospital, 1743.
[47] W. Brocklebank, *Portrait of a Hospital, 1752–1948* (1952), p. 23.

Infirmaries ruled that out-patients might be discharged for non-attendance at out-patient clinics on two successive occasions, or for failing to bring back their vials and gallipots for filling up with fresh medicines.

The relationship of the infirmary to the local community was a sensitive one, not least because of its financial dependence on subscriptions.[48] The eighteenth-century infirmary was serviced largely by traditional patterns of face-to-face charity; subscribers nominated poor individuals for in-patient treatment whom they already knew from their household, parish or workplace.[49] In return they paid an annual subscription of two or three guineas. The necessity for good public relations therefore meant that out-patients were enjoined not to loiter outside the hospital gates or to beg from passers-by, and that after medical treatment was completed in-patients were expected to give thanks to God for their providential recovery in the local parish church.

Hospitals were very highly selective in whom they admitted as in-patients; such rigorous policies of exclusion meant that scarce resources could be targeted on those whom medical knowledge could benefit. Generally excluded were the pregnant; those suffering from mental disorders or epilepsy; people with infectious disorders such as smallpox, the itch (or, in the case of Taunton, measles); and those considered incurably or terminally ill – often those with cancer, TB or developed dropsies. Children under seven (or in the case of Leeds and Norwich under six) were also excluded from general hospitals. Sufferers who would gain equal benefit from out-patient care were not given beds. And those chosen for in-patient care were supposed to be limited in their hospital stay (two months was the usual period before discharge), although in practice discharge was not necessarily on so strict a basis. In selecting from out-patients those suitable for treatment, hospital physicians and surgeons were also motivated by their desire for clinical interest.

The hospital marked a shift in the power relationship between doctor and patient, and the poor had the uncertain honour of first becoming such patients. Foucault has suggested that there was a 'hidden contract' being formed between the hospital where the poor were being treated and the clinic where doctors were being trained.[50] That this was not universally the case is indicated by a detailed study of one atypical infirmary, that of the Edinburgh Infirmary by Risse;

[48] Porter, 'The Gift Relationship', p. 157.
[49] Fissell, 'Sick and Drooping Poor', p. 36.
[50] Foucault, *Clinic*, p. 83.

here requirements of teaching did *not* predominate over the interests of patients.[51] More generally, in-patients' 'free' treatment was paid for by their becoming clinical objects. This, as Foucault perceptively suggested, was 'the interest paid by the poor on the capital that the rich have invested in the hospital', since the latter benefited from the increased medical knowledge obtained from such treatment.[52] The Anatomy Act of 1832, which allowed the unclaimed bodies of deceased hospital patients to be used for demonstration or dissection in medical schools, was only the most obvious illustration of this process.[53] Predictably, it caused hostility by the poor towards the medical profession.[54] In lying-in wards the practice of making entry conditional on being delivered by students also made clear the non-monetary payment being extracted. Less obvious perhaps were the clinical benefits for society as a whole to be obtained from the serial observation of hospital in-patients, with enhanced opportunities for more careful diagnosis, for empirically determined treatment, and for more accurate prognosis. And in the long term the poor themselves also benefited from this improved clinical knowledge.

This overall impression of the poor being regarded increasingly as clinical objects was a consequence of one of the hospital's functions in providing clinical material for the medical profession. The veritable 'production lines' of poor patients lined up for bleeding, as occurred at one infirmary, vividly illustrated the routinisation involved in handling them:

On the days when the bleedings were numerous, the pupil for the week would often arrange five or six of these patients in a row, side by side; first fix a bandage round the arm of each, and give them a pewter bleeding dish to hold in the other hand; then beginning at one end, open the vein of each in succession, and, when finished with the last, go back to the first, ready to remove the bandage.[55]

Teaching procedures involved a further loss of dignity for poor patients on the wards. A medical student recorded how his instruction proceeded on a Scottish hospital ward, with the physician standing at the bedside, interrogating the patient in a very loud voice so that all the class of students could hear, whilst the student acting as the clerk repeated the patient's reply in an equally loud voice, and his peers

[51] Risse, *Hospital Life*, pp. 178, 250.   [52] Foucault, *Clinic*, pp. 84–5.
[53] R. Richardson, *Death Dissection and the Destitute* (1988). See also, for example, Barnes Medical Library, University of Birmingham, School of Medicine Minute Book, 1831–8, minute of 27 July 1832 for how quickly medical schools availed themselves of this.
[54] Marland, *Medicine and Society*, pp. 519–20.
[55] Marland, *Medicine and Society*, p. 189.

recorded the exchanges in their notebooks.[56] A humiliating loss of
individuality was involved in the way in which bedside teaching
reduced the patient to a case:

> Some of my happiest hours were those during which I was occupied in the
> wards with my pupils around me, answering their queries, explaining the
> cases to them at the bedside of the patients, informing them as to the grounds
> on which I formed my diagnosis, and the reasons for the treatment I
> employed, and not concealing from them my oversights and errors.[57]

This reduction of the patient from a subject to an object found its
logical culmination in public operations on patients who, in the days
before anaesthetics, were strapped or held down on tables in the
centre of a lecture theatre surrounded by rows of ascending seats
filled with medical students. Where post-operative open wounds were
concerned, there was great risk of cross-infection so that even if the
original complaint was treated successfully in the infirmary, a possibly
far more serious one succeeded it. The most notorious incidence of
this was that of puerperal fever in the lying-in wards. The founding
statement of the Westminster General Dispensary conceded that poor
patients' fears of contracting contagious diseases in hospitals were
'well-founded'.[58]

How effectively were the interests of the poor served by hospital
treatment? The material conditions of diet, bedding, ventilation,
warmth and nursing care were generally far superior in the institution
than in the home, so that care and recovery were facilitated. The small
numbers of cases trying fraudulently to gain admission or treatment
may at first sight also suggests the attractiveness of the infirmary to
the poor.[59] But care needs to be taken to distinguish the varied kinds
of motivation involved: for comfortable living; for attention but not
actual treatment; or for unnecessary medication and even surgery. It is
likely that more assiduous observation was given the poor patient in
the infirmary than to other patients because their history-taking was
difficult, so that doctors had to rely on their own perceptions.
However, the kind of procedures performed on hospital in-patients
partook of the ideas of the age – with blistering and bloodletting as the
most common therapies – so that there was not much class differenti-

---

[56] J. D. Comrie, *History of Scottish Medicine* (1927), p. 130.
[57] *Autobiography of Brodie* (1865), pp. 185–6.
[58] RCPL, MS 629, Minutes of Governors of Westminster General Dispensary, vol. 1.
[59] 'With hospital patients, sailors, soldiers etc, there are but two classes – the really sick,
     suffering from an affliction of a well marked type, and malingerers' confidently
     stated a professional guide (de Styrap, *Practitioner*, p. 39).

ation.[60] Little reliance can be placed upon published 'cure' rates, since these were increased by as much as one-third for publicity purposes. In any case 'cure' did not necessarily mean recovery.[61] Infirmaries also proclaimed that patients were well treated; patients were 'in all respects as well provided and attended to as persons of affluence in their own homes.'[62] Early institutions attempted to build in administrative safeguards against abuse. Not all patients found that these were satisfactory.[63] In 1784 Chester Infirmary discharged 'John Jones and Elias Lloyd ... for a complaint about their meat, which upon enquiry appeared to be groundless,[64] whereas in 1826 patients at the Leicester Infirmary complained that 'many have seen no medical gentlemen but the house surgeon for several weeks together.'[65] The official house visitors and, through them, the infirmary's governors, were an ultimate safeguard against *prolonged* neglect on the part of hospital staff. But the ways in which treatment was administered were less amenable to bureaucratic safeguards. In reality, the day-to-day experiences of poor patients varied with the individual medical staff with whom they came into contact; they were not protected – as were the affluent – by the doctor's hope of a fee, and were therefore dependent on a sense of professional propriety and honour. Some doctors undoubtedly treated the poor with as much care, attentiveness and skill, as they did their private patients; the Surgeon, J. G. Crosse, at the Norfolk and Norwich Hospital in the 1830s and 1840s, and the Senior Physician, Andrew Carrick at the Bristol Infirmary in the 1820s, were instances of this. But their colleagues were less disinterested. S. T. Taylor, Physician at Norwich and a later colleague of Crosse's, wrote revealingly of 'contriving to finish them all off [sic] before 12 a.m.', when referring to his hospital out-patients. And at Bristol one of Carrick's colleagues was Dr H. H. Fox, whose 'chief aim in seeing his in- and out- patients at the Infirmary was, apparently, to get through the work as quickly as he could.'[66]

A poor patient's dilemma in deciding on whether to resort to

---

[60] Risse, *Hospital Life*, p. 203.   [61] Risse, *Hospital Life*, p. 230.
[62] Wilts. RO J8/110/1, Auditors Reports 1774–5.
[63] W. B. Howie, 'Complaints and Complaints Procedures in the Eighteenth century and Early Nineteenth Century Provincial Hospitals in England', *MH*, 25 (1981), pp. 345–62.
[64] Chester RO, H1/5, Chester Royal Infirmary Minutes, 26 October 1784.
[65] Leics. RO, Leicester Infirmary House Reports, 1826–52, Minute 4 May 1826. Further complaints occurred on 29 October 1827.
[66] Crosse, *J. G. Crosse*, p. 132; H. Alford, 'The Bristol Infirmary in My Student Days, 1822–1828', *Bristol Medical and Chirurgical Journal*, September 1890, pp. 170–1, 174–5; RCPL, MS 2437, Medical Diary of S. T. Taylor, 1882–8, 19 May 1882. Andrew Carrick (1767–1837), was an MD Edinburgh (*Eighteenth Century Medics*, p. 102).

hospital care might have centred on the consequent loss of autonomy and possibility of cross-infection as against the advantage of a necessary operation being performed. On first reading, a poem left by Joseph Wilde suggests the way in which the values of an ideal patient had been internalised during a stay at the Devon and Exeter Hospital in 1809. Further reflection suggests that its customary expressions of gratitude may well have been ironic – thus indicating Wilde's awareness of the mercantilist calculation that had provided for his 'free' treatment.[67]

Medical charities

The perceived balance of advantage against drawback of voluntary hospitals casts some light on the objectives of those founding dispensaries. Hospitals were seen by the Westminster General Dispensary, for example, as disadvantaged both by the medical danger of cross-infection and the social drawback of being unattractive to those poor with 'a decent pride'.[68] This dispensary saw those with infectious disorders as being well served by an institution, like itself, that was organised to treat them in their own homes. Since dispensary patients did not need the letter of recommendation required by a voluntary hospital, this would also have the advantage of preventing harmful delays that might have been associated with obtaining letters from hospital subscribers, thus aiding early treatment and recovery.

The Westminster Dispensary had been set up in 1774 to serve the borough of Westminster. It had been preceded by the General Dispensary in Aldersgate of 1770 (which focused on the City of London), and was followed in 1783 by the Carey Street Dispensary, (which operated in the Lincoln's Inn Fields area.) The 'small beginnings' of the General Dispensary[69] thus gradually widened out so that the dispensary movement became a national one.[70] The instrumental social philosophy that motivated the General Dispensary was described by its founder and first physician, J. C. Lettsom, in these terms:

67 J. Wilde, *The Hospital, a Poem in Three Books, Written in the Devon and Exeter Hospital, 1809* (Norwich, 1809). See also W. B. Howie, 'Consumer Reaction: a Patient's View of Hospital Life in 1809', *BMJ*, 3 (1973), pp. 534–6, and Porter, 'The Gift Relation', for differing interpretations.
68 RCPL, MS 629, Minutes of the Governors of the Westminster Dispensary, vol. 1, original statement of aims.
69 J. C. Lettsom, *Medical Memoirs of the General Dispensary* (1774), p. xv.
70 I. S. L. Loudon, 'The Origins and Growth of the Dispensary Movement in England', *BHM*, 55 (1981), pp. 322–342.

The poor are a large, as well as a useful part of the community; they supply both the necessary and ornamental articles of life; and they have, therefore, a just claim to the protection of the rich ... This mutual obligation between the rich and the poor, [is such that] neither ... could long subsist without the aid of the other.[71]

The Carey Street Dispensary also saw its target clientele as this same class of 'industrious poor'.[72] It aimed to serve them by the regular attendance of a physician and a surgeon at the dispensary, and also by the services of an apothecary resident there. Medical treatments appear to have ranged from the simple to the sophisticated, since an inventory of instruments listed not only catheters, a scarificator and cupping glasses, but trepanning and amputating instruments, and also an electrical machine.[73] Of particular importance, however, were the dispensary's domiciliary visits, developed because 'many of the patients from the nature of their complaints must necessarily be confined at home, where they are often in danger of perishing miserably through indigence and improper treatment.'[74] Such home visits comprised about one-quarter of the poor that were attended.[75] Willan, the physician, wrote of 'the great pressure of business' at this dispensary, whilst Thomas Hodgkin who officiated at the North London Dispensary indicated how time-consuming was such visiting of patients in their own homes.[76] The bedside manner practised there was of a different character from that practised with the affluent. Percival wrote revealingly of the fact that 'greater *authority* and greater condescension will be found requisite.'[77]

Domiciliary visits alerted the medical profession to the full enormity of the public health problems posed by urbanisation. 'The miserable courts and alleys' in which the poor lived[78] were perceived to be a major cause of those alarming statistics of urban morbidity and mortality that were beginning to be collected on a more regular basis. The dispensary movement thus became intimately involved in the growth of specialist institutions to treat diseases from which the poor suffered. For example, those involved in administering the London

[71] Lettsom, *Medical Memoirs*, p. v.
[72] RCPL, MS 2509/1, Plan of the Publick Dispensary in Carey Street, 1783, p. 3.
[73] RCPL, MS 2508D, Carey Street Dispensary Accounts, 1782–93, Inventory of Apothecary, 1789.
[74] RCPL, MS 2509/1, p. 3.
[75] RCPL, MS 2468, Minutes of the Carey Street Dispensary; annual *Reports* giving attendance and visits, 1794–1801.
[76] RCPL, MS 2468, minute of 13 December 1803; Friends Library, microfilm 180 of Hodgkin MSS, undated letter.
[77] T. Percival, *Medical Ethics* (Manchester, 1803), p. 9.
[78] Lettsom, *Medical Memoirs*, pp. viii–ix.

dispensaries, with the Society for Bettering the Condition of the Poor, helped set up a Fever Institution in 1802, inspired by earlier initiatives including that of Haygarth in Chester during 1784.[79] The public good argument was the overriding rationale for such specialist fever hospitals and Houses of Recovery. By segregating poor patients (who were in any case excluded from voluntary hospitals), infectious disease could be reduced in the whole community since contagion could be prevented from spreading by good management. The work of the Fever Institution in London had so removed contagious fevers that they had 'nearly ceased to exist within the precincts of this institution', and this was attributed to the fact that 'many of the sources and receptacles of contagion have been purified.'[80] The utility to other classes in society was important in that the institution was thought to prevent contagion from 'diffusion among the other classes of the community ... [and] affords the higher ranks an open and comfortable asylum for their domestics, when attacked by contagious fever.'[81] Purification as a concept involving moralistic as well as public health measures informed contemporary reports on these houses of recovery as well as early statistics on public health.[82] The inter-penetration of medical and moral ideas was well-illustrated by the Quaker, Dr Willan, first Physician to the Carey Street Dispensary, and one of the founders of the London Fever Institution. He published a pathbreaking set of statistics and observations on the diseases of London.[83] However, he also held strong views on the dreadful effects of drinking spirits which, in his view, had been 'more destructive to the labouring class ... than all the injuries accruing from unhealthy seasons, impure air, [and] infection.'[84]

The poor may have laboured under the moral exhortations of their betters but also benefited from an extension of specialist facilities. A good example of this was the opportunity given poorer members of society to partake of spa treatment or sea bathing. The chronically sick London poor were sent to the Sea-bathing Infirmary at Margate, after their 'inveterate maladies had long resisted the faculties' art.'[85] Spas,

79 RCPL, MS 2468D, Carey St Dispensary, minute 9 June 1801; *Extract from an Account of the Proposed Institution to Prevent the Progress of Contagious Fever in the Metropolis* (1801).
80 RCPL, Ms 2509/1, Reports of the Public Dispensary in Bishop's Court (formerly Carey St), report for 1805.
81 *Reports of Society for Poor* (1798–), vol. 5, p. 180.
82 *Reports of Society for Poor* (1798–), vol. 2, p. 359.
83 R. Willan, *Miscellaneous Works* (1821) includes his Reports on the Diseases in London, 1796–1800.
84 *Reports of the Society for the Poor*, vol.3, pp. 23–4.
85 Wellcome, AL 67615, John Anderson to Rev John Pridden, 3 October 1790.

which are usually seen as the preserve of polite society, also catered for the poor.[86] At the spa at Buxton ordinary people paid their penny to drink water at the well, and during the 1820s and 1830s about 15,000 poor had free use of Buxton Charity Baths of whom four-fifths had allegedly been 'cured or much relieved.'[87]

The large extent of individual lay philanthropy directed at improving the health and treating the sicknesses of the poor is easy to underestimate. Much of the evidence for it has disappeared, whilst other material lies scattered in a myriad of household accounts and diaries. It is clear, however, that particularly in rural areas looking after the household servants when ill, assisting a sick tenant, or giving a helping hand to a poorer member of the community were everyday events. Women played a particularly significant role here: through financial assistance if they belonged to the propertied classes; through home-made medicines or nutritious food for the sick if they were less well endowed; and for women of all social ranks through personal visiting or attendance – especially during confinements. For example, Lady Cardigan's early-eighteenth-century account book contained varied entries suggesting the range of financial assistance that was given:

Paid Mrs Lambert for a nurse to attend sick people, 10s; Mary Bradley, £4.5s.0d for nursing Thomas Lee, postillion, for four weeks; Paid the woman that cured Roger White's child; Paid Maiching the surgeon for Widow Hawe's cure 15s.; To Mr Baker, for physic for poor people . . . £11.15s.0d'[88]

The matter-of-fact brevity of many of the entries itself suggested the routine nature of the activity. More than a century later this same tradition still flourished, as can be seen from the Victorian charity book of the Le Strange family.[89] And, more rarely, lay charity and medical altruism combined to good effect in the private sphere: as with the partnership between Lord Crewe and Dr John Sharpe in County Durham, which led to the creation of a small hospital; or that between William Fellowes and the surgeon, Benjamin Gooch, in erecting a cottage hospital in Shotesham, Norfolk.[90] In addition, zeal on the

---

[86] R. Cruttwell, *The Stranger's Assistant and Guide to Bath* (Bath, 1773), pp. 49–50; *A Narrative of the Efficacy of the Bath Waters in Paralytic Disorders* (Bath, 1787), pp. xii–xiv: *Cases of Persons Admitted into the Infirmary at Bath under the Care of Doctor Oliver* (Bath, 1760); R. W. Falconer, *The Bath Mineral Waters* (1861).

[87] Granville, *Spas*, pp. 29, 35–6.

[88] J. Wake, *The Brudenells of Deene* (second edn 1954), p. 217.

[89] Norfolk RO Le Strange Collection, Account Book of Charities to the Sick and Poor.

[90] C. J. Strange, 'The Charities of Nathaniel Lord Crewe and Dr John Sharpe 1721–1926', Durham Cathedral Lecture, 1976. I am indebted to Dr Alan Heeson for this reference. See also, A. Batty Shaw, 'Benjamin Gooch, Eighteenth Century Norfolk Surgeon' *MH*, XVI (1972), p. 44.

part of individual medical practitioners created a tremendous range of specialist hospitals, many of them targeted on the poor. Lying-in charities and eye infirmaries were commonly found in provincial towns whilst specialist facilities to treat diseases of the skin, chest, and rectum, or to provide orthopaedic treatment, were concentrated in metropolitan centres.[91] In some areas the extent of these voluntary medical charities exceeded that of the statutory poor law.[92]

The New Poor Law

The New Poor Law provided a more uniform system of medicine than had the Old Poor Law, but there were worsening terms for doctors, and some deterioration in the quality of care given to outdoor paupers. Since an escalation in poor rates had been a major cause of reform in 1834, economy became a powerful force. Instead of the previous custom of appointing a doctor in each parish, the aggregation of parishes into unions under the New Poor Law facilitated the creation of much larger medical districts. In some rural areas districts were so large as to make it insuperably difficult for even the most conscientious medical officer to operate efficiently. In addition, during the first years of the new system a minority of parishes appointed doctors by tender, which meant that cost rather than adequate qualification became the driving force. The worst of these features was addressed in the General Medical Order of 1842 which laid down a maximum medical district of 15,000 acres for a single medical officer, and insisted on a double qualification in both medicine and surgery for poor-law medical officers. But – as so often in poor-law affairs – prescription did not necessarily lead to compliance; in the 1860s medical districts of up to 100,000 acres could be found, while even though a well-qualified doctor had been formally engaged as medical officer, an unqualified assistant might do the actual work in caring for the poor.[93] By the end of our period there were some four thousand poor-law doctors of whom rather more than one in five had a poor-law institution as their responsibility. (See Plate 12 and Table 4.1.)

Driven by a cost-cutting engine and informed by a deterrent social philosophy, the system set up under the 1834 act loaded the dice against the development of an adequate system of medical care, whilst

91 L. Granshaw, 'Fame and Fortune', in Granshaw and Porter, *Hospital*, pp. 206–7.
92 Marland, *Medicine and Society*, p. 543.
93 M. W. Flinn, 'Medical Services under the New Poor Law' in D. Fraser, ed., *The New Poor Law in the Nineteenth Century* (1976), pp. 54–5.

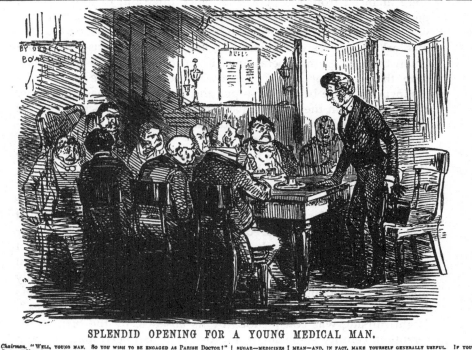

SPLENDID OPENING FOR A YOUNG MEDICAL MAN.

Chairman. "WELL, YOUNG MAN, SO YOU WISH TO BE ENGAGED AS PARISH DOCTOR?" | SUGAR—MEDICINES! MEAN—AND, IN FACT, MAKE YOURSELF GENERALLY USEFUL. IF YOU
Doctor. "YES, GENTLEMEN, I AM DESIROUS——" | DO YOUR DUTY, AND CONDUCT YOURSELF PROPERLY, WHY—AH—YOU—AH——"
Chairman. "AH! EXACTLY. WELL—IT'S UNDERSTOOD THAT YOUR WAGES—SALARY I | [*Punch.* "WILL PROBABLY BE BOWLED OUT OF YOUR SITUATION BY SOME HUMBUG, WHO
SHOULD SAY—IS TO BE TWENTY POUNDS PER ANNUM; AND YOU FIND YOUR OWN TEA AND | WILL FILL IT FOR LESS MONEY."]

Plate 12   'Splendid Opening for a Young Medical Man' (*Punch*, 1848)

the tensions inherent in operating such a medical service were almost impossible to resolve satisfactorily. The clearest example of this was the issue of what were termed 'medical extras'.[94] In the Wimborne Union in Dorset, for instance, Dr Parkinson would order two pounds of mutton and eight ounces of wine, or half a pint of porter daily, in order to build up his patients.[95] Typically, this kind of order was seen by the board of guardians as a usurpation of their role, since this was not medication, but relief. Another factor in the predilection of poor-law doctors for medical extras over medicine was that the cost of the more expensive drugs came out of their own pockets whilst extras

[94] Digby, *Pauper Palaces*, pp. 176–7; *SC on Medical Relief*, PP 1844, IX, QQ 9720–1, evidence of Sir John Walsham, poor-law inspector.
[95] Dorset RO, PE/WM OV 18/3, Register of Medical Relief in the Wimborne District of the Wimborne Union, 1861–3.

were financed from the poor rate. Since three out of four cases of pauperism in the mid-nineteenth century involved sickness, this issue was a central one for poor-law administrators. They suspected that medical officers were inadvertently helping to pauperise the population through giving liberal relief in aid of sickness. A comparison with the Old Poor Law is instructive here since one of the few distinctions made between pauper and independent patients before 1834 had been in the less expensive medical extras prescribed by the doctor, although in the earlier era such orders had not been challenged by the parish overseer.

Within the workhouse of the New Poor Law tensions affecting the sick poor were less obvious, but resource constraints were more prominent. In rural areas the sick continued to be cared for in sick wards located in workhouse buildings that had been erected in the 1830s or even earlier. A survey in the early twentieth century revealed that there were three hundred rural workhouses with less than fifty sick beds in each.[96] Inevitably, these became progressively more out of step with modern thinking on hospital design and amenity. But during the mid-nineteenth century care in the wards was usually given by other pauper inmates, who might be only marginally less infirm than the patient, and were untrained in nursing procedures.[97] Night nursing was conspicuous by its absence. By the turn of the twentieth century some slight improvement had been made in both respects; the use of pauper nurses had been prohibited in 1897, but difficulties in recruitment remained. A poor-law inspector described how advertising a post of workhouse nurse at twenty pounds a year typically produced no trained applicant, so that an ex-maid had to be appointed. He pondered 'how much suffering may her willing ignorance cause to the patients', and to illustrate what might happen, cited a couple of cases he had encountered:

A confinement where the doctor declared that the 'nurse' had never seen a confinement before and had no idea what to do; and ... another where the 'nurse' being told to take a temperature in the course of the evening put the clinical thermometer, which the doctor had left with her, into the chamber utensil; and a third case where, in endeavouring to pass a catheter, she caused the death of a patient.[98]

In urban areas there was much greater variety in poor-law medicine. In the sick wards of town workhouses numbers of beds varied from

[96] S. and B. Webb, *The State and the Doctor* (1910), p. 92.
[97] For example, the Strand Union in mid-century (J. Rogers, *Reminiscences of a Workhouse Medical Officer* (1889), p. 4).
[98] PRO, MH 32/102, Final Report on Yorkshire by H. G. Kennedy, 10 February 1900, fo. 6.

50 to 400, and with some institutions having a resident medical officer. Specialist infirmaries had also been built which were estimated to take one-third of poor-law institutional cases. These took not just chronic and incurable cases customary under the poor law but acute ones as well.[99] Trained nurses were employed, with an improved ratio of nurses to patients, and in addition there were a few night nurses. The standard of medical care to be found in the new poor-law urban infirmaries was sufficiently good for patients to be attracted into them. After 1885, when receiving poor relief in time of sickness no longer carried a voting disqualification, much of its stigma was removed. The practice of physically distancing the infirmary from the workhouse reinforced this perception, so that the infirmary eventually came to be regarded as little different from a general hospital. So much was this the case that traditional fears of pauperisation through 'generous' social provision were voiced, 'There seems to be no limit to the number of sick who are willing to avail themselves of the medical skill and good nursing provided in connection with modern workhouse infirmaries.[100] Indeed, the standard of such provision meant that the gap between the poor-law sector and the voluntary hospitals was narrowing; the Royal Commission on the Poor Laws of 1905–9 considered that the best infirmaries were equal to the general hospitals, although the perceived stigma of such institutions continued into the interwar period.[101]

Standards of medical care for the outdoor poor showed far less improvement. There is some evidence that the low calibre of the first medical appointments under the new system inhibited the working class from seeking help; in Manchester, for example, it was said that the poor avoided them because they considered that the poor-law doctors were deficient in skill.[102] The outdoor poor suffered delays in treatment because of the bureaucratic procedures of the New Poor Law: an application had to be made to the relieving officer to obtain an order authorising treatment, which then had to be taken to the home of the union medical officer. The problem of tracking down first a busy relieving officer and then an active rural practitioner, created long delays during which medical problems could be seriously aggravated. In these circumstances misunderstandings and allegations of neglect were predictable. An experienced poor-law inspector analysed this:

[99] Webb, *State and Doctor*, pp. 95, 104–6.
[100] PRO, MH 32/101 Report of H. Jenner Fust, 23 May 1896, fos. 4–5.
[101] *Majority Report of the Royal Commission on the Poor Laws*, Cd 4499, p. 273: B. Abel Smith, *The Hospitals, 1800–1948* (1964), pp. 97, 131–2, 202–3.
[102] *Lancet*, 28 April 1838; SC on Medical Relief, PP, 1854, xii, QQ 2195–7.

Suppose there is a *prima facie* case of neglect, and that a pauper appears to have had no medical attendance when it was desirable that should have been given without delay, it generally turns out that a message had been sent down by the poor person to the medical officer; that he was not at home; that the message was left with a servant; and that when asked why this poor person had not the medical relief that was due, the medical officer rejoins, 'I got no order; I heard nothing of it.' The poor person, who is brought forward, declares the message was sent; the medical man rejoins, 'I never got the message; I know nothing about it.' Such a case is relatively of very common occurrence.[103]

In the event, fewer cases of negligence were actually brought than were discussed in numerous guardians' minutes but, given these circumstances, even these fairly horrific instances were difficult to prove. A few cases from the mid-nineteenth century illustrate some of the difficulties in assessing evidence on the adequacy of medical care. In the Wisbech Union one of the medical officers, Dr John Hemming, was found guilty of serious neglect by the Poor Law Board in 1863. On two successive days he had failed to visit a terminally-ill woman patient, who lived only ten minutes away from his own home, restricting his ministrations to giving medicine to the patient's husband to take home to his wife. The doctor was not dismissed because he had given ten years without prior complaint in his office. However, there was a further complaint against Hemming in 1868, when a pregnant woman in his care died, at a time when Hemming was away for several days and had left only an unqualified assistant to mind his practice. No action was taken against Hemming because he argued that an alternative medical officer was available for the poor to consult.[104] In the Sherborne Union in Dorset a clergyman was active in 1854, and again in 1863 in alleging medical neglect of his parishioners by the Medical Officer, a surgeon named White. In the first instance the guardians got so far as admitting that White was 'not wholly free from blame' but managed to defend their officer by concluding that the relatives had not made clear the patient, Mary Mitchell's 'alarming state'. Once White had visited her he was praised for doing 'all in his power to relieve her', but it was acknowledged that by then it was too late for human agency. So the guardians closed ranks against the outsider in concluding that the Rev Harston's claims were not 'fully or clearly substantiated.'[105] Nine years later the board of guardians did not even bother to investigate further allegations of neglect made by

---

103 *SC on Medical Relief*, PP 1844, IX, Q 9717, evidence of Sir John Walsham.
104 Greer, *Tubbs*, pp. 55–6, 62.
105 Dorset RO, BG/SH A1/12 Sherborne Union Minutes of 15 November and 2 December 1854.

the same cleric, but White was sufficiently incensed to take legal action against Harston![106] Even when cases were proved against medical officers the difficulty of getting a better replacement might lead to a continuance in office after reprimand, as in Norfolk in the 1840s, or even (as in Huddersfield in 1848) to reappointment after dismissal.[107] As to the adequacy of the treatment the outdoor pauper received, before 1847 Hodgkinson estimated that at least one medical officer per year was dismissed for gross neglect, although much good work was also accomplished.[108] Even medical officers disagreed amongst themselves as to the quality. A surgeon for sixteen years in the Wells Union considered in 1854 that the poor did not get sufficient attendance, whilst another with ten years experience of the same job, this time in the Stowe Union, concluded that such attendance was as efficient as that given to private or club patients.[109]

Medical altruism

That treatment of the poor was as good as it was owed much to medical altruism, and this section deals not only with that by surgeon-apothecaries and GPs but by physicians as well. Informing this was a nice balance between the calculated pursuit of self-interest and philanthropy. Credence must be given to genuinely idealistic, charitable, religious and humanitiarian impulses behind it. But it is necessary to look not just at elevated rationales but also at the practicalities of treating poor patients. The bottom line, although hardly one that was trumpeted loudly, was that there was little alternative to giving a considerable amount of free treatment to the poor. The lawyer could turn away a poor but litigious-minded individual, but a Georgian doctor – working broadly within the ethical tradition of the Hippocratic oath and influenced by the paternalistic social philosophy of the day – was unlikely to refuse to treat a destitute, accident case. To some extent such medical philanthropy did bring more than its heavenly reward, since practice amongst the poor was considered to lead to an extension of that among the propertied classes, whilst taking on such responsibilities might also keep out unqualified medical competition. An honorific post as Surgeon or Physician at a voluntary hospital

---

[106] Dorset RO, A1/16 Sherborne Union Minutes of February to May 1863; D/48/18/25, Legal papers of White and Harston.
[107] Digby, *Pauper Palaces*, p. 168; Marland, *Medicine and Society*, p. 79.
[108] R. L. Hodgkinson, 'Poor Law Medical Officers of England, 1843–1871', *JHM*, xi (1956), p. 312.
[109] *SC on Medical Relief*, QQ, 3079, 2410.

brought direct contact with the county families who were its governors or subscribers. The even more onerous, unpaid work in similar positions at dispensaries might have a similar if more indirect result, since the high profile of such office publicised the names of doctors to subscribers and other townspeople. Such offices became the subject of intense competition for this very reason.[110] However, attitudes to less elevated public posts changed during the course of the nineteenth century as the divisions between social classes widened. Chapter 4 suggested that a post as medical officer to a poor law union was later seen as a drawback in recruiting affluent patients. Clinical advantages were also an important element in medical altruism; opportunities for advancing professional knowledge were present both in the private and public treatment of the poor. One doctor commented enthusiastically towards the end of the nineteenth century, for example, that in the voluntary hospitals 'the clinical material is simply overflowing, especially in the surgical and gynaecological wards.'[111] And it was for the same reason that, during the early nineteenth century, ambitious, young practitioners used to see the poor early in the morning at their own homes to widen their experience sufficiently to become consultants.[112] An entrepreneurial drive led doctors to found specialist hospitals, many of which in their early days were focused on the poor; Granshaw has estimated that the proportion of notable surgical members of the profession who were involved in specialist institutions rose from about one-fifth in the 1850s to nearly three-fifths by the 1890s.[113]

The earliest form of charitable treatment by the profession for impoverished members of the community was, however, through individual practitioners in private practice who were practising what was seen as an important ethical strand in medicine. John Bell advised that 'Our profession, by making us feel whatever man can feel, by giving us a direct and daily interest in the sufferings of our fellow-creatures, carries with it ... the purest principles of charity and benevolence.'[114] In London, Quaker doctors such as Fothergill and Lettsom became renowned for the numbers that they attended freely, with the poor coming to the doctor's house very early in the morning.[115] In the provinces this charitable kind of activity was also performed: Erasmus

[110] Marland, _Medicine and Society_, p. 202.   [111] Keeteley, _The Student's Guide_, p. 65.
[112] For example, Brock, _Astley Cooper_, pp. 12–3.
[113] Granshaw, 'Fame and Fortune', p. 212; the criterion for notability was inclusion in Plarr's Fellows of the Royal College of Surgeons.
[114] John Bell, _Letters on Professional Character and Manners_ (Edinburgh, 1810), p. 41.
[115] T. Hunt, _The Medical Society of London, 1773–1973_ (1972); Lettsom, _Medical Memoirs_ (1774), p. xvi.

Darwin gave medical advice freely to the Georgian poor in Lichfield; as did Richard Wilkes and his colleagues in Wolverhampton. Their Exeter contemporary, Dr Glass, treated poorer patients for nothing, and on being asked his fee replied, 'Your recovery will be my recompense'.[116] This custom continued in the early nineteenth century, and surgeon-apothecaries might advertise this service as did W. Lewis in Wolverhampton, and Henry Hickman in Tenbury.[117] Sometimes, what had been done earlier in this private sphere was then shifted into the public one, as a result of a later involvement with a dispensary.[118] Such dispensary service was extremely onerous. Dr Willan, for instance, served the Carey Street Dispensary for twenty-one years as its first physician, receiving only occasional gratuities for attending three times a week at the dispensary and, in addition, during the winter and spring seeing as many as half of the patients in their own homes. When he eventually resigned, the governors of the charity thanked him for what they significantly termed his 'parental solicitude', as well as for the 'unwearied zeal and attention' he had displayed in his office.[119]

What were the boundaries of medical altruism and to what extent is it possible to discern any changes in attitudes toward philanthropic practice? Practical limitations existed for the practitioner in that medicine was a business. Dr Chambers, a physician in eighteenth-century Hull was reputed to have died poor, because he 'frequently returned one half of the money which his patients thought he deserved, but which he thought them imprudent in giving.'[120] And it was said of one Victorian family doctor that 'unfortunately his large-heartedness was too large for his means, and he ... failed in practice.'[121] Whilst a Georgian practitioner expressed a commonplace in 1790 in suggesting that for doctors 'Distress and Poverty have ever an allowed claim to their assistance, independent of all pecuniary reward',[122] revealingly he went on to complain to the Trustees of the Bath Casualty Hospital. 'I was induced to offer you my services *gratis* from the circumscribed state of its finances, and I meant to continue them, as long, and as

[116] Wellcome MS 5005; King-Hele, *Erasmus Darwin*, p. viii; P. M. G. Russell, *A History of the Exeter Hospitals, 1170–1948* (Exeter, 1976), p. 31.
[117] *Wolverhampton Chronicle*, 11 October 1826; W. D. A. Smith, 'A History of Nitrous Oxide and Oxygen Anaesthesia IVE: Henry Hill Hickman in his Time', *British Journal of Anaesthesia*, 50 (1978), pp. 855, 859.
[118] Willmott, *Journal of Dr John Simpson*, p. 26.
[119] RCPL, MS 2468, 13 December 1803.
[120] Holmes, *Augustan England*, p. 225.
[121] Clarke, *Autobiographical Recollections*, p. 95.
[122] Wellcome MS 1094, Bath Royal United Casualty Hospital Rules and Orders, Letter to the Trustees from James Norman, MD.

often, as it should be so circumscribed; but when advanced to a state of ability, may I not reasonably expect a gratuity?' He ended by referring to the 'Interest of the Profession', and it was to this interest that doctors appealed increasingly during the nineteenth century.

Percival warned against wealthy physicians giving free advice since he thought it was 'an injury to his professional brethren.'[123] Colleagues used this rationale to deprecate Thomas Hodgkin's indifference to charging what his colleagues regarded as adequate fees,[124] in contrast to the admiration that such action had elicited when performed by an earlier generation of Quaker doctors. Hodgkin's friend, William Stroud, was also viewed with suspicion by his colleagues because it was said that 'he practises in a curious manner. He will not take fees. I do not understand it.'[125] This difference in attitude was the result of narrow professional changes being reinforced by broader social ones; after 1815 the economic prospects for an individual doctor in an increasingly crowded profession had worsened, whilst the New Poor Law signalled that social attitudes towards the poor had hardened. Thus, by mid-century those who did not charge, or who were indifferent to the size of the fee they received, were viewed with hostility by their professional brethren. It was significant that a standard guide to the profession warned in 1857 that the physician should consult his colleagues before indulging in medical altruism. 'He must be careful not to trench on the practice of those who may by such gratuitous practice become ... his ... greatest enemies.'[126]

During the Victorian and Edwardian periods calculation rather than sentiment became more prominent as a result both of the doctors' increasing economic struggles and society's exploitation of them. H. W. Rumsey, a persuasive advocate on the subject of the medical profession's humanity, reckoned that in some cases 'Legal medical relief reached little more than one-sixth of the destitute sick, nearly five-sixths being left to the charitable feelings of a profession which certainly does not luxuriate in the marrow of English opulence.'[127] In 1836 practitioners complained of the 'vast amount of gratuitous assistance' given in out-patient clinics in voluntary hospitals, which was

---

123 C. D. Leake, *Percival's Medical Ethics* (Baltimore, 1927), p. 105. See also page 60 above.
124 G. E. Foxon, 'Thomas Hodgkin, 1798–1866. A Biographical Note', *Guy's Hospital Reports*, 115 (1966), p. 246.
125 Friend's Library, microfilm 178 'Memoir of William Stroud' by Thomas Hodgkin (1858). Stroud (1789–1859) was an Edinburgh graduate and licentiate of the Royal College of Physicians.
126 Thomson, *Profession*, p. 163.
127 *SC on Poor Law Medical Relief*, PP 1844, IX, Q 9119, evidence on the position in Newark.

reducing the amount of general practice. The most sensitive issue, however, was the extent to which the profession's altruism was voluntary rather than enforced. The degree of professional bitterness that this aroused can be appreciated if doctors' justified feeling of continued exploitation under the New Poor Law,[128] is juxtaposed with their anger at the organised consumer-power of the working class in friendly societies.[129] Low-paid contracts of an open-ended character were involved both with these so-called clubs and with poor-law practice. Another central concern of Victorian practitioners – although one that was probably less well-grounded in fact – was the extent to which people were falsely claiming to be poor in order to qualify for medical charities; from the mid-nineteenth century this professional perception that there was widespread abuse of out-patient facilities by non-indigent people grew.[130] The next chapter indicates that pressure on medical incomes resulted both in a search for new sources of income, and in hostility to non-traditional entrants to the medical profession.

[128] *BMJ*, 14 July 1883, p. 64.
[129] Bartrip, *Mirror of Medicine*, p. 53; M. A. Crowther, 'Paupers or Patients? Obstacles to Professionalization in the Poor Law Medical Service before 1914', *JHM*, 39 (1984), pp. 45–6.
[130] Abel Smith, *Hospitals*, p. 104; *Lancet*, 1840–1 (ii), p. 373; 'Report on Out-Patient Departments', *BMJ*, 22 February 1913, p. 173.

9

Expanding practice with women and child patients

'The successful management of the diseases of women is the key to general practice and forms a large portion of your work', was the advice given to medical students in 1885.[1] It was the key to Victorian general practice since although midwifery was generally regarded by the profession as under-paid, childbirth gave an entrée to the household and then to employment as both the woman's doctor and the family doctor. And, for the more specialist practitioner, the expanding field of gynaecology offered substantial rewards. Estimates suggested that the proportion of practice made up by women and children was as high as three-quarters – although in my view this was an over-estimate.[2] One of the main arguments used by feminists who wanted to see medical employment opened up to women in the second half of the nineteenth century was the central role of women patients in general practice. Drs Elizabeth and Emily Blackwell argued in 1860 that 'More than half of ordinary medical practice lies among women and children.'[3] This chapter discusses the experience of women and children as patients, and the professional rivalries of male and female practitioners associated with them.

Income from obstetrics

That 'most practices were built up on a reputation for skill in obstetrics', was a commonplace by the end of our period.[4] What were the immediate rewards – as opposed to the longer-term strategic goals – to

[1] J. H. Aveling, gynaecologist, quoted in J. M. Kerr, ed., *Historical Review of British Obstetrics and Gynaecology, 1800–1950* (Edinburgh, 1954), p. 317.
[2] S. Gregory, *Female Physicians* (London, 1864), p. 1.
[3] 'Medicine as a profession for women', *English Woman's Journal*, v (May 1860), p. 27.
[4] Cox, *Doctors*, p. 53.

Table 9.1. *Recommended schedules of midwifery fees, 1819–1874*

Type of midwifery	Class 3 patient	Class 2 patient	Class 1 patient
1819 (Blackburn)			
Ordinary	15/-	21/-	
1865 (Manchester)			
Ordinary	21/-	21–63/-	42–84/-
1870 (National)			
Ordinary	15–21/-	21–63/-	42–105/- (and up)
1874 (National)			
Ordinary	15–21/-	21–63/-	42–105/- (and up)
Difficult	Fee and a half		
Administration of chloroform 10/6–21/- 21/-31/6 21–42/-			
Use of forceps	Extra half fee		
Turning	Extra half fee		
Embryotomy	Extra full fee		
Caesarian	210–315/-	210–420/-	315–630/-

Notes:
(1) In 1819, the patients in a lower-paying class were said to be labourers, servants, and weavers whilst those in a higher-paying class were said to include those in a trade or profession, and thus included patients who would later be placed in a higher class.
(2) In 1865, those living in houses with rentals of more than £100 had a separate band of charges.
(3) In 1874 and 1879 patients in class 3 had house rentals of £10–25 in 1870 and £15–25 in 1874; those in class 2 had rentals of £25–50; and those in class 1 had rentals of £50–100.
Sources:
Rules and Regulations Agreed and Entered into by the Medical Gentlemen of Black-burn (Blackburn, 1819); *Lancet* 29 July 1865; *A Tariff of Medical Fees Recommended by the Shropshire Ethical Branch of the BMA* (Shrewsbury, 1870, 1874).

be obtained from midwifery fees? Midwifery fees charged in the late eighteenth century were generally half a guinea, fifteen shillings, or one guinea, with only a few billed at one to three guineas for more affluent patients.[5] A fashionable London accoucheur was in a different league, charging ten guineas a delivery or more.[6] During much of the nineteenth century scales of charges for midwifery give a clear idea of the relatively static nature of midwifery fees. Table 9.1 indicates that

---

[5] Loudon, *Medical Care*, pp. 94–7.   [6] Bynum and Porter, *Wiliam Hunter*, p. 40.

the lowest *recommended* fees were fifteen shillings or one guinea, whilst the upper end of the range went up to five guineas. The lower half of the table also indicates that by the 1870s practitioners had attempted to operate with greater economic efficiency for time spent in difficult or complicated operative procedures.

However, these fees probably indicated aspiration rather than achievement. For instance, a meeting of London accoucheurs in 1845 had recommended that all practitioners should 'abandon the habit of attendance on a midwifery patient at so small and unreasonable a sum as half a guinea, excepting as an act of charity'.[7]

More plentiful information on later fees is available. John Pickles of Leeds had a local reputation in obstetrics and his delivery book contained some 2700 mothers' names. Earning £800 per annum in the 1880s he may be said to have built up a 'good' general practice. The much younger Alfred Cox, also practising in a northern town at the turn of the century, but attempting to build up a viable practice, attended nearly 200 midwifery cases a year. He blessed the fact that confinements (at half a guinea to fifteen shillings a case) meant cash down for a hard-pressed practitioner.[8] However, even when an immediate cash down-payment was demanded, payment for midwifery could still be troublesome. During the 1870s and 1880s a Lincolnshire practitioner, Frederick Hall of Wragby, made poorer mothers put five or ten shillings down, and then pay off the remaining five shillings in instalments. Revealingly, some had not managed to repay their debt within a year.[9] This showed continuity in practice difficulties, since a century earlier a surgeon-apothecary practising in the same area also demanded a down-payment.[10] Table 3.1 also indicates that some GPs were sufficiently incensed by the late or non-payment of midwifery fees that they imposed a penalty for this. And as one surgeon perceptively commented at the turn of the nineteenth century, 'I know of no surgeon who would not willingly have given up attending midwifery cases provided he could retain the family in other respects.'[11]

Advertisements of practices for sale in the *BMJ* in the late Victorian and Edwardian periods give a more structured insight, although unfortunately the sample is small. Whilst midwifery apparently offered a steady income it was also an onerous business, so that the better sort of practices limited the number of cases and elevated the

[7] *Lancet*, 1 November 1845.   [8] Cox, *Doctors*, p. 53.
[9] Lincs RO, MS Don 477, Ledger of Lincolnshire Surgeon, 1875–85.
[10] Lincs RO, Flinders MS.
[11] Richard Smith of Bristol, quoted in Loudon, 'Family Doctor'.

charges. A handful of superior practices even boasted that they either declined or discouraged midwifery. A few rural practices suggested that this type of work was 'chiefly attended by the assistant.'[12] Sound practices saw the lowest charge as one guinea; 'nothing under a guinea' became a badge of a respectability. Only the struggling urban practices, or those with a substantial component of working-class patients, admitted to charging only fifteen shillings. Similarly, the well-founded practice appears to have restricted the number of midwifery cases to about 40 per year, whereas those with less secure finances would take up to 130 or even 140 cases annually. Only a tenth of practices were located at the 'upper end' of midwifery where charges were between five and ten guineas per case. Tables 9.2 and 9.3 indicate both the narrow range of charges, and the small amount of movement in them during several decades. Indeed, the usual charge at the inception of the National Health Service in 1948 was still only three guineas.[13]

This data indicates that practice income from midwifery was around £100 per year, and thus constituted around ten per cent of a good practice's income and proportionately more for a struggling one, so that as much as one-quarter to one-third might come from this one source alone. This estimate is based on the assumption that those with good general practices took fewer patients at higher fees, whereas those less fortunate economically charged lower fees but took more patients. This gives credence to the commonplace that midwifery provided the 'jam' on the 'bread and butter' of the general practice. A survey in 1869 indicated that the decision whether to employ the GP or a female midwife depended crucially on the mother's income. In the wealthier West End of London only 2 per cent or fewer made use of a midwife, whereas in the less affluent East End between 30 and 50 per cent did so, and in large manufacturing towns the figure might be as large as 90 per cent.[14] GPs' fees therefore needed to be kept low in a competitive market.

How did GPs' fees compare with those charged by women as midwives? It is possible that payment in kind survived longer in female midwifery than in other areas of practice, whilst evidence on midwives' monetary charges is fragmentary. In the eighteenth century professional female midwives in London commanded a fee of five shillings, or seven shillings and sixpence for a difficult case, whereas the man-midwife would charge a guinea for complicated cases. Village

[12] For example, *BMJ*, 14 July, 13 October 1877.
[13] C. Webster, *The Health Services since the War* (1988), vol. 1, pp. 117–8.
[14] Aveling, *English Midwives*, pp. 164–5.

Table 9.2. *Minimum midwifery fees charged by practices, 1877, 1899, 1909*

Fees	1877 %	1899 %	1909[a] %
1 guinea or under	72	83	75
2 guineas or under	91	100	94
N	66	53	178

Source: Analysis of figures in practice advertisements in the *BMJ Advertiser*, 1877, 1899 and April – June 1909

Table 9.3. *Maximum midwifery fees charged by practices, 1877, 1899, 1909*

Fees	1877 %	1899 %	1909 %
1 guinea or less	41	21	9
2 guineas or less	41	56	41
3 guineas or less	51	81	65
5 guineas or less	89	93	89
N	37	43	120

Source: Analysis of figures in practice advertisements in the *BMJ Advertiser*, 1877, 1899 and April – June 1909.

midwives at this time had lower charges of two shillings and six-pence.[15] For 'old wives', who provided a service on demand for neighbours, this sum of half a crown apparently continued as the standard payment throughout the period. But more regular female practitioners in midwifery had increased their charges from this to around four shillings by the 1870s, and to seven shillings and sixpence or even ten shillings by the end of the period. More experienced or trained female midwives could always command a premium; those working for established charities could charge from 15 shillings to four guineas. And for midwives trained under the 1902 Midwives Act, a range of from 10 shillings to 21 shillings per case was possible.[16] Thus,

---

[15] J. Donnison, *Midwives and Medical Men. A History of Inter-Professional Rivalries and Women's Rights* (New York, 1977), p. 208, n. 66; J. Towler and J. Bramall, *Midwives in History and Society* (1986), p. 114.

[16] E. Roberts, *A Woman's Place. An Oral History of Working-Class Women, 1890–1940*, (Oxford, 1984), p. 225; J. Lewis, *The Politics of Motherhood* (1980), p. 141; Donnison, *Midwives and Medical Men*, p. 216 n. 37, p. 59; Towler and Bramall, *Midwives*, p. 172;

old wives were cheaper than professional female midwives, and the latter were cheaper than male doctors, the so-called man-midwives. In part this was because, as Moscucci argues, medical practitioners had been concerned to keep midwives out of the better remunerated practice.[17] Not only relative fees but other factors need to be brought into the analysis when looking at the choices that mothers made as to which type of practitioner to choose for the birth of their baby.

Women as patients

Before discussing the evidence it is useful to look briefly at some of the issues posed in an extensive literature. The historiography of women as patients has tended to become polarised: medical histories emphasised clinical progress, heroic endeavours of male doctors, and ensuing benefits to women,[18] whilst modern feminist accounts have highlighted the sexual politics of sickness and the exploitative, self-interested nature of doctors' interventions.[19] Early feminist work was valuable in indicating that the supposedly neutral values of positivistic medicine were laden with cultural as well as scientific assumptions, but as the complexities of the historical record have become more apparent a more nuanced and balanced interpretation is beginning to emerge. Here women are not mere victims or male doctors simple oppressors.[20] This part of the chapter attempts to contribute to this third category of historical writing by using a liberal feminist viewpoint to look at three topics; childbirth, surgery and invalidism. Why have these been selected? Childbirth was an ambiguous event at the conjunction of the natural/physical, the healthy/ill, the social/cultural. In a radical feminist interpretation the incursion of the male accoucheur has been depicted as a 'cultural subjection of women', in

---

F. B. Smith, *The People's Health* (1979), p. 44; M. Chamberlain, *Old Wives Tales* (1981), p. 111.

[17] O. Moscucci, *The Science of Women. British Gynaecology 1849–1890* (Cambridge 1990), p. 71.

[18] For example, H. R. Spencer, *The History of British Midwifery, 1650–1800* (1927) and J. M. Kerr et al, *Historical Review of British Obstetrics and Gynaecology 1800–1950* (Edinburgh, 1954).

[19] For example, B. Ehrenreich and D. English, *For Her Own Good. 150 Years of the Experts' Advice to Women* (1979); H. Roberts, ed., *Women, Health and Reproduction* (1981); A. Oakley, *The Captured Womb* (Oxford, 1984).

[20] For example, Moscucci, *The Science of Women*; A. Wilson, 'Participant or Patient? Seventeenth-Century Childbirth from the Mother's Point of View', in R. Porter, ed., *Patients and Practitioners. Lay Perceptions of Medicine in Pre-Industrial Society* (Cambridge, 1985).

which reproductive autonomy is surrendered.[21] Here, an alternative historical interpretation is suggested that, whilst offering a critique of certain aspects of male medicine, yet recognises some strengths, and also acknowledges the role that women themselves played in such medicalisation. The second topic selected for discussion, that of breast cancer, was the most frequent kind of major surgery attempted before anaesthesia, and in extreme form offers an opportunity to test a view of woman as clinical object. The third selected topic, female invalidism, is of obvious relevance in this chapter's wider discussion of woman as practitioner, since the cultural construction of female frailty was relevant to contemporary attempts to open the medical profession to women.[22] My interpretation suggests that whether as patron, participant or patient, women's roles were complex; common situations dictated by gender, when mediated through variable status, income and class, might result in highly differentiated experiences. Female perceptions of health or sickness and medical diagnoses of women's illness were not necessarily congruent. Lay and professional perspectives clashed most obviously over childbirth; greater symmetry was evident over surgery, while the ambiguous area of female invalidism illustrated interconnecting interests, that were as much harmonious as antipathetic. Neither the medical conspiracy models of much feminist writing, nor the unproblematical accounts of medical progress as seen in traditional historiography, provide adequate explanatory models for these three topics.

Returning to the first theme – that of mothers in childbirth – it is clear that attitudes of genteel women became increasingly favourable to male practitioners assisting at the birth of their children. In 1812 it was reported that 'Anne Norma is in the family way ... she wishes to have every thing done in the newest and most approved style. She is determined on employing Henry as her accoucheur.'[23] Why was there this decided preference amongst some women for male assistance? In part it seems to have been a self-sustaining trend. The consultant midwife, Sarah Stone, wrote as early as 1737 that it had become customary for 'pregnant women to bespeak them, [i.e. men] so that it is become quite a fashion', and she blamed this on credulous midwives who called in male help when no such assistance was needed, thus

---

21 For example, A. Oakley, *Women Confined. Towards a Sociology of Childbirth* (New York, 1980), pp. 7–9.
22 A. Digby, 'Women's Biological Straitjacket' in S. Mendus and J. Rendall, eds., *Sexuality and Subordination* (1989).
23 Somerset RO DD/8AS TN 54, Letter from Henry Norris to his sons, 4 March 1812.

devaluing their own skills.[24] Certainly, women having a difficult childbirth did call in the male doctor. In 1785 Mary Noel wrote that Lady Gally 'has been terrible bad, and in the greatest danger, which I myself in my private opinion attribute to her having an old woman at first.' Then 'the most excruciating pain' forced her to send for the esteemed male accoucheur Dr Denman, who also called in another fashionable colleague, Dr Ford, to help him.'[25] The perception that male doctors were superior to female midwives was founded on a belief that the former could intervene more effectively, if difficulties arose, through their ability to use forceps. Was this belief justified?

The basis of the claim for male participation in midwifery came from their monopoly of surgical instrumental skills. During the seventeenth century these had been used to deliver dead babies, but during the following century an improved forceps enabled them to deliver live ones with abnormal positions, thus substantially increasing the potential practice of the eighteenth-century surgeon. Georgian midwives criticised surgeons for their alleged enthusiasm for forceps intervention: Elizabeth Nihell considered that they were operating 'weapons of death', whilst Sarah Stone concluded that 19 out of 20 women delivered with forceps could have given birth without their aid.[26] During the Victorian period statistics suggest that there were considerable differences among male practitioners. In mid-nineteenth-century Norfolk, for example, the Norwich surgeon, J. G. Crosse, used the forceps for 1 in 55 cases, whilst a Cromer colleague, Earle, deployed them in only 1 in 135 cases. In contemporary maternity institutions less use was apparently made of them: 1 in 472 births in the Edinburgh Maternity Hospital or 1 in 322 in the Royal Maternity Charity, London. However, the figures may not be a valid basis for comparison, since the Norfolk surgeons were likely to have been called to attend more difficult domiciliary labours, whereas the institutional figures were likely to cover a more even spread of normal and difficult cases.[27]

Paradoxically, in view of the allegations made against men-midwives by female midwives, eminent Georgian male practitioners – Smellie, Denman, Hamilton and Hunter – tried to discourage their

[24] S. Stone, *A Complete Practice of Midwivery* (1737), pp. ix–x.
[25] M. Elwin, *The Noels and the Millbankes. Their Letters for 25 Years* (1967), p. 269.
[26] J. H. Aveling, *English Midwives, their History and Prospects* (second edn, 1967), pp. 109, 122.
[27] E. Copeman, ed., *John Green Crosse. Cases in Midwifery* (1851) pp. 7, 9; W. O. Storer, ed., *J. Y. Simpson's Obstetric Memoirs and Contributions* (2 vols., Edinburgh, 1855) I, p. 854. These figures relate only to forceps intervention and therefore exclude use of the crochet etc.

pupils from an over-zealous use of instruments in normal childbirth.[28] William Hunter warned his students, 'my opinion is 19 out of 20 [cases] had been better left alone. For my practice I have not taken with me a pair of forceps for these ten years.'[29] Students were also advised that it was the parturient mothers themselves who begged for surgical intervention.[30] Surgeons varied in their response to this situation, as a comparison of the late-eighteenth century case notes of the Lincolnshire surgeon, Matthew Flinders, with those of his Essex contemporary, Richard Paxton, indicates.[31] It is also instructive to compare the practice of Paxton with that of the experienced Somerset midwife, Sarah Stone. Stone used manual methods in her consultancy practice in the Bristol area between 1702 and 1736, whereas Paxton deployed instruments. In other respects their case notes showed similar responses to such difficult occasions as breech presentations, and each showed sensitivity in having regard to the wishes of the mother.[32] For example, Paxton wrote of a case where he was summoned to a dying woman who had been three days in childbirth. 'The poor woman herself begged to be delivered, and after giving such an opinion it ought not to be ignored ... She bore the whole with great resolution and expressed great pleasure at being delivered.'[33] Stone repeatedly refers to 'poor women' under the care of ignorant midwives, and gave advice to her 'sisters professors in the art of midwifery.' For one case of normal childbirth she described how 'I put the woman on a stool ... [for] I don't approve of compelling women to any particular place against their inclinations.'[34]

In acquiring a more intimate knowledge of the mother a midwife was advantaged by her gender. A male practitioner was sensitive to the delicacy of his new position, and professional manuals warned that he must 'never violate the trust reposed in him, so as to harbour the least immoral or indecent design'.[35] The English position in child-

---

28 W. Radcliffe, *Milestones in Midwifery* (Bristol, 1967), p. 38; T. Denman, *Aphorisms on the Application and Use of Forceps* (fourth edn, 1793), pp. 9–12; A. Hamilton, *Elements of the Practice of Midwifery* (1775), Introduction.
29 Wellcome MS 2966, Lectures of W. Hunter on obstetrics.
30 Denman, *Aphorisms*, p. 12.
31 Wellcome MS 3820 Case book of Richard Paxton; Lincs. RO, Flinders MS.
32 Wellcome MS 3820 and Stone, *Complete Practice*. Since Paxton recalled only some of his more interesting cases, and Stone selected forty of hers that were most instructive to her readership, it is not possible to make anything other than an impressionistic comparison.
33 Wellcome MS 3820, fos. 50–1, 4 February 1764.
34 Stone, *Complete Practice*, pp. xiv, 133.
35 W. Smellie, *A Treatise on the Theory and Practice of Midwifery* (3 vols., 1752–64), p. 440. See also, Leake, *A Lecture Introductory to the Theory and Practice of Midwifery* (1782), p. 57.

birth, with delivery on the left side, was influenced by prudery and gave less opportunity for observation than did the birth-stools of female midwives.[36] Manuals advised the male accoucheur that 'the pillows ought to be placed in such a manner that the face of the woman, when she is on her left side, may be turned away from where the practitioner is to sit'.[37] Concern over possible accusations of sexual impropriety made Georgian accoucheurs reluctant to propose a vaginal or abdominal examination, or their early Victorian successors to utilise a stethoscope to detect foetal heartbeat.[38] Inability to thoroughly examine the female patient contributed to misdiagnoses. (See Plate 13.) Some female patients were harmed by having 'a pregnancy' confirmed when, in reality, a serious illness was involved. At the turn of the nineteenth century, Lady Charlotte Erskin still had had no child after ten months but continued to be plagued by sickness and backache, whilst Sophia, Lady Curzon was diagnosed belatedly as not *enceinte* but terminally ill.[39] 'To mistake a tumour for pregancy or *vice versa* is one of the most mortifying and personally damaging errors of judgement that can well be', ominously warned one late-Victorian manual. An earlier one cautioned against another misdiagnosis in that pregnant 'women have been supposed to be dropsical and actually tapped.'[40] Practitioners who made such errors were disadvantaged in their practices, as report soon spread. Harriet, Countess Granville, wrote of her prospective accoucheurs, Sir Walter Farquhar and Sir Richard Croft, 'I fear Farquhar and Croft as I do viper and vixen and I shall expire of fright at being left at their mercy.' Since the former had a poor record in managing his aristocratic female patients, and the latter was in charge when Princess Charlotte later died in childbed, such lack of confidence was well-founded.[41]

Given continued social concern about the delicacy of their situation in a lady's chamber,[42] and their reluctance to use their distinctive forceps technique in childbirth, male practitioners were all too conscious that successful competition with female midwives must

[36] Denman, *Introduction to the Practice of Midwifery* (2 vols., second edn, 1794), I, p. 340; Radcliffe, *Midwifery*, p. 91.

[37] A. Hamilton, *A Treatise on the Management of Female Complaints* (seventh edn, Edinburgh, 1813), p. 129.

[38] J. H. Young, 'James Hamilton (1767–1839) Obstetrician and Controversialist', *Medical History*, 7, (1963), p. 72.

[39] Scottish RO GD 253/143/3; Elwin, *Noels*, pp. 187–8.

[40] de Styrap, *Practitioner*, p. 123; R. Gooch, *An Account of some of the Most Important Diseases Peculiar to Women* (1829), pp. 198–9.

[41] B. Askwith, *Piety and Wit* (1982), p. 73.

[42] See, for example, J. Stevens, *Man-Midwifery Exposed* (1862); W. Talley, *He or Man-Midwifery* (1863).

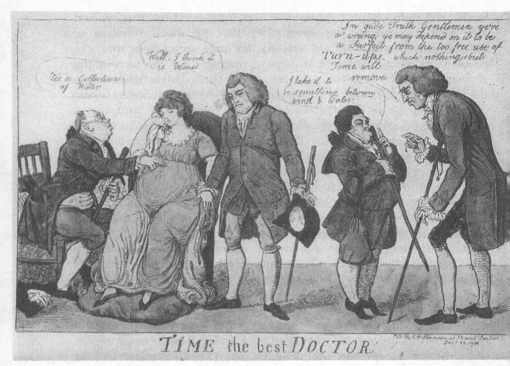

Plate 13　I. Cruikshank, 'Time the Best Doctor' (1804)
The physician prodding the woman's stomach is saying ''tis a collection of
water', another taking her pulse retorts, 'well I think it is wind.' The short
physician says 'I take it to be something between wind & water', and the taller
physician with tartan breeches replies 'in gude truth gentlemen ye're a'wrang,
ye may depend on it to be a surfeit from the too free use of "Turn-ups" which
nothing but time will remove.'

depend in large part on their social skills and professional demeanour.
'The method of pleasing ... ought therefore to make no inconsiderable
part of his character', wrote John Leake in his manual on midwifery of
1782.[43] He suggested that the accoucheur should be 'sober, patient,
and discreet; polite and easy in his address, and of modest and
humane disposition; yet possessed ... of resolution.' Earlier, William
Smellie had emphasised the need for 'natural sagacity, resolution, and
prudence ... together with that humanity ... agreeable to the distressed patient.'[44]

[43] J. Leake, *A Lecture Introductory to the Theory and Practice of Midwifery* (1792), p. 52, 55.
[44] W. Smellie, *A Treatise on the Theory and Practice of Midwifery* (third edn, 1756), p. 440.

The 'art of management' of lying-in women was a topic that took up an increasing amount of space in midwifery manuals of the Georgian and Victorian eras. It is instructive to notice the changing emphasis from a general delineation of the accoucheur's desirable moral qualities, such as those already quoted, to practical instructions on the social niceties to be observed in the lying-in chamber. Whilst it is, of course, impossible to know to what extent this prescriptive advice was heeded, it gives insight into contemporary values. Manuals emphasised the necessity for a confident command of every eventuality. James Blundell advised that if the male accoucheur was visiting his patient for the first time, he should not go straight into the bed chamber but enter an adjoining room and await the nurse. Once he had been admitted, he must use his own judgement as to when it was expedient to remain or to withdraw, but it was essential to stay in the house lest 'you may lose the confidence of the patient.'[45] Significantly, it was suggested that the practitioner should 'regard the feelings of the parturient woman in a degree only secondary to her safety.'[46]

Retaining the patient's confidence might be difficult, since the female lying-in chamber was a foreign land in which language and customs were distinctive; male practitioners had to acquire familiarity with them before attempting to mould the practice to their own preferences. Underlining this sense of gendered space was the custom of referring to the nurse's function as 'guarding the bed'. The young surgeon learned that 'touching' meant a preliminary examination, and 'taking or trying a pain' involved a later one, whilst 'making safe' was removing the placenta, and the bandage tied round the stomach was termed 'a safeguard'. Having acquired this strange language he was then equipped to assess and overturn the alien rituals of traditional childbirth including those of: excluding fresh air, keeping the room warm and dark, or providing 'spiceries'.[47] Having thus taken control of the lying-in chamber, 'It is the province of the accoucheur to assist nature, not to interrupt or counteract her.'[48] However, it was important to be seen to be active, so that, as William Hunter counselled, 'in most cases tho' I pretend to be doing something yet I do very little for them and hardly anything more than to take off one reproach of doing

[45] T. Castle, *The Principles and Practice of Obstetricy by James Blundell* (1834), pp. 214–5.
[46] F. H. Ramsbotham, *Principles and Practice of Obstetric Medicine and Surgery* (1841), pp. 149, 153, 181.
[47] Ramsbotham, *Principles and Practice*, p. 189; T. Castle, ed., *The Principles and Practice of Obstetricy by James Blundell* (1834), p. 217; W. S. Playfair, *A Treatise on the Science and Practice of Midwifery* (1876), p. 338.
[48] Hamilton, *Practice of Midwifery*, p. 273.

nothing at all.'[49] A useful resort in this situation was with 'easy good-tempered firmness' to give orders to the nurse.[50] By Victorian times, she was seen as an assistant to the doctor, rather than a principal in her own right, as earlier midwives had been.

A central aspect of this incursion into the lying-in chamber by male accoucheurs thus involved interprofessional rivalry. Georgian midwives repaid with interest any accusations against them, as in this accusation of 1787. 'Almost every young man, who hath served his apprenticeship to a barber-surgeon, immediately sets up for a man-midwife; [and although] ... much ignoranter, than the meanest woman of the profession ... puts on a finished assurance that their knowledge exceeds any woman's.'[51] Contemporary evidence indicated that inexperienced young surgeons might learn by practising, but with no guarantee of eventual proficiency. A country surgeon wrote in 1775 'Obliged to use the forceps which after several slippings at last proved effectual, she has done well. This is the first case I have had in that end, [i.e. manner] and 'tis likely to produce me some others.'[52] Male practitioners buttressed their own self-esteem by denigrating midwives as lacking proficiency and anatomical knowledge.[53] There may have been some substance in this claim, since it has been calculated that earlier country midwives would have had so few cases that little skill would have been acquired.[54] And leading midwives themselves indicated that ignorance amongst midwives, especially in country areas, was a serious problem.[55]

Midwifery as a skill among male practitioners was even less developed. Social prejudice against it was an important reason for this. Henry Halford, with characteristic snobbery, stated to the Select Committee on Medical Education of 1834 that midwifery:

is considered rather as a manual operation, and ... we should be very sorry to throw any thing like a discredit upon the men who had been educated at the Universities, who had taken time to acquire their improvement of their minds in literary and scientific acquirements, by mixing it up with manual labour.[56]

[49] Wellcome MS 2966, Lectures on Obstetrics.
[50] D. Davies, *Elements of Obstetric Medicine* (1841), p. 189.
[51] Stone, *Complete Practice*, pp. xi-xii.   [52] Lincs RO Flinders MS, fo. 4, March 1775.
[53] For example, Wellcome MS 5103, Thomas Young's lectures on midwifery; J. Leake, *A Lecture Introductory to the Theory and Practice of Midwifery* (1782), p. 54; Copeman, *Midwifery*, pp. viii-ix.
[54] A. Wilson, 'Childbirth in Seventeenth and Eighteenth Century England' (University of Sussex PhD thesis, 1984), p. 125. Wilson suggests annual case loads of twenty in seventeenth-century East Anglia.
[55] Stone, *Complete Practice*, pp. vi-vii.
[56] *Report from SC on Medical Education*, PP 1834, Part 1, p. 17.

Thus persistent prejudice against it as an ungentlemanly subject helped inhibit its inclusion as an examination subject until 1841 at London, 1859 at Cambridge, and 1860 at Oxford. It is salutary to appreciate that midwifery was not an element in nineteenth-century examinations for membership of the Royal College of Surgeons nor for licentiates of the Royal College of Physicians. Indeed it was not until the Medical Amendment Act of 1886 that the subject was included as a necessary qualification to practise. Yet even then, the rules on the number of labours that should be attended during courses could not be complied with in practice, because of shortage of maternity beds and labour cases. Earlier, training opportunities were even more limited, although eight lying-in charities or lying-in hospital wards in London and seven in Edinburgh that were established in the second half of the eighteenth century provided clinical experience. In Georgian London experience could only be gained through becoming a pupil of a leading hospital physician-accoucheur, such as Leake at the Westminster, or Denman at the General Lying-In, Hospital. It followed from this dearth of training that much learning, both clinical and social, was done in later practice. An inexperienced surgeon recorded of a case in the 1760s:

The attempt in this case, made to deliver, it must be confessed, tho' the woman did well, was premature ... could he have commanded the patience of the woman and those about her, he believed he should have waited much longer, but wanting the authority of an old practitioner, he was in some measure forced to act too soon and contrary to his judgement.[57]

Another young surgeon recorded in the following decade that 'I wish I could remember always to turn the head with the forceps 'ere extracting, as I think it would be accomplished easier.'[58]

The range of competence among midwives at least equalled and probably exceeded that amongst surgeon-apothecaries, encompassing as it did not only the skilled and the moderately competent, but the ignorant as well.[59] Britain's provision for the schooling of midwives was less well developed than in France, but in both countries qualified midwives were few in number.[60] An English professional midwife and consultant such as Sarah Stone had a six-year training under her

---

57 Wellcome MS 3820, Paxton casebook, fo. 61.
58 Lincs. RO Flinders MS 1, fo. 4, 18 April 1775. That Flinders used the forceps in 4 out of 44 cases in 1775 may suggest that the leading members were wise to emphasise in their teaching the need for practitioners to refrain from over-enthusiastic intervention in childbirth.
59 For cases of midwives' limititations, see, for example, Wellcome MS 3820, Paxton cases of 4 February 1764.
60 Radcliffe, *Midwifery*, p. 22; Ramsey, *Professional and Popular Medicine*, p. 24.

mother, a practising midwife. In publishing her cases and observations upon them for others to study, she hoped 'that midwives of the lowest capacity may be able to deliver their women, without calling in, or sending for, a man, in every seeming difficulty.'[61] Her London colleague, Martha Mears, also wrote a handbook that was influenced by the teaching of Leake, Smellie, Denman and other male accoucheurs in her criticisms of the customs surrounding traditional childbirth such as spicy caudles and windows shut to fresh air. But she was critical of them in emphasising that birth was a natural event and not 'a state of indisposition or disease.'[62] Lectures were also available to Georgian midwives, like those given by Mrs Margaret Stephens, midwife to Queen Charlotte's Hospital, who offered anatomical instruction and practice on specially constructed 'body machines'. Large provincial towns had similar facilities.[63] Some male practitioners also developed instruction for female midwives, as did John Leake at the Westminster Lying-in Hospital and James Hamilton, Professor of Midwifery at Edinburgh. Hamilton also wrote *A Treatise of Midwifery* specifically for midwives. It was not until 1902, however, that it was enacted that all new midwives must take examinations to become certified, enabling them to become registered and thus authorised to practise.

During the Victorian period midwives had made even slower progress than male practitioners towards professional training, registration and control of entry, and this was due in large part to the latter's opposition.[64] Economic self-interest dictated this hostile stance, although earlier, when medical practitioners were less confident of their competitive power, a *rapprochement* with midwives had seemed a better way both of resolving interprofessional rivalries and, at the same time, of achieving some benefit to the cash ledger. In 1782 Leake cautioned that browbeating of midwives could result in a 'loss of business',[65] and Smellie argued that an uncritical approach would make the female midwife 'more apt to call for necessary assistance on future occasions, and to consider the accoucheur as a man of honour and a real friend.'[66] However, this kind of *modus vivendi* operated only at a personal level. Collectively, male practitioners remained critical of

---

[61] Stone, *Complete Practice*, pp. xvi.
[62] M. Mears, *The Pupil of Nature* (1797), pp. 3–4, 50, 92–3.
[63] Donnison, *Midwives*, pp. 25–8, 40; J. H. Aveling, *English Midwives, their History and Prospects* (second edn, 1967), p. 168.
[64] Donnison, *Midwives*, pp. 177–8.   [65] Leake, *Practice of Midwifery*, p. 33.
[66] A. H. McClintock, ed., *Smellie's Treatise on the Theory and Practice of Midwifery* (3 vols., New Sydenham Society, 1876), p. 432.

female midwifery.[67] The competition of midwives remained unwelcome, and Table 3.1 indicated that confinements where a midwife
had been in attendance earlier were charged double the usual rate by
GPs. (The high charge was also a suitable recompense for what were
often difficult and prolonged cases.)

Male practitioners regarded midwifery with some ambivalence. If
things went well there were, as one Georgian practitioner recollected,
'tedious laborious labours' requiring 'patient management'.[68] But even
'a good natural labour' meant that, as Flinders recorded, 'I got home by
2 in the morn', whilst a difficult one resulted in the surgeon being
'much fatigued, as I had not been in bed or my boots off for 40 hours.'[69]
Despite this, midwifery was recognised as a reliable component in
practice income; time spent in midwifery was a good investment, both
clinically and economically. Medical students were advised that
'Women ... enjoy, and always find time for gossip with one another ...
the ... practitioner ... who has been successful will have the trumpet of
fame sounded with extravagant force.'[70] Equally, the unsuccessful
midwifery practitioner faced professional disaster. Maternal mortality
was very sensitive to the effects of the quality of medical intervention.[71] 'Best estimates' of maternal mortality by Roger Schofield are
of rates that were just under 16 per 100 in the late seventeenth century,
just over 10 in the early eighteenth century, and between 5 and 6 by
the early nineteenth century.[72] In Eccles' view, major causes of a
relatively high rate in the late seventeenth century had been mothers
undelivered because of 'ante-partum haemorrhage, convulsions, dis-
proportion and pelvic deformity, difficult presentations and uterine
inertia', all conditions that female midwives would have been unable
to deal with.[73] Obstetric developments in the Georgian period, notably
the forceps, helped reduce mortality in some of these situations. This
was offset, however, by growing risks of sepsis arising from instrumental intervention, and by increased risks of puerperal fever in
deliveries in hospitals. Florence Nightingale in 1871 criticised a situation where, 'for every two women who would die if delivered at

---

[67] For example, Norfolk RO MS 20795 Letters of J. G. Crosse, 1830–46, fos. 13–5, 26
where horrific cases are described.
[68] Wellcome MS 3820, fos. 58–61, 20 February 1765.
[69] Lincs RO Flinders MS I, fos. 2 an 4, 1775.
[70] The influential gynaecologist, J. H. Aveling, in 1885, quoted in Kerr, *Historical Review*,
p. 317.
[71] I. Loudon, 'Deaths in Childbed from the Eighteenth Century to 1935', *MH*, 30 (1986),
p. 27.
[72] R. Schofield, 'Did the Mothers really Die?', in L. Bonfield, P. Laslett, and R. Smith,
eds., *The World We Have Gained* (Cambridge, 1985), pp. 232, 250.
[73] A. Eccles, *Obstetrics and Gynaecology in Tudor and Stuart England* (1982), p. 125.

home, 15 must die if delivered in Lying-in Hospitals.'[74] Statistics indicated that maternal mortality rates remained at a plateau of between 4 and 5 per 1000 births from 1847 to 1934, before a steep, sustained decline set in. Standards of obstetric practice were crucial in influencing maternal mortality, whilst further improvement awaited the introduction in the 1930s of sulphonamides for the control of puerperal fever.[75]

The actual risks of mothers dying in childbed were not as high as their apprehensions led them to suppose. Traditionally, the mother had been supported by other women in the lying-in room, whereas the employment of a male doctor cut her off from these female networks. Birth had been an all-female occasion in which the husband was excluded, the external world sealed off with every aperture blocked and curtained, and the mother attended by a small group of 'gossips'.[76] This custom was resilient as is shown by a continued attempt by popular medical manuals to supersede it with a situation in which the male doctor was central.[77] Female midwives, such as Margaret Stephens put the case for a retention of lay control, and the preservation of decorum in a traditional female occasion, 'Ladies have been induced to dispense with that delicacy which was their greatest ornament, by the insinuations of designing men, who taught them to believe they endangered their own lives, and that of their children, by employing women.'[78] Interestingly, once the gossips had been displaced from the lying-in chamber, more husbands ventured there; a practice made fashionable among the aristocracy and gentry by Albert's presence at Queen Victoria's accouchements.[79] It was Victoria, too, who had anaesthesia during childbirth and thus encouraged its spread.

Anaesthesia for childbirth had been introduced by J. Y. Simpson in institutional deliveries amongst poor women at the Edinburgh Maternity Hospital in 1847. He had argued that 'the degree of actual pain usually endured during common labour is as great, if not greater, than

---

[74] F. Nightingale, *Introductory Notes on Lying-In Institutions* (1871), p. 68.
[75] Schofield, 'Did Mothers really Die?', p. 254; I. Loudon, 'On Maternal and Infant Mortality 1900–1960', *Social History of Medicine*, 4 (1991), pp. 34–6, 72.
[76] Wilson, 'Participant or Patient?', pp. 129–44.
[77] T. Bull's *Hints to Mothers* (1837) went through 14 editions and emphasised the need to exclude gossiping women.
[78] Quoted in Aveling, *English Midwives*, p. 128.
[79] P. Jalland and J. Hooper, eds., *Women from Birth to Death* (1986), pp. 155–61. W. S. Playfair commented that 'the husband's presence must be left to the wishes of the patient.' (*Midwifery*, pp. 325–6).

that attendant upon most surgical operations.' Some mothers opposed it at first on the grounds that pain during childbirth had been enjoined upon them by Scripture. But most women welcomed this clinical innovation and, according to Simpson, 'set out like zealous missionaries, to persuade other friends to avail themselves of the same measure of relief.'[80] By then, a working-class mother giving birth in hospital had become a patient within a medical institution, and the clinical interests of doctors had become dominant.

Institutional deliveries had been started in order to give medical students and other practitioners clinical knowledge of childbirth. In choosing accommodation and diet that was superior to that in their own homes, with care informed by accumulated expertise, many poor women were likely to have been ignorant of the risks of infection, and hence of the nature of the trade-off they were making.[81] Doctors too were ignorant of both cause and treatment of puerperal fever. Dr Young wrote poignantly of cases of puerperal fever in the Edinburgh Infirmary in 1774 that 'the women were in good health before they were brought to bed.'[82] Women in the infirmary experienced humane treatment, in which sensitivity was shown in making patients comfortable, indulging their requests, and relieving their pain. Most were liberally supplied with opiates, since medical orthodoxy regarded 'the distress and pain which women often endure while they are struggling through a difficult labour ... [as] *beyond* all description.'[83] Once in an institution, mothers might be reluctant to take on the sick-role that was expected in a hospital ward, as is suggested by an unusually detailed description of 40 deliveries in the lying-in ward at Edinburgh. For instance, Ann G., mother of six, clearly felt that giving birth was more a natural than a clinical event. Her case notes read:

This patient was a remarkably strong woman. Within two hours after she had been put into bed and laid quiet after delivery [on 3 January 1794] she was found sitting by the fireside smoking tobacco, notwithstanding the remonstrance of a nurse.

5 January ... Has been out of bed repeatedly since delivery.[84]

[80] RCPL, Royal Maternity Hospital Indoor Case Book; Priestley and Storer, eds., *Simpson*, II, pp. 580, 587, 598, 608.
[81] Between 1757 and 1832 the Dublin Lying-In Hospital had 1488 deaths out of 132,979 deliveries and between 1749 and 1824, the British Lying-In Hospital had 433 deaths out of 33,627 delivered (R. Lee, *Lectures on the Theory and Practice of Midwifery* (1844), pp. 2–3).
[82] C. White, *The Management of Pregnant and Lying-In Women* (1773), letter to C. White in appendix.
[83] T. Denman, Introduction to Midwifery (fifth edn), p. 377.
[84] RCPL, Hamilton MS 9, case of Ann Galloway, January 1794.

Another patient was described as 'so well in every respect that she disappeared from the ward and was found in the wash house washing her own and the child's linen.'[85] These extracts suggest that poor mothers did not share in the medical view of them as patients, and thus were not deemed compliant.

Some other working women also appear to have used medical institutions for their own ends. With only a few pieces of ambiguous evidence, the historian can only speculate about the numbers of spurious patients. A deliberate choice of a sick-role is indicated by two surgical cases at Guy's and St Thomas' Hospitals in the late eighteenth century. Susannah Lee, aged 27, was admitted in October 1785 having stated that in falling downstairs a needle had stuck into her leg, and that she was in great pain because of this. Despite the application of poultices, and an operation to cut tendons to ease her suffering, she continued to ask for her leg to be amputated to stop the pain. The doctors grew suspicious:

1786 The patient wish'd much to have her leg off: from many circumstances it was thought she was an imposter and wished to be got into some charitable house where she might live without labour, and she was therefore discharged.[86]

A few years later, a female patient complained of the stone and 'was tied [down] for the operation', but the surgeon, on examining her, 'found her vagina full of pieces of coal, introduced for the purposes of imitating the presence of calculus in the bladder.'[87] Given that these two women were volunteering for very painful and high-risk surgical operations, performed without the benefit of an anaesthetic, some 'hysterical' elements (later termed Munchhausen's syndrome), may well have been present. The existence of 'hysterick' admissions – as entries in the patients journals of eighteenth-century hospitals, and these more plentiful amongst women than men – may possibly indicate similar cases.[88]

---

[85] RCPL, Hamilton MS 9, case of Mary Smith.
[86] Brotherton Library, University of Leeds, MS 560, Notes of Richard Hey, 1785–6.
[87] RCSL, MS of Alexander Marcet (1804–17).
[88] For example, Devon RO, HR1, Patients Journal, Devon and Exeter Hospital, 1753–61; RCPL, MS 4337, Notes taken at St Bartholemew's Hospital, 1778–81, entry for Jane Wray. Hysteria was such an ambiguous state that contemporary practitioners disagreed both as to its nature and its treatment. Contrast, for instance, Denman's view of 'an hysteric affection not worthy of regard', with Hamilton's assertion that hysterical complaints were a 'very curious disease [which] appears in such a variety of modifications in different individuals.' (T. Denman, *Midwifery*, p. 304 and Hamilton, *Female Complaints*, pp. 46–7) See also J. M. Peterson, 'Dr Acton's Enemy: Medicine, Sex and Society in Victorian England', *Victorian Studies*, 29 (1986), p. 577.

Reluctance to contemplate more than minor surgery was common before the mid-nineteenth century, when anaesthesia made operations more bearable. Medical manuals emphasised that the end of the childbearing years marked a time when tumours and cancers of the breast became more common.[89] Surgery for breast cancer was the most frequent of the few major operations attempted before anaesthesia,[90] so that it is a topic that gives good insight into women's relationships with surgeons. Significantly, in view of the stereotypical view of the surgeon as interested in technique but viewing patients as mere clinical material, objects more than subjects, surgeons seem to have recognised the special dread that breast cancer posed for women. A sympathetic surgeon reflected that 'we know the patient's mind is always anxious about any tumour situated there, and she is always attending to it and handling it.'[91] Surgeons might also be distracted by women's cries of agony during mastectomies.[92]

Georgian surgeons preferred conservative treatment using a variety of caustics to dissolve the tumour, and applying soothing salves, or anodynes to relieve the pain. Even when the practitioner might consider surgery a more suitable course, these were occasionally persisted with, because of the fears of the patient. Monro recorded that;

she absolutely all the while refused to let it be cut off ... all the very bad symptoms of an ulcerated cancer [appeared] which in a short time made her so miserable, that she was content to submit to the amputation of the breast, which was done successfully.[93]

The relatively high failure rate of these postponed operations led to a change in medical opinion which increasingly favoured surgery as a first option. Disagreement persisted over whether it was best that the tumour should be excised, or the whole breast cut off, but by the Victorian period there was a preference for a mastectomy.[94] By this time what had earlier been seen as orthodoxy was now interpreted as quackery. A Norwich surgeon wrote irritably of a woman who had placed herself under an 'ignorant fellow (a labourer) in Horstead who applied caustics and brought the disease into its present formidable state.'[95]

Whether through ignorance, dread of major surgery, fear of de-

---

[89] S. Mason, *The Philosophy of Female Health* (1845), p. 3.
[90] Crosse, *J. G. Crosse*, p. 55.
[91] Norfolk RO MS 20789, fos. 179–80, Crosse's surgery cases.
[92] *Works of Monro*, II, p. 49.
[93] *Works of Monro*, p. 485.
[94] D. Davies, *Elements of Obstetric Medicine* (second edn, 1841), p. 526.
[95] Norfolk RO MS 20795, Crosse correspondence, fo. 81.

formity, or apprehension of painful terminal illness, women preferred to ignore indications of their predicament. Of women admitted to the Middlesex Hospital Cancer Ward with breast cancer between 1805 and 1916, only seven per cent were seen within six months of discovering their condition, and a further 22 per cent between six and twelve months of this. Amongst the remainder, 12 per cent delayed action for more than five years.[96] In the 1860s Elizabeth Woodhouse was described by a house surgeon at the Norfolk and Norwich Hospital as a 'jolly fat looking woman with an enormous tumour of the right breast which has been growing 15 years', and was now the size of her head. Also to the same hospital came a mother of six, Hannah Parsons:

About 12 months since she noticed a small knot at the upper part of the left breast ... in six months it increased to the size of a nut and became extremely painful and has gradually attained its present size which is that of a large egg.[97]

Surgeons disagreed on the prognosis for those who had undergone a mastectomy.[98] It was easy to give an over-optimistic picture since all too often surgeon and poor patient lost contact, whilst hospital records typically recorded the outcome as 'cured' or 'relieved', without reference to a more long-term outcome. Occasionally, a fuller picture was given, and this is illuminating in showing that readmissions occurred for further removal of nodules and tumours.[99] Surgeons thought it important to spell out risks (even when antisepsis and anaesthesia had reduced them) and get the patient's informed consent to an operation, as in this case of 1879:

The woman, her husband, and her friends having been informed of the dangers of the operation, but that an operation was the only curative means that could be employed, expressed her wish to have the operation.[100]

In the era before anaesthesia, accounts of public mastectomies of poor women in hospital suggest the rapidity of the operation, the professional self-confidence of the surgeon, and the endurance of the patient. Harriet Melville, operated on by Benjamin Brodie in 1822, sent

96 H. J. G. Bloom, W. W. Richardson and E. J. Harries, 'Natural History of Untreated Breast Cancer', *BMJ*, 11 (1962), p. 215.
97 Norfolk RO MS 49/5, Michael Beverley's House Surgeon's Notes.
98 For example, James Hill disagreed with the pessimism of his old teacher, Alexander Monro, I, (J. Hill, *Cases in Surgery* (Edinburgh 1772) pp. 18–19 and *Alexander Monro*, pp. 490–1).
99 Norfolk RO MS 49/5 Michael Beverley's Notes on Anne Brand, Susan Chapman and others.
100 Wilts. RO J6/196/3, Surgeons and Doctors Consultations at Savernake Cottage Hospital, 1873–9, case of Mary Ann Orchard, 3 October 1879.

a cousin into hysterics and drove her husband out of the house, with her 'awful screams'.[101] In 1811 Fanny Burney had felt 'condemned' to a mastectomy and that her doctors had 'pronounced my doom'. During the twenty-minute operation she 'began a scream that lasted unintermittently during the whole time of the incision'; so 'excruciating was the agony' as 'the dreadful steel was plungd into the breast.' For months afterwards she felt sick whenever she recollected her ordeal.[102] It thus took a particularly depressed individual, such as Alice James, to actually welcome a diagnosis of breast cancer after an adult life of continuous invalidism.[103]

Social and medical perceptions of the division between female health and sickness were not so much a finite boundary as a broad zone whose fluid, permeable extent was shaped as much by expectation, fashion and individual circumstance as by objective, scientific knowledge. Between the Georgian and Victorian period medical men changed their views on this frontier; a more robust view of women's health tended to be displaced by a biological reductionism that identified femininity with invalidism. The interpretation of one well-known Victorian medical manual was that a woman's life was 'a long chain of never-ending infirmities.'[104] Economic pressures – particularly evident when there was an overstocked medical profession – provided a sectional rationale for this, whilst limitations of medical knowledge inadvertently reinforced it. A more general social assumption followed in that 'every woman is … more or less an invalid.'[105]

Earlier, during the second half of the eighteenth century, Georgian practitioners had adopted a confident tone in arguing that what the female sufferer might construe as illness could, by effective management, soon be translated into health. In London, William Hunter took a comparable line in lecturing medical students that 'hysterics are best managed by strengthening medicines … try everything that tends to brace and strengthen.'[106] In the Lake District, William Brownrigg treated both Mrs Christian and Mrs Milham along lines which, in addressing both psychological and physical symptoms, aimed to restore each to a vigorous health. And in the Midlands, Erasmus

[101] E. M. Thornton, *Marianne Thornton. A Domestic Biography* (1956), p. 134.
[102] J. Hemlow, ed., *'Journals and Letters of Fanny Burney'* (Oxford, 1975), vol. v, pp. 600–8. Since Burney survived for 30 years after the operation, some have questioned whether her tumour was benign, rather than malignant.
[103] L. Edel, *The Diary of Alice James*, (New York, 1964), p. 14.
[104] E. J. Tilt, *On the Preservation of the Health of Women* (1851), p. 70.
[105] J. M. Allen, 'On the Differences in the Minds of Men and Women,' *Journal of the Anthropological Society of London*, 7 (1869), p. cxcc.
[106] Wellcome MS 2966, Lectures on Obstetrics, 1775–83.

Darwin had earlier prescribed a comparable regimen for Miss Ryder's debility, morbid feelings and hypochondria in advocating that 'all those means should be used, which can strengthen her general system [and] . . . whatever can amuse [or] employ her.'[107] Of the nervous and digestive ailments of Mrs Cochrane, the Scottish consultant William Cullen stated that 'I am persuaded that by good management such trouble may be prevented or, when it happens, easily cured', Good management involved exercise, warm clothing, sensible rest and a moderate diet suited to the peculiarities of her digestion, and Mrs Cochrane 'must by this time know her own [digestion] and govern herself accordingly.' Similarly, Mrs Innes's fears of uterine cancer were dismissed as merely 'nervous or hysteric', Cullen arguing that 'with a little good management she may enjoy very good health.'[108]

In counselling one young patient to adopt a healthy regimen Cullen suggested to her that 'I would have her avoid physicians and apothecaries who will give her drugs.'[109] Whilst this reflected Cullen's well-known preference for regimen over physic, it may also have been an early warning signal that medical practitioners were stimulating female hypochondria and invalidism from financial self-interest. This was to become all too obvious later and to attract censure from the Victorian medical élite. Sir Anthony Carlisle, President of the Royal College of Surgeons, stated that obstetrics 'leads to *unlimited power* in every family and thence to lucrative ends. Women are peculiarly exposed, during the most important office of their existence, to the menaces of more knowing persons.'[110] And Sir Thomas Allbutt indicted some gynaecologists in 1884, 'Arraign the uterus and you fix in the woman the arrow of hypochondria it may be for ever.'[111] Twelve years later, Allbutt and another leading specialist in women's diseases, Playfair, went further in referring to the 'adventurousness' and 'unbalanced zeal' that had led to 'injudicious practice' by specialists in gynaecology.

Frequent childbearing did place immense strains on many women's health, and there is no suggestion here that the physical justification for medical intervention was lacking. Reading about Georgian cases (when doctors were not concerned to inculcate but rather to combat invalidism) provides convincing evidence of this. They indicate the

---

107 King Hele, *Erasmus Darwin*, letter to Lady Harrowby, 21 May 1796; Carlisle Library E 104, Case Book of William Brownrigg, 1737–41, cases of Mrs Christian and Mrs Milham in the 1740s.
108 RCPE, Cullen 30/1, fos 28–30, 39.
109 RCPE, 31/2, correspondence, June–October 1775.
110 Quoted in Talley, *Man-Midwifery*, p. iv.
111 Quoted in H.D. Rolleston, *Sir Thomas Allbutt. A Memoir* (1929), p. 87.

kind of problems that female sufferers faced, which contributed to their decision to become patients. For example, 'her constitution . . . has been much debilitated by the further pregnancies and abortions [i.e. miscarriages] which she has experienced.' Or, from Scotland, 'her Ladyship has borne her children [so] fast that she has ... never recovered her former strength' and ran 'a most imminent risk of totally ruining her constitution.'[112] Medical support might be welcomed in such cases, and be beneficial to the patient. What was problematical, however, was the extent to which some Victorian medical men encouraged women to adopt a superfluous invalid role.'[113] I have argued elsewhere that this was evident in the practice of some Victorian and Edwardian gynaecologists and psychiatrists.[114]

Vigorously promoted views of innate female incapacity produced a general psychological climate in which women doubted their own physical capabilities, and hence the possibility of engaging in a more demanding role in society. One wrote:

I think those who insist on ignoring the very weakness which you so fully allow, are really running counter to Nature's clearest indications and are perverse in wishing women to go at men's work till they drop, or at any rate till their poor babies and homes come to grief.[115]

Some gifted women were probably adversely affected by this social climate. Beatrice Webb had constant self-doubts about her health and energy, 'feeling my health diminishing every day', whilst Bessie Rayner Parkes felt that she 'laboured under mountains of difficulty', and George Eliot despaired of her 'want of health and strength.'[116] However, some more robust spirits managed to reject medical orthodoxy:

CAN A NATURAL STATE BE CALLED A STATE OF INVALIDISM? – I have just been glancing at a modern American book, bearing the name of a well-known physician, and treating of the functions and diseases of women, and I have shut it in disgust on finding . . . that women's natural state is that of invalidism, and that all her peculiar natural functions are unavoidably attended with inconvenience and disability.[117]

---

112 Wellcome MS 67582, Dr Baillie to Mr Woolett about his Monmouthshire patient, Mrs Molyneux, 29 October 1807; Scottish RO GD 253/143/2/12 and 52x Letter to Lady Hope, March 1770 and undated note to Sir J. Pringle.
113 Quoted in Rolleston, *Allbutt*, p. 87.
114 Digby, 'Women's Biological Straitjacket'.
115 British Library MS 46235, fo. 240, Lucy Cavendish to Mary Drew, 27 November 1858.
116 N. and J. MacKenzie, eds., *The Diary of Beatrice Webb, 1873–92* (1982), vol. I, pp. 22, 42–3, 73–4, 91, 121–2, 154, 193, 259: quoted in Ponsonby, *Diaries*, pp. 406–7; Parkes Papers, Girton College Cambridge, BRP Box v/62 15 April 1852 and Box v/106. I am indebted to Jane Rendall for references on Bodichon.
117 E. B. Duffey, *What Should Women Know* (1873), pp. 43–4.

Less common was a strategy of utilising the artificial creation of an invalid state to serve an individual's own social objectives, with ensuing collusion between patient and doctor to maintain it. An invalid state had attractions for a woman who wished to create a private space to escape from the pressures of bourgeois society, with incessant demands of family life involving responsibilities for childcare or household management. Florence Nightingale's adoption of the sick-role on her return from the Crimea was a deliberate device to isolate herself from her family, thus enabling her to carry on her professional work. That of Elizabeth Barrett may well have been an unconscious response to unendurable family tensions.[118] These women achieved an invalidism that was socially approved, not only because such a role was compatible with Victorian bourgeois ideals of femininity but also because it was financed privately. In contrast, working women's attempts to adopt a voluntary sick-role tended to fail; not only did this go against social perceptions of their destiny but, in utilising public funds for personal ends, it was regarded as fraudulent.

This discussion of women as patients suggests that medical practitioners had a genuine concern for their female patients, although their strong financial and clinical interests translated people into cases. (See Plate 14.) Women patronised male medical practitioners to an increasing extent, but might be reluctant to avail themselves of advances in medical technique on the terms offered to them: in childbirth, women wished to benefit from forceps deliveries but showed some reluctance either in the domestic lying-in chamber or in institutions to change from participant to patient in ceding control to the male practitioner. Women sufferers with breast cancer showed a preference for conservative medical methods over radical surgical ones, but found less space to negotiate their viewpoint in the professional terrain of operative surgery. However, surgeons showed sympathy with their patient's feelings and clearly did not regard them simply as clinical material. In invalidism, shared ignorance, and therefore a less unequal relationship, made possible a variety of encounters that ranged through deception by the patient to manipulation by the practitioner, and on to the possibility of mutually beneficial collusion. Gender dictated common situations for women, but their social class differentiated the treatment that they received. This did not always discriminate against the poor woman, since she could benefit from

---

[118] C. Woodham Smith, *Florence Nightingale, 1820–1910* (1950), pp. 303–4; E. Berridge ed., *The Barrettts at Hope End. The Early Diary of Elizabeth Barrett Browning* (1974), pp. 18, 41–2.

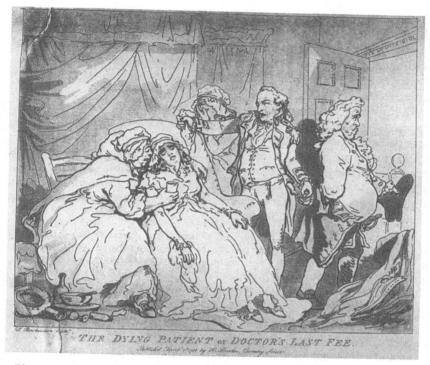

Plate 14   T. Rowlandson, 'The Dying Patient or Doctor's Last Fee' (1786)

earlier hospital facilities, which were often associated with those for children.

Children as patients

Children were seen as a desirable part of a medical practice by the mid-to late-nineteenth century, making up as much as one-third of the Victorian practitioner's patients.[119] However, this situation was comparatively recent; earlier, parents viewed practitioners as ill-qualified for dealing with their offspring, whilst in turn doctors viewed the child as a particularly difficult subject. Whereas a case history could be developed through questioning an adult patient, for the young patient the doctor was forced to formulate a diagnosis from examination, close

[119] C. West, *Lectures on the Diseases of Infancy and Childhood* (London, 1848), p. 1. West was Senior Physician to the Royal Infirmary for Children, and one of the founders of the Great Ormond Street Hospital.

observation, and comparison with similar cases. Whether children had distinct diseases, or merely needed different treatment, was a subject of continued speculation and debate. The necessity for extreme care with dosages of powerful drugs was also recognised, whilst certain drugs and applications were acknowledged to be unsuitable for children.[120]

There was a well-founded perception that children were neglected by the Georgian medical faculty.[121] George Armstrong, who in 1769 founded the first dispensary for sick children in Europe, wrote that 'I know there are some of the physical tribe who are not fond of practising among infants' because 'they are not capable of telling their ailments; and therefore, say some, it is working in the dark.'[122] Such anxieties persisted, and Charles West warned his medical audience in 1848 that they would encounter:

a difficulty that disheartens many, and makes them abandon in despair the study of children's diseases. Your old means of investigating diseases will here to a great degree fail you, and you will feel almost as if you had to learn your alphabet again ... You cannot question your patient; or if old enough to speak, still, through fear, or from comprehending you but imperfectly, he will probably give you an imperfect reply.[123]

What reassurance could specialists in childhood diseases offer their colleagues? Armstrong assured his colleagues in 1771 that 'the very symptoms themselves will, for the most part, speak for them, in so plain a manner as to be easily understood.'[124] In 1830 Miles Marley counselled a reliance on close observation in making a diagnosis of the young, 'they have a language which may always be interpreted ... such are the countenance, the expression of the eye, the numerous gestures and cries ... the appearance of the tongue and skin, the secretions, excretions etc.'[125] As with female patients, practitioners felt

---

120 J. F. Goodhart, *The Diseases of Children* (third edn, 1888), p. 13. Goodhart was Physician to the Evelina Hospital for Sick Children. Such recommendations had a wider currency in household manuals, for example, *The Household Encyclopaedia or Family Dictionary* (1858), vol. 1, p. 426. See also Dr Robert Darwin's prescriptions in the Receipts and Memoranda MSS of the Darwin Family, in Cope, *Invalid*, pp. 150–1.

121 W. Buchan, *Domestic Medicine* (second edn, 1772), p. 6. See also, J. Clarke, *Commentaries On Some Of The Most Important Diseases Of Children* (1815), p. 31 for similar sentiments.

122 G. Armstrong, *An Essay on the Diseases Most Fatal To Infants* (second edn, 1771), pp. 4–5. The first edition of the essay appeared in 1771, and the third in 1808, which indicates its continued popularity. See also, F. N. L. Poynter, 'A Unique Copy of George Armstrong's Printed Proposals for Establishing the Dispensary for Sick Children, 1769', *Medical History* (1957).

123 West, *Lectures on Childhood*, p. 2.   124 Armstrong, *An Essay on Infants*, p. 7.

125 M. Marley, *On the Nature and Treatment of the Most Frequent Diseases of Children* (1830), p. iv.

that within the sickroom of the child patient they were entering a foreign territory. 'You will feel ... as if, entering a country whose inhabitants you expected to find speaking the same language ... you observe manners and customs such as you had never seen before.'[126] In consequence – as with female patients – a distinctive 'bedside manner' for children was developed. Medical students in 1888 were advised not to frighten the child: to take time so that the child became accustomed to the doctor, and also so that the child could play with an instrument before it was used.[127] Even more persuasively, a specialist advised that 'if you are not fond of little children' you would not be successful. The practitioner needed to cultivate a gentle and quiet way of approaching and talking to the young patient. Good management, good temper and patience facilitated accurate observation; for example amusing the child with a watch whilst performing a brief examination.[128] Several visits were needed where one would have sufficed for an adult patient. These concerns are remarkably similar to those of modern paediatricians except that now more reliance is placed on questioning the parent during the examination of the child, and on eliciting more details about the child's family and environmental background.[129]

Perceptions of childhood illness and knowledge about it developed rather slowly in England.[130] This was not only a result of the practitioners' tardy recognition of their ability to treat children, but also because of British social custom. Until the end of the eighteenth century and beginning of the nineteenth century, wet-nursing practised away from the home for infants of the affluent meant that early childhood illnesses were not a matter of immediate anxiety to the parent, and thus did not result in the doctor being called into the household.[131] In addition, few Georgian hospitals would treat very young children, although dispensaries would see them.[132] However, there were five paediatric texts written by British authors in the seventeenth century and more followed in the eighteenth. In some of

---

[126] West, *Lectures on Childhood*, p. 2.   [127] Goodhart, *Diseases of Children*, p. 3.
[128] West, *Lectures on Childhood*, pp. 4–5.
[129] See, for example, H. Jolly, *Diseases of Children* (third edn, 1976) Chapter 1 *passim*.
[130] The first children's hospitals in Europe preceded those in England by several decades in the nineteenth century, whilst even in the twentieth century professional organisation lagged behind that in Europe and the USA; the British Paediatric Association was not founded until 1928.
[131] V. Fildes, *Wet Nursing. A History from Antiquity to the Present* (Oxford, 1988) p. 190; V. Fildes, *Breasts, Bottles and Babies* (Edinburgh, 1986), pp. 121, 182.
[132] J. B. Davis, *A Cursory Inquiry into some of the Principal Cause of Mortality Among Children* (1817), p. 25. Davis was *inter alia* the founder and Physician to the Universal Dispensary for Sick Infant Cildren, St Andrew's Hill, London.

Table 9.4. *Deaths of children aged 1–14 years from certain causes, in 1911–15 and 1970–74*

Illness	1911–15 Rate per million	1970–74 Rate per million
Pneumonia and bronchitis	1464	43
TB	887	1
Diphtheria	447	0
Accidents	353	133
Measles	936	2
Whooping cough	385	0
Gastroenteritis	488	9
Appendicitis	76	3
Cancer[a]	46	69
Diseases of the ear	48	1
Rheumatic fever[a]	67	0
Scarlet fever	189	0

Note: [a] In the case of rheumatic fever the figures are not strictly comparable because of changes in classification, and in the case of cancer, it is possible that this was under-diagnosed at the earlier date.
Source: *Fit for the Future. The Report of the Committee on Child Health Services* (1976), vol. 1, p. 41.

these texts Georgian doctors tried to make sense of infant disease by postulating a common cause for them: this was glandular secretions in Armstrong's view, or acid stomach in Cadogan's.[133] Diseases were sometimes conflated together: commonly measles and scarlet fever were confused, as were the lesions of congenital syphilis with scurvy or rickets. Many of the conditions of children appear to have been as common in the past as the present (such as thrush or colic), whilst familiar problems such as dentition might cause serious anxiety, since concurrent convulsions arising in reality from another illness might be conflated and thus the death of the infant be attributed to teething problems. Other common afflictions in the past such as worms are, however, much less familiar today.[134] The most striking difference was, however, the large impact of infectious diseases on childhood mortality in the Georgian and Victorian ages, a scourge that has been greatly diminished during the mid-twentieth century. Table 9.4 shows

[133] Armstrong, *An Essay on Infants*, p. 20; W. Cadogan, *An Essay upon the Management of Children* (tenth edn, 1777).
[134] S. X. Radbill, 'Paediatrics', in A. G. Debus, ed., *Medicine in the Seventeenth Century* (Berkeley, 1971), pp. 250–1, 257–63, 270, 272.

Table 9.5. *Deaths^a in infancy and childhood, in 1911 and 1974*

	Age Under 1	Age 1–4	Age 5–9	Age 10–14
1911	130.1	17.68	3.42	2.05
1974	16.3	0.65	0.31	0.28

Note: ^a Rates for those under 1 year are per 1000 live births and, for those above that age, they are per 1000 population.
Source: Fit for the Future. The Report of the Committee on Child Health Services (1976), vol. 1, p. 41.

the very marked decline in the impact of infectious diseases upon the death rate in childhood between the end of our period and the 1970s. Table 9.5 indicates very strikingly the decline in deaths in infancy and childhood during the twentieth century. Without these figures it is difficult to appreciate just how much of a historical problem was serious illness in infancy and early childhood.

As medical students, Georgian and early Victorian doctors gained only a partial insight into childhood diseases. Lectures on this topic followed those on obstetrics, and were seen as an adjunct to midwifery rather than an independent specialism.[135] For example, W. Hunter dealt in this way with rickets, red gum, sore eyes, gripes, fits and convulsions, inoculation, teething, and 'scabby face'. By the mid-nineteenth century such cursory treatment was thought to be inadequate by paediatric pioneers, such as Charles West, to whom the illnesses of childhood were a medical specialism. He gave a series of lectures solely on the diseases of infancy and childhood.[136] The advent of specialist children's hospitals advanced knowledge of paediatrics. The Physician to the Samaritan Free Hospital of Women and Children wrote of the clinical interest of young patients in so far as they facilitated an ideal pathology, 'seeing disease, as it were, unrestrained and free', and without the complications of worn adult tissues and organs.[137]

Broader social, cultural and economic changes had by this time led to a growing value being placed upon child health. Mercantilist fears about a possible population decline in the mid-eighteenth century had

[135] For example, Wellcome MS 2966, W. Hunter's Lectures on Obstetrics and Royal College of Physicians, Edinburgh, James Hamilton MS 5, Heads of Lectures on the Diseases of Infancy and Childhood, 1815.
[136] West, *Lectures on Childhood*, p. 2.
[137] W. H. Day, *Essays on the Diseases of Children* (1873), pp. 1–2.

led earlier to anxieties over the high mortality of children. The modernization process involved a requirement for better general health care of a more scientific nature, and a reliance on specialists to provide it, had contributed to the growth of medical philanthropy. Specialist foundations for children were outside the mainstream of the institutional foundations; Armstrong's Dispensary for the Relief of the Infant Poor lasted only until 1782, and closed because of 'lack of public interest and support.'[138] That dispensaries for children met a longer-term need, however, is suggested by their growth. In the metropolis there were the Dispensary for the Relief of the Infant Poor (1769), J. B. Davis's Universal Dispensary for Sick Infant Children (1816),[139] the Royal Western Infirmary for Children (1820), and the Kensington Dispensary and Children's Hospital (1840), and in the provinces a dispensary for women and children was founded in Cheltenham (1817), and others in Manchester (1829), and Liverpool (1851).[140]

In a sentiment ahead of its time, Armstrong had preferred an out-patient dispensary to an in-patient hospital because it meant that a child would not be separated from a parent which would 'break its [sic] heart immediately.'[141] It is interesting to see that an institution which apparently bridged the earlier dispensary movement with the later specialist children's hospitals – the Kensington Dispensary and Children's Hospital (founded 1840) – allowed visiting of its in-patients on any day between 2pm and 4pm. However, this concern to preserve the contact of parent and child was not generally shown by later Victorian hospitals for children which (driven by a confidence in medical hegemony reinforced by fears of cross-infection, or of upsetting the child), usually limited visiting to the same very restricted hours applicable to those of adult patients. By the end of our period, for instance, the Hospital for Sick Children in Great Ormond Street allowed visiting only from 2 pm to 3.30 pm on Sundays, whilst the East London Hospital for Children stated that 'No visiting allowed except in cases of grave illness.'[142] This may have contributed to parental boycotts.[143]

138 Loudon, 'Dispensary Movement', *BHM*, 55 (1981), p. 323; E. Sadler, 'An historical survey of children's hospitals', in Granshaw and Porter, *Hospital in History*, p. 184.
139 This later was built in 1902 as the Royal Waterloo Hospital for Children and Women, and is now part of St Thomas's Hospital.
140 A. W. Franklin, 'Children's Hospitals' in F. N. L. Poynter, *Hospitals*, pp. 114–15. In 1857 the Liverpool Dispensary expanded and took in-patients, thus becoming a children's hospital.
141 G. Armstrong, *A General Account of the Dispensary for the Relief of the Infant Poor* (1769), p. 13.
142 *Burdett's Hospitals and Charities* (1919), pp. 267, 265, 253.
143 M. Newby, 'Children's Nursing in the 19th century', paper given at the Wellcome Unit, Oxford, 10 March 1988.

Not until the 1930s were mothers allowed to stay with their children in hospital.[144]

Even before the inception of specialist child institutions general hospitals had provided in-patient treatment, but only on a restricted basis. Guy's Hospital admitted children to the women's wards from its foundation in 1722, and in 1833 created a children's ward.[145] Others had taken children, but only those over the age of six in the case of the Norfolk and Norwich Hospital or, more usually, at seven (the age adopted at Exeter, Chester, Taunton and elsewhere).[146] For accident and surgical cases, however, these rules were relaxed. For example, Alfred Hubbard, aged two years, had a cataract removed in the Norfolk and Norwich Hospital in May 1827.[147] And child accident cases were admitted in quite large numbers as in-patients by hospitals.[148] It was partly through the perceived inadequacies of meeting the special needs of children in a general mixed institution, and partly the example given by European pioneering hospitals, that contributed to the inception of specialist hospitals for children in mid-nineteenth century Britain.[149] Table 9.6 indicates that most English children's hospitals were built within a few decades between the 1850s and the 1880s. Significantly, this period witnessed the height of medical entrepreneurialism in the foundation of specialist institutions of all kinds. These were seen as a good way to advance individual doctor's career prospects, when posts at general hospitals were difficult to obtain.[150] The creation of the Children's Hospital at Great Ormond Street in 1852 provided a model and stimulus for imitation.[151] The difficulties that had been encountered in general hospitals were not immediately overcome for child in-patients in specialist establishments, however,

---

[144] The first institution to allow this was the Babies Hospital in Newcastle (U. Ridley, *The Babies Hospital, Newcastle* (Newcastle, 1956), p. 15).

[145] *Fit for the Future. The Report of the Committee on Child Health Services* (HMSO, 1976), p. 60.

[146] Norfolk RO, MS 564, Rules and Orders for the Norfolk and Norwich Hospital, 1804, rule XLVIII; Devon RO, HS 1, Statutes and Rules of the Devon and Exeter Hospital, 1743; Chester RO, H1/316, T. Crane, *The Statutes of the General Infirmary at Chester* (1763); Somerset RO, D/P/bh/13/10/3/SAS TN 54, Annual Reports of the Taunton and Somerset Hospital, 1828, 1832; *Rules and Orders of the Hospital for the Small-Pox and Inoculation* (1786), pp. 12–3.

[147] Norfolk RO, MS 20789, Norfolk and Norwich Hospital Surgical Cases, 1826–8.

[148] For example, 'the vast numbers of boys injured by machinery' stated to be in the Leicester Infirmary in 1850 (Leicester RO, Leicester Infirmary House Visitors Reports, 1826–1850, entry 2 December 1850), or those admitted to the Walsall Cottage Hospital under Sister Dora's care (J. Manton, *Sister Dora* (1971), pp. 240–1).

[149] Sadler, 'An historical survey', pp. 185–8.

[150] Granshaw, 'Fame And fortune' in Granshaw and Porter, *The Hospital*, p. 206.

[151] C. West, *On Hospital Organisation with Special Reference to the Organisation of Hospitals for Children* (1877).

Table 9.6. *The growth of children's hospitals*

Dates of foundation	London	Provinces
Before 1850	2 (2)[a]	1
1850s	1	5 (3)
1860s	6 (1)	8 (1)
1870s	3	5
1880s	2	4 (1)
1890s	1 (1)	1
1900s	1	-

Note: [a] Figures in brackets refer to the number of children's institutions which also catered for women patients.
Source: Analysis of entries in *Burdett's Hospitals and Charities* (1919).

especially in problems of infection. There was also a continued short-age of children's nurses who could provide the high ratios necessary in a patient-orientated specialism.[152] This influenced the age of entry as an in-patient in the new children's hospitals, with two years as the most common lower limit, although a few had infancy or one year.[153] It is interesting to see that one outcome of their success in treating young children was that general hospitals began to take children from two years of age, and also began to set up children's wards, as at Exeter in 1860.[154] A few children's hospitals with paediatric specialisms followed.[155]

Unlike the general hospitals for the adult population, those for children did not rely on subscribers' letters as a means of limiting the numbers of their patients. Instead they either admitted on the basis of the urgency and/or seriousness of the illness, as did the Edinburgh Infirmary, or enquired into the financial means of the family, as did Birmingham.[156] It is also important to appreciate that in several crucial respects children's hospitals were similar to adult hospitals in that they treated the *poor*, and that they had much larger numbers of out-patients than in-patients. Children's hospitals, aware of the prevent-

152 Birmingham Children's Hospital (founded in 1862) found that it had to set up its own Nurses training Institution for this purpose in 1868 (R. Waterhouse, *Children in Hospital. A Hundred Years of Child Care in Birmingham* (1962), p. 91).
153 *Burdett's Hospitals and Charities* (1919). A patient ceased to be a child at twelve years in most institutions, but there was a range from ten to fifteen, and with girls commonly being taken up to an age two years beyond that specified for boys.
154 Davis, *A Cursory Inquiry*, p. 25; Russell, *Exeter Hospitals*, p. 68.
155 A. W. Franklin, 'Children's Hospitals', pp. 118–19. The Infants Hospital later became part of Westminster Hospital.
156 Waterhouse, *Children in Hospital*, pp. 40–1.

able nature of much childhood illness, used out-patient clinics as a valuable means of educating mothers. They issued 'Rules for the Management of Children' which stressed the need for cleanliness, warmth and fresh air, and gave guidance on infant feeding and weaning.

The forty specialist hospitals for the care of children created during the nineteenth century had important implications for professional prospects. Over 500 posts, most of them consulting or visiting ones, were attached to these institutions by the end of the Edwardian period. In the provinces each hospital had – on average – some nine posts attached to it, whilst in London that number doubled.[157] Some of these posts were held by those having office at the local general hospital. For example, S. T. Taylor, who was at the Norfolk and Norwich Hospital, also saw child patients at the Jenny Lind Hospital for Children. 'Saw 15 patients at Jenny Lind and 7 at the Hospital' was a typical entry in his medical diary.[158] Most children's hospitals found difficulty in recruiting specialist physicians, as did Birmingham, so that GPs were employed.[159] Offices at a hospital were divided between the few resident medical officers, who were salaried young doctors, and the majority of unpaid, honorary positions to which more senior members of the profession were elected.

An honorary appointment at a children's hospital could have a beneficial impact on the growth of private practice in treating children of middle- or upper-*class* families. Practice with children, as has been indicated above, might be expected to make up one-third of a general practitioner's workload, not least because of the youthfulness of society. *Census* returns show that in 1851, 40 per cent of the population of England and Wales was aged fourteen or under, compared with only 22 per cent a century later.[160] However, it might be thought that the decline in completed family size from 6 children (for those marrying in the 1860s) to 3 (for those marrying in the 1900s) would have had a major impact on midwifery. That this was not the case towards the end of our period was the result of a continued general population increase.[161] And the illnesses of infancy continued to pose a very real threat to life. Infant mortality remained obstinately high: the infant

---

[157] Analysis of entries in *Burdett's Hospitals and Charities* (1919).

[158] Norfolk RO, MS 2437 Medical Diary of S. T. Taylor, 1882–8, fo. 26.

[159] Waterhouse, *Children in Hospital*, p. 83; H. Rolleston, 'The Changes in the Medical Profession and Advances in Medicine during the last 50 Years', *BMJ* 23 July 1932.

[160] Mitchell, *British Historical Statistics*, p. 12.

[161] D. Gittins, *Fair Sex. Family Size and Structure, 1900–1939* (1982), p. 188. The population of England and Wales increased from 20.1 million to 36.1 million between 1861 and 1911.

mortality rate was 148 deaths per thousand in 1860–12, and still 146 in 1900–2, before eventually beginning the modern decline and falling to 110 in 1910–2. (For comparison, the figure in 1986 was 9.4).[162] Thus, a central reason for the importance of paediatrics in general practice was the character and frequency of childhood illness.

Charles West (later one of the founders of Great Ormond Street Hospital for Sick Children), told his medical students in 1848 that the seriousness of children's diseases meant that 'one child in five dies within a year after birth, and one in three before the completion of their fifth year.'[163] Smallpox, measles, scarlet fever, whooping cough, convulsions, gastroenteritis and TB were then serious and common afflictions of early childhood. West counselled his students 'You must visit your patient very often ... New symptoms succeed each other in infancy and childhood with great rapidity ... The issues of life and death often hang on the immediate adoption of a plan of treatment ... Do not wait, therefore, for symptoms of great urgency before you visit a child three or four times a day.'[164] Household budgets give a good indication of the financial implications of this since it was mainly in households with young children or with pregnant and nursing mothers that, in middle-class households, regular and specific sums for the doctors' visits were included in the annual budget. This testifies to the importance of the child patient in a medical practice's economic viability.

The vulnerability of infant or child health caused continued concern to parents and doctors responded to this by providing attendance, strategic interventions, and advice manuals. Doctors both allayed such fears, and were able to benefit from them professionally, by offering prescriptive advice. Georgian practitioners suggested, for example, 'Avoid giving any Quack Medicine – for fear of bringing on decline or sudden death.'[165] They were also adamant about when – in the course of advancing illness in the child from bad breath, through restlessness, and loss of appetite, to the onset of definable ailments – it was thought essential to specify the occasions 'that require all the skill of the good physician.'[166] Apart from the normal attendance given to a child patient, doctors were also active strategically in matters of public health; notably their activity in inoculating – and later vaccinating –

---

[162] R. Mitchison, *British Population since 1860* (1977), p. 50; *Social Trends* (HMSO, 1989), p. 117.
[163] West, *Lectures on Childhood*, p. 1.   [164] West, *Lectures on Childhood*, p. 10.
[165] 'Rules for Domestic Management of Young Children', caution number vi, in J. B. Davis, *A Cursory Inquiry, into some of the Principal Causes of Mortality among Children* (1817).
[166] Cadogan, *An Essay*, p. 8.

Expanding practice with women and child patients   289

children against smallpox.[167] Practitioners varied the charges according to the income of their patients. In 1819, Blackburn doctors agreed to charge from five shillings to one guinea for vaccination, whereas in the 1830s practitioners in Newcastle and Gateshead were recommended to charge from five shillings to two guineas.[168] Later, as vaccination became more commonplace, fees appear to have diminished since the BMA's recommended scales in the 1870s were from two shillings and sixpence to three shillings and sixpence for the poorer patient and then up to one guinea for the wealthiest.[169] Whereas the parents of middle- and upper-class children were convinced of the utility first of inoculation and later of vaccination, popular prejudice among the poor continued, so that public interventions were needed. After the success of the Sutton family in inoculation during the 1760s, some Georgian surgeon-apothecaries were employed by parish poor-law overseers to inoculate groups of children, although the geographical extent of this practice remains problematical.[170] The Victorian state legislated to remedy the low take-up of vaccination in 1853, when it became compulsory for infants before the age of three months. Fees of from 1s 6d to 2s 6d per head paid from this mass vaccination became a significant item in the remuneration of those doctors who served as medical officers under the New Poor Law.

Another source of employment and income for doctors came from appointment as school medical officers. The development of free and compulsory attendance for elementary schoolchildren between 1870 and 1891 had meant that the indifferent health of many children came fully into public focus for the first time. How could such unhealthy children benefit from public schooling? These anxieties were reinforced by Social Darwinist concerns for national efficiency and hence the health of the nation – more specifically the physique of the young. As a result of these concerns a Medical Officers of Schools Association was created in 1884, and in 1907 a national School Medical Service was established. In three out of four local education authorities the office of School Medical Officer was combined with that of MOH and, in one in four, it was held in conjunction with that of Public

---

[167] Lincs RO, Flinders MS, fo. 27, December 1777; RCSL, Edward Rigby to Charles Murray, 13 January 1812.
[168] *Rules and Regulations Agreed and Entered into by Medical Gentlemen of Blackburn* (Blackburn,1819); *Lancet* 15 January 1830.
[169] *Tariff of Medical Fees* (Shrewsbury 1870 and 1874).
[170] Razzell and Thomas argue that inoculation was a relatively widespread practice. See P. Razzell, 'Population Change in Eighteenth-Century England: a Reappraisal', *Economic History Review*, 18 (1965); E. G. Thomas, 'The Old Poor Law and Medicine', *MH*, 24 (1980).

Vaccinator.[171] Salaries for this part-time employment as School Medical Officer ranged from £50 to £150 per annum;[172] a useful supplement to the basic income derived from being MOH, or from private practice. More significantly, the influence of the medical profession was correspondingly enhanced. The duties of School Medical Officers ranged from a minimalist situation in some areas (where they only inspected a minority of children to check whether they were really unfit to attend school), to that in others (where all children were inspected periodically with attention being given to eyes, ears, teeth and general physique.)[173] The School Medical Service was one area to which female entrants to the Edwardian medical profession turned.

Women in the profession

One of the principal objections to women's incursion into Victorian medicine was 'What is to become of the men, if women crowd into this already overcrowded profession?'[174] (See Plate 15.) Not only did medical women appear to have a natural affinity for the care of young children, but contemporaries also suggested that women would prefer to be treated by one of their own gender.[175] Why was this? Not only were there moral arguments concerning delicacy, but claims that 'doctresses' possessed greater manual dexterity, and also caused less anxiety than would a male physician when dealing with female patients.[176] In this context it is important to appreciate the *economic* implications for male colleagues of women entrants to what was an increasingly over-stocked medical market in the late nineteenth century. It was the threat to the pocket, as well as the challenge to patriarchal ideas on the fit and proper place of bourgeois women in Victorian England, that made the arguments against female entrants to the profession so heated. At a meeting of the Obstetric Society of London, which turned down Garrett Anderson's application for membership, J. H. Aveling roundly declared that 'if there is one occupation for which they are less fitted that another, it is that of attending to the

---

171 *Annual Report of the Chief Medical Officer of the Board of Education for 1910*, Cd 5426, PP 1910, xxIII, pp. 192–3. *The Report on British Health Services* of 1937 indicated that at this date only 275 of 1458 school medical officers were full-time appointments.
172 *Interdepartmental Committee on Inspection and Feeding of Children*, Cd 2779, PP 1906, xLVII, Appendix v, pp. 406–35.
173 *Committee on Feeding of Children*, p. 13.
174 E. Davies, 'Medicine as a Profession for Women', a paper read at the Social Science Congress, June 1862, reproduced in C. A. Lacey, *Barbara Smith Bodichon and the Langham Place Group* (1987), p. 412.
175 For example, E. Davies, Female Physicians, *English Woman's Journal*, May 1862.
176 A London Physician, *Men-Midwives and Female Physicians* (1864), pp. i, v, vi.

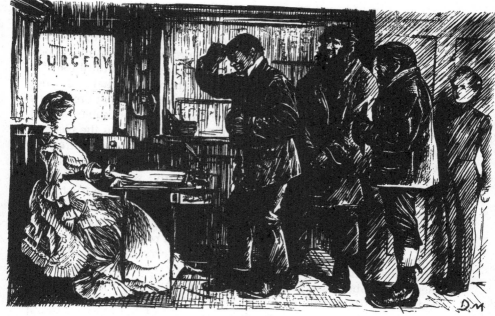

OUR PRETTY DOCTOR.

Dr. Arabella. " WELL, MY GOOD FRIENDS, WHAT CAN I DO FOR YOU ¦"
Bill. " WELL, MISS, IT'S ALL ALONG O' ME AND MY MATES BEIN' OUT O' WORK, YER SEE, AND WANTIN' TO TURN AN HONEST PENNY HANYWAYS WE CAN; SO, 'AVIN' 'EARD TELL AS *YOU* WAS A RISIN' YOUNG MEDICAL PRACTITIONER, WE THOUGHT AS P'RAPS YOU WOULDN'T MIND JUST A RECOMMENDIN' OF *HUS* AS NURSES."

Plate 15   'Our Pretty Doctor' (*Punch*, 1870)

emergencies of obstetric practice.'[177] This warmth of feeling was
mirrored in professional handbooks which spoke of 'the profane
attempt of ambitious women to enter the sacred precincts of the
medical profession', and of the way in which medical women had
'opened the door to further trouble and given grave offence.'[178] In
turn feminists accused male doctors of restrictive practices. Frances
Power Cobbe declared that 'Never, indeed, has there been a more
absurd public manifestation of trades-unionism than this effort to
keep ladies out of the lucrative profession of physician and crowd
them into the ill paid one of nurses.'[179]

The attempts by women to acquire formal medical training in the

[177] *Transactions of the Obstetric Society of London*, 16 (1875), p. 75.
[178] Rivington, *Medical Profession*, pp. 135–6; Dale, *Medical Profession*, p. 5.
[179] Cobbe, 'Medicine and Morality', p. 323.

1860s and 1870s have been well documented.[180] Much less appreciated is that opposition continued to be felt in relation to choice and progress in women's later medical careers. One indication of this was the tardy recognition of women as doctors in professional groups, which preferred to keep such bastions as male preserves. It took until 1892 for the British Medical Association to modify its rules so that it did not exclude women,[181] and until 1908 for the Royal Colleges of Physicians and Surgeons to admit females.[182] There was a noticeable lack of women on hospital boards, boards of examiners, and on the General Medical Council. Handbooks advising entrants to a medical career were masterpieces of professional doublespeak in discussing it as a possible career for women. Most significantly, women graduates' attempts to gain worthwhile employment continued to be frustrated. For example, when Miss Murdoch Clark was appointed as Junior House Surgeon to the Macclesfield Infirmary in 1902, six honorary surgeons resigned from the infirmary. After six months, in which time it proved impossible for the infirmary to carry on surgically, the unfortunate Clark was forced to give up her post.[183] Not only were there notorious cases like this but, more routinely, women had to endure discrimination. In public health women had lower pay and worse conditions of service, whilst those wishing to enter general practice normally could do so by taking assistantships at a very low salary, or for room and board.[184]

An early female MD, Louisa Martindale, considered that the 'chief disability' of women in medicine was 'professional isolation'.[185] How then did medical women cope with this situation? First they formed professional groups and started professional journals specifically for women. These not only acted as support groups for building up solidarity and an *esprit de corps*, but also gave an opportunity for airing grievances and sharing problems, as well as giving an opportunity for older, more successful professional women to give helpful advice to their younger colleagues. They also gave an opportunity for women to discuss clinical matters of interest, since they found it difficult to receive serious attention in the mainstream journals. Examples of

---

180 For example, J. Manton, *Elizabeth Garrett Anderson* (1965); E. Moberley Bell, *Storming the Citadel* (1953); P. Chambers, *A Doctor Alone: a Biography of Elizabeth Blackwell* (1956).
181 It had inadvertently admitted E. Garrett Anderson and then altered the regulations in 1878 so as to specifically prohibit women.
182 *Medical Women's Journal*, 18 (December 1908), p. 258.
183 *Women's Medical Journal*, 12 (January 1902), p. 8.
184 *Medical Women's Journal*, 28 (December 1921), p. 307; *Medical Women's Federation Newsletter* (July 1928), pp. 85-6.
185 L. Martindale, *The Woman Doctor and her Future* (1922), p. 85.

professional journals included the *Medical Women's Journal,* and the *Medical Women's Federation Newsletter.* Of equal importance was the formation of the Association of Registered Medical Women of the UK.

All-female institutions such as the New Hospital for Women, which was founded in 1872, were important in offering posts for pioneering women in specialisms that were difficult to enter in male-dominated institutions. Elizabeth Garrett Anderson, for example, undertook surgical (as well as medical) work there, operating 'in a variety of gynaecological cases, fibroid of uterus, prolapsus, cancer, imperforated vagina, mammary abcess, ovarian tumour, and fistula.'[186] Significantly her first public post was at the St Mary's Dispensary for Women and Children that she had been prominent in founding.[187] Other early institutions that offered a monopoly of employment to legally-qualified medical women included medical charities in Notting Hill, West Kensington, Manchester, Leeds and Edinburgh.[188] One may speculate that such institutions were also important in providing an environment in which women could be comfortable and relaxed professionally, and where they were not perpetually having to 'prove themselves' to sceptical male colleagues.

Women GPs specialised in the treatment of female and child patients. Yet few women were able to enter general practice. One may conjecture that this was partly because of male principals' prejudice against female partners, and also because medical women themselves preferred other options, especially work in the community. Elizabeth Garrett Anderson, when reviewing the employment of 144 women on the *Medical Register* of 1892, suggested this when she hoped that women 'had given good service to the community.'[189] Their choices of career was more limited than that of their male counterparts. Table 9.7 illustrates this in giving the appointments of a small sample of Edinburgh medical women. They entered public medical positions in large numbers; predominantly these were those with low prestige and low salaries. It is interesting to see that one-fifth of these appointments were in institutions catering solely for women or children. And, even when posts were obtained in more general establishments, it is probable that women specialised in treating female patients, as in lunatic asylums or medical missions. Arguably, at least one in three public

---

[186] Manton, *Garrett Anderson,* p. 230.
[187] Also significant was the fact that Garrett Anderson was the first woman to hold an honorary hospital post and that this was in the East London Hospital for Children.
[188] *Report of RC into Medical Acts,* PP 1882, xxix, p. 442 (evidence of E. Garrett Anderson).
[189] *Westminster Review,* March 1893.

Table 9.7. *Employment of Edinburgh medical women graduates, 1902–4*

Type of employment	Number of posts	% of posts
Private practice	2	5
Work with women	3	7
Medical missions	4	9
Work with children	5	12
Lunatic asylums	5	12
MOH	6	14
General hospitals	9	21
Specialist institutions[a]	9	21
N	43	101

Notes: [a] Specialist institutions included dispensary (2), hospice (2), sanatorium (1), isolation and fever hospital (3), and workhouse (1).
Source: Analysis based on recent appointments of Edinburgh medical graduates reported in *Women Students Medical Magazine* (Edinburgh 1902–4).

appointments taken up by medical women had a paediatric or female specialism. Interestingly, an analysis of Glasgow women medical graduates' first posts in 1898–1900 and 1908–10 revealed a similar concentration of appointments in asylums, dispensaries and poor-law infirmaries.[190] Women soon established a reputation in public appointments so that demand sometimes exceeded supply, as had occurred by 1900 with graduates of the School of Public Heath at the London School of Medicine for Women.[191] They thus moved swiftly into expanding openings in public medical services that were so characteristic of the late nineteenth and early twentieth centuries. One of these offices was that of School Medical Officer, created in 1908. Table 9.8 indicates their numbers in England one year after the post was created; six female appointments were to that of principal School Medical Officer, and a further 62 appointments were to assistantships. Thus, one in eight of the total 986 were at this time held by women.[192] This enthusiasm for the school medical service among women further increased the weighting of their work with child patients.

The first woman to qualify in England, Garrett Anderson, skilfully reviewed the situation in 1896:

---

[190] W. Alexander, *First Ladies of Medicine. The Origins, Education and Destination of Early Women Medical Graduates of Glasgow University* (Wellcome Unit for the History of Medicine, Glasgow, 1987), p. 43.
[191] London School of Medicine, *Annual Report*, 1900.
[192] *Interdepartmental Committee on the Inspection and Feeding of Children*, Cd 2779, PP 1906, XLVII, pp. 192–4.

Table 9.8. *Female assistant school medical officers, 1909*

Type of area	Full-time	Part-time	Total
Counties	23	13	36
County boroughs	10	5	15
Non-county boroughs	5	1	6
Urban districts	5	-	5
N	43	19	62

Source: Annual Report of the Chief Medical Officer of the Board of Education, Cd 5426, PP, 1910, XXIII, p. 194

About thirty-five years ago a movement was initiated which had two objects in view. It aimed at enabling women to obtain, if they desired it, medical advice from qualified practitioners of their own sex, and at enabling such women as were able and willing to go through a long and severe professional training to earn their living in a way not hitherto open to them ... The two things hung together, if medical women were welcomed they would be employed, and if employed a new and large field of professional work would be open to women.[193]

Garrett Anderson's own career in her work as a consultant and GP indicated the unmet demand for women in this role. Personal recommendation from one family to another operated with her, as it had traditionally done with male colleagues. Female patients were reassured in presenting their intimate ailments to another of their own gender. But, irrespective of sex, the success of a doctor was the outcome of personality as well as of technical skills, and Garrett Anderson scored highly in terms of good judgement and a warm humanity.[194] She thus met the social expectations of patients. Mindful of this she ironically instructed students at the London School of Medicine for Women that 'the first thing that women must learn is to behave like gentlemen.'[195] Female practitioners only gradually established themselves but, by the early twentieth century it was stated somewhat over-optimistically that, 'In every large, provincial city we find her established, busy and respected, and of her occupying positions as honorary physician or surgeon on the children's or women's hospital.'[196]

[193] *Times*, 11 December 1896.
[194] Manton, *Garrett Anderson*, pp. 264, 266.
[195] Garrett Anderson's dictum as Dean of the School, quoted in Manton, *Garrett Anderson*, p. 311.
[196] Martindale, *Woman Doctor*, p. 84.

PART IV

Synthesis

Reflections

This final chapter selects important topics that have been discussed earlier in separate chapters and attempts to synthesise and interpret them. In order to place this in a wider perspective some additional empirical material is introduced and new conceptual material also assists in arriving at an overall interpretation.

The control of the medical market by practitioners was crucial in the process of professionalisation, as Friedson has emphasised.[1] In this context, what has been called 'patient-centred medicine' as well as 'illness-centred medicine' was of importance.[2] Medical sociologists have criticised present-day doctors in their encounters with patients for their preference for illness-centred medicine. This has allegedly resulted in a lack of 'deep-listening' to what the patient is actually trying to communicate, an exclusive attention to the symptoms being presented, and hence an outcome in the form of a diagnosis of physical illness, with the doctor's accompanying hope of a speedy cure.[3] In the past, doctors were patient-centred to a much greater degree and this was linked to more limited therapeutic power.[4] It was also related to their need to win acceptance and trust by the patient in a medical market where there was an abundance of practitioners and a paucity of paying patients. Patient-centred medicine attached great value to the art of healing; patients were perceived as more than malfunctioning systems or diseased organs. Encounters – more specifically those with more affluent patients – were less a process than a relationship, which involved a matching of doctor and patient

---

[1] E. Friedson, *Profession of Medicine* (New York, 1975).
[2] M. Balint, *The Doctor, His Patient and the Illness* (1964).
[3] Balint, *Doctor*, pp. 121–4, 257; E. J. Cassell, *Talking with Patients* (2 vols., MIT, 1985), I, p. 14; P. S. Bryne and B. E. Long, *Doctors Talking to Patients* (DHSS, 1976), pp. 5–7.
[4] Shorter, *Bedside Manners*, pp. 21–3.

expectations in the nature and outcome of the consultation. Rapport, sensibility, empathy and effective communication characterised a doctor skilled in the art of medicine, who was thus enabled to win the patient's confidence. The 'traditional' patient responded with trust, truthfulness, and compliance. But this stereotype effectively ignores the time-pressures the doctor encountered with most patients. In perpetuating a view of an unequal power relationship between doctor and patient, it also underplays the patient's autonomy in choosing from a wide range of strategies in maintaining health or overcoming sickness.

A crucial conceptual distinction between the patient-role (in which professional help is sought) and the sick-role is relevant here. Adopting a sick-role usually meant exemption from normal social or work obligations and, in this context, some have argued that patients are deviant since, in becoming sick or dysfunctional, they are not fulfilling their role in society. Towards the end of the period the doctor took on important 'gatekeeping' reponsibilities in policing such a system, through providing certification for insurance companies, friendly societies, or the national health and unemployment insurance scheme. However, a sick-role may be claimed without seeking the aid of a doctor. Historians of medicine have argued that there is a key distinction to be made between sufferers and patients. Whether sufferers decided to become patients and place themselves under regular practitioners was influenced historically by an evolving state of medical authority.

Expectations of patient and doctor were not necessarily symmetrical, although the most well-known models of their relationship emphasise precisely this aspect of the encounter. Complementary expectations and attitudes between doctors and patients arising from their respective professional and lay backgounds were postulated in Parsons' structuralist view.[5] A more individualistic model by Szasz, Hollander and Knott was one that advanced a hypothesis influenced by psychoanalytical insights. This interpretation put forward an evolutionary view with the earliest stage being one of activity by the doctor, and passivity by the patient; a second stage also posited unequal powers, with guidance and leadership allegedly provided by the doctor and obedience and admiration by the patient; and the third

[5] T. Parsons, *The Structure of Social Action* (New York, 1949); *The Social System* (1951); 'Illness and the Role of the Physician: a Sociological Perspective', *American Journal of Orthopsychiatry*, 21, (1951); T. S. Szasz, W. F. Knott, and M. H. Hollander, 'The Doctor-Patient Relationship in Historical Context', *American Journal of Psychiatry*, 115 (1958), p. 525.

stage – reached at the turn of this century – was one of mutual participation and interdependence between practitioner and patient.[6] This interpretation is poorly defined historically but the specification of relationships between doctor and patient is of use here.

This model will be applied to the material discussed in *Making a Medical Living* in order to gauge how well it fits the complexity of past problems. Other interpretations are also tried to see whether these are more realistic historically. In the context of this volume, it is obvious that the encounters postulated in the model are too neatly complementary, a feat achieved through over-emphasising the patient's passivity. This ideal type most forcibly outlined in the first type of doctor activity and patient passivity, broadly corresponds to the kind of encounters discussed in Chapter 8, in which poor patients (male and female) – dependent on charitable, voluntary or statutory bodies for their medical welfare – were usually (although not invariably) compliant. But even in the hospital, where the poor were viewed as clinical objects, patients showed a reluctance to obey institutional rules and attempted to manipulate doctors, indicating that social control was not wholly effective. However, the child patients discussed in Chapter 9 fit more easily into this category of patient passivity, as do adult patients undergoing major surgery, discussed in Chapters 8 and 9. In contrast, the activity of affluent patients correlates more positively with that of the third, or modern model of doctor-patient relationships. Nevertheless, it was suggested in Chapter 7 that the doctor was more capable of independent initiative in encounters with élite patients than a simple patronage model indicated. Class is important in looking at female patients where middle- and upper-class patients fit most appropriately into the second type of relationship put forward by Knott, Szasz and Hollender – that of guidance and cooperation. This cooperation between women and their doctors is one that has been relatively neglected in feminist analysis which, particularly in its earlier phases, has preferred to emphasise the economic exploitation of female bodies by male practitioners.[7] Chapter 9 argued that in reality other therapeutic benefits for patients were involved, but also acknowledged that within a medical market a financial imperative was important in the expansion of practice with women (as with child) patients.

[6] T. S. Szasz and M. C. Hollender, 'A Contribution to the Philosophy of Medicine. The Basic Models of Doctor-Patient Relationship', *AMA Archives of Internal Medicine*, 97 (1956), pp. 585–92.
[7] Ehreneich and English, *For Her Own Good*, p. 115.

Sufferers and medical authority

The social and cultural context of medical practice is of obvious importance. Earlier Whiggish and medical-centred perspective depicted a 'rapid growth of science during the eighteenth and nineteenth centuries [which] led to the development of the doctor as the expert engineer of the body as machine.'[8] This reflected the contemporary statements of doctors as medical knowledge increased. The *Lancet* remarked optimistically in 1878, for example, that 'The doctor, with the advance of civilisation and of medical science, becomes more and more indispensable.'[9] Viewed from a modern perspective this approach assumes too much about the doctor's curative power, and thus underestimates the importance of the doctor's *caring* role. Until the mid-twentieth century limited healing potential perforce highlighted practitioners' social and empathetic qualities. Expectations and assumptions were important in medical encounters, as Kunitz has pointed out:

We shall never know whether the *placebos* given to our ancestors measurably lengthened or shortened their lives, but surely all the dosing, purging, cupping and bleeding they endured encouraged them to believe that something was being done for them. At least as important, these therapeutic activities allowed physicians to believe that they were effective.[10]

Earlier, in Chapter 3, doctors' self doubts – expressed in the privacy of their casebooks – were cited to indicate that practitioners were not as confident therapeutically as their demeanour to their patients might have indicated. A test of the authority of medicine, however, was the confidence that doctors had in therapeutics when role reversal occurred and they became patients. Henry Sigerist remarked that 'Physicians as a rule, are poor patients, they know too much.'[11] During the eighteenth and early nineteenth centuries doctors were conscious that they knew too much only in the sense that they knew that they knew too little. When sick, their informed calculation of the ration of pain to gain made them reluctant to trust themselves as patients to their colleagues.

Dr Haygarth noted that 'Medical practitioners are exposed to ... danger. They visit patients ill of infectious fevers. Two of my patients,

---

8 Szasz, Knott, and Hollander, 'The Doctor-Patient Relationship', p. 525.
9 *Lancet*, i, 1878, 19 January 1878.
10 S. J. Kunitz, 'The Personal Physician and the Decline of Mortality', in Schofield, Reher and Bideau, *The Decline of Mortality*, p. 249.
11 Quoted in M. Pinner and B. F. Miller, eds., *When Doctors are Patients* (New York, 1952), p. 3.

who were physicians ascribed their infection to short exposure to the poison'.[12] In such a situation practitioners might adopt a therapeutic nihilism. Alexander Monro I, for example, preferred in 1739 to endure what he himself termed such paroxysms of 'sharp pain' on the right side of his face that 'the tears rushed out,' but 'the hope of each fit being the last, made me suffer these periodical pains ten days, without trying to remove them by medicine.'[13] Crosse of Norwich provided the rationale for this in stating that 'It is a matter of common observation, that medical men have, of all persons, the least confidence in physic, no doubt because they have the best opportunities of observing how little it has the power to accomplish.'[14] Doctors were thus intolerant of others' professional inadequacies. Jenner, for instance, grumbled to a colleague that his doctor had been unable to bleed him because he had broken his cupping glasses, together with the points of his lances, and his leeches had died in the cold weather. He concluded, 'Thus, dearest doctor am I treated, worse off by far than a parish pauper.'[15] This self-pity was trumped by Dr Fothergill, who, in similar vein, found the prospect of 'two anatomists' inspecting him quite 'terrible to think of', but bore his ill-health philosophically, 'I am yet alive, tho' not quite well.'[16] In cases of terminal illness in particular, the practitioner needed to compensate for his inability to produce a satisfactory outcome, by bustling activity. Medical practitioners were conscious that drastic therapy in terminal illness was better avoided when they were themselves patients, if not for others in the same predicament. Two days before his death in 1841 Astley Cooper informed the two physicians and three surgeons then in attendance upon him: 'My dear sirs, I am fully convinced of your excellent judgement and of your devotion to me, but your good wishes will not be fulfilled in my case, and you must excuse me, for I will take no more medicines.'[17]

Lay sufferers also did not perceive questions of sickness or of recovery as being in the sole gift of the professional but gave continuing importance to self-management. Remedies were eagerly sought by the literate in journals such as the *Gentleman's Magazine*.[18] With an informed lay public, role reversal could and did occur. For

---

[12] J. Haygarth, *A Letter to Dr Percival on the Prevention of Infectious Fevers* (1801), pp. 40–3.
[13] *Works*, p. 641.
[14] Norfolk RO, MS 470, letter from Crosse to Mr Butter of Kenninghall, 10 April 1825.
[15] RCSL, Jenner correspondence, letter from Jenner to Baron, 7 April 1821.
[16] RCSL, Hunter correspondence, Fothergill to Hunter, 23 July 1778.
[17] Brock, *Astley Cooper*, p. 162.
[18] R. Porter, 'Lay Medical Knowledge in the Eighteenth Century: the Evidence of the *Gentleman's Magazine*', *MH*, 29 (1985), p. 147.

example, in 1793 Samuel Johnson, 'bullied, and bounced and compelled the apothecary to make his salves according to the Edinburgh
dispensatory, that it might adhere better. I have two on now of my
own prescriptions.'[19] He also acted as medical adviser to his relatives,
'I have just now read a physical book, which inclines me to think that
a strong infusion of the bark would do you good.'[20] Indeed, this was a
continuation of an older tradition in which, as Paul Slack has suggested, one use of a vernacular medical literature in Tudor times was
for the lay person to judge physician's expertise and instruct the
physician.[21] In the Georgian period, Enlightenment values emphasising individualism reinforced a propensity to manage one's own
health.[22] Whilst this continued to be seen within a Galenic tradition, in
which the environment was an important influence upon health,
Enlightenment values encouraged a greater readiness by the bourgeoisie, as well as by more élite groups, to enquire into its action.[23]
Every reader of Georgian letters, journals and diaries will be familiar
with their recurrent anxieties about the weather, with sickly summers
preceding ague-prone autumns, which were then followed by wither-
ing winters. Popular prescriptive manuals on domestic medicine also
reflected the same concern. Buchan's ever-popular *Domestic Medicine*
admonished:

Particular constitutions not only dispose persons to peculiar diseases, but
likewise render it necessary to treat these diseases in a peculiar manner ...
Attention ought likewise to be paid to the place where the patient lives, the air
he breathes, his diet, occupation.[24]

Whilst the thrust of manuals was broadly financial, emphasising the
economy to be gained from home management an important outcome
was sustaining the centrality of a home-based regime in health and
sickness. An illustrative extract from the end of our period stated that
'It is quite absurd to suppose that every slight attack of cold or cough
must demand and receive the care of a physician.'[25]

Given the perceived limitations of medical authority, many suffer-

[19] Letter to H. Thrale, 19 June 1783 quoted in J. Wain, *Johnson on Johnson* (1976), p. 190.
[20] Birkbeck Hill, *Johnson*, I, p. 75.
[21] P. Slack, 'Mirrors of Health and Treasures of Poor Men: the Uses of the Vernacular
    Medical Literature of Tudor England' in Webster, *Health, Medicine, and Mortality*,
    p. 260.
[22] R. Porter, 'Medicine and the Enlightenment in Eighteenth Century England', *Bulletin
    of the Society for the Social History of Medicine*, 25 (1979), p. 38.
[23] W. Coleman, 'Health and Hygiene in the *Encyclopédie*. A Medical Doctrine for the
    Bourgeoise' *Journal of the History of Medicine* 29 (1974), pp. 399–421.
[24] W. Buchan, *Domestic Medicine* (second edn, 1772), p. 168.
[25] Walsh, *Domestic Economy* (1890), p. 744.

ers preferred client-led therapeutics. A strong lay culture of healing, with popular faith in a spectrum of remedies, gave confidence in the ability of the sufferer to discriminate appropriately amongst them. Two relatively well-known cases will bear re-examination in this context – Nicholas Blundell in the early eighteenth century and Charles Darwin in the mid-nineteenth century. Their self-management of health involved a highly selective use of orthodox practitioners, side-by-side with an individual set of choices that involved self-medication, use of regimen, and recourse to alternative practitioners. This therapeutic range indicated an absence of confidence in orthodox medicine as the solution to all the ills of the body, and thus a cautious reluctance to cede authority to the practitioner.

Health was perceived as a very serious affair in the Blundell family during the early eighteenth century; it was health not sickness that was central in longer-term concerns. Bleedings, blisterings, sweats and vomits were administered routinely, very much as service checks designed to keep the body ticking over; believing that the body built up a superfluity of toxic humours the Georgian response was to get rid of them periodically through vigorous therapeutic interventions. In the Blundell household bleeding might be done by a layman on a physician's instructions (as for a time by Richard Cartwright, the butler) or by a surgeon or surgeoness.[26] Chronic ailments or a generalised feeling of malaise also merited short trips for sea bathing or journeys to a spa. Significantly, in relation to the family's adherence to an older set of religious beliefs, the Blundells also patronised a holy well in Flintshire. Health maintenance was clearly too vital to be reserved solely for the professionals. Nicholas Blundell recorded that he had 'advised with the doctor about going to the spaws' by which he meant that he had solicited advice but retained his autonomy as a free agent.[27] Like many of his contemporaries, his freedom of action was shown in the apothecary's shop or medicine cupboard in the household, complete with a prescription and recipe book containing some twenty-nine recipes for his eye problems, and the requisite number of gallipots and bottles to house other medicaments. From this store Nicholas treated himself, making up his own eye wash and ointment for his chronically afflicted eyes. He not only treated himself and his immediate family, but also his neighbours and tenants as well.[28]

[26] M. Blundell, ed., *Blundell's Diary and Letter Book, 1702–1728* (Liverpool, 1952), pp. 62, 103–4.
[27] *Great Diurnall*, vol. II, p. 198.
[28] *Great Diurnall*, vol. II, 17 November 1713, 9 September 1714; vol. III, 29 May 1725.

The experience of Nicholas Blundell had strong parallels with that of Charles Darwin, and both were good examples of client-led therapeutics. Darwin was the grandson and son of doctors and had completed two years of a medical training at Edinburgh, all of which seemed to have impressed him with medicine's limitations. Although he made a medical confidant of Dr Hooker and had some initial confidence in doctors, he later became more sceptical. 'I have great faith in [water] treatment, and no faith whatsoever in ordinary doctoring', he remarked in 1856.[29] He stated of his water-cure specialist in 1849, 'I much like and think highly of Dr Gully.'[30] He also asserted that 'Dr Gully feels pretty sure he can do me good, which most certainly the regular doctors could not ... I feel certain that the water-cure is no quackery.'[31] Living with a chronic complaint, however, Darwin became aware that medicine could not effect a cure. Significantly, he commented about Lane that 'in one respect I like him better than Dr Gully, viz that he does not believe in all the rubbish which Dr Gully does; nor does he pretend to explain much which neither he nor any doctor can explain.'[32] His impression that the water cure possessed financial as well as therapeutic dimensions steadily increased. 'Dr Smith ... is very careful in bad illness but he constantly gives me the impression as if he cared much more for the Fee and very little for the Patient', he wrote.[33] Darwin consulted many doctors, but a repetitive pattern developed in which trust and confidence was replaced by doubt and disillusionment.[34] Darwin's growing reservations about the medical faculty meant that increasingly he undertook the self-management of his health. From 1849 to 1855 he kept a *Diary of Health*, which enabled him, through self-observation, largely to undertake his own treatment and management. His diary entries revealed his everyday martyrdom from gastric flatulence and less frequently commented on his boils and other skin eruptions, his headaches, and colds. Typically, there were other less specific comments on his general state of health, such as 'weak and languid', 'poorly', 'goodish' and 'well'. Darwin recorded his daily routines: hydropathy, several walks, and the occasional self-medication. He was ready to try out almost any medicine: taking a great variety of bitters and tonics for his stomach;

29 F. Burkhardt and S. Smith, eds., *The Correspondence of Charles Darwin* (6 vols., Cambridge, 1985), VI, p. 238, Letter to W. D. Pox, 3 October 1856.
30 Colp, *Invalid*, pp. 4, 5, 31, 41, 58.
31 Letter from C. Darwin to J. D. Hooker quoted in F. Darwin, ed., *The Life and Letters of Charles Darwin* (1888), I, p. 373.
32 Darwin to his cousin Fox, 30 April 1857, quoted in Colp, *Invalid*, p. 60.
33 Darwin to Fox, 16 November 1859, quoted in Colp, *Invalid*, p. 67.
34 Darwin to Huxley, 5 December 1873, quoted in Colp, *Invalid*, p. 89.

and trying arsenic, 'Mr Startin's muddy stuff', and tartar emetic oint-ment. And the Darwin household (like the Blundell's and many others) had its own Receipts book, with medical prescriptions culled from various sources.[35]

Did patients prosper?

Sufferers could thus take it or leave it; they could see medical advice as money-grubbing meddling on the one hand, or alternatively as a judicious intervention. Once the sufferer became a patient, however, the preceding chapters suggest considerable diversity in encounters and relationships with doctors. Joint management of chronic disorders by affluent patients and their physicians indicated that relationships attained a mutually satisfactory equilibrium in which lay patronage was counterbalanced by professional experience and insight. Although within the competence of lay sufferers practitioners were not slow to make regimen and the taking of spa waters into technical medical fields, nor were sufferers necessarily reluctant to accept such pretensions and thereby constitute themselves as patients. Medicali-sation also operated with poor patients in a growing range of institu-tional provision. When the poor became patients a more unequal encounter ensued since other people's interests determined the nature of the relationship. Whether they were viewed by surgeons and physicians as interesting clinical material, by lay philanthropists as a promising moral opportunity, or by New Poor Law administrators as objects of social control, poor patients found themselves constituted more as objects than subjects. Women too might be seen as mere accidents of their diseases, although a more complex spectrum of relationships ranged from collusion through compliance to rejection of the doctor's ministrations. As well as gender and class, age increased the variety of medical encounters. Recapturing the experi-ence of child sufferers and patients is only possible to a limited extent through indirect evidence, but it appears that this experience shared certain characteristics with poor patients in that children commonly were viewed rather as the accident of their diseases, and therefore as objects to be treated institutionally. In other respects, children had a comparable experience to that of women in that they were seen as the 'other', as differentiated from the norm of the adult male patient in ways which – while treated – were only gradually understood.

What was the quality of care that patients received? Two forms of

[35] Colp, *Invalid*, pp. 43, 35–51, 53, 101, 147.

quantitative evaluation would be to estimate the number of times the
doctor saw the patient each year, and the time taken for each consultation. This kind of data is available only for the period after the one
with which we are concerned. Retrospectively, however, it gives a
revealing insight into patient care.

At the inception of the National Insurance Scheme in 1911, a critical
view of allegedly deteriorating standards of care was estimated on the
basis of list size and the length of the working day. In this calculation
panel doctors could only devote three and a quarter minutes to each
insurance patient in the surgery, and four minutes when on visits to a
patient's home.[36] (Interestingly, this was not too different from
modern studies which found that only five to six minutes was provided for the patient's consultation with the doctor in National Health
Service surgeries).[37] That the panel experience was taken as an indi-
cator of declining standards by sections of the medical profession
reflected a certain class blindness, since the implicit comparison
appeared to have been the more time-consuming work which a
private practitioner would have done earlier in a middle-class practice. In contrast, previous standards in a working-class branch surgery
by the so-called 'sixpenny doctor' would have meant an even briefer
consultation. Typically, this would have resulted in a predictable
outcome in that one of the few standard coloured bottles of medicine
available in the surgery would have been given. In reality there would
have been strong elements of continuity between the pre- and post-
1911 eras, except that in insisting on a prescription for a specific type of
medicine (and later of a restricted upper limit to the number of panel
patients) the National Health Insurance Scheme led to an improvement – rather than the contemporary allegation of a deterioration – in
standards of medical care.

This conclusion is reinforced when the number of times that practitioners saw their patients is reviewed. In the first year of the new
insurance system, panel practitioners on average saw 66 per cent of
their panel rather than the 30 per cent that they had been expecting,
whilst in the poorest districts the figure rose to 90 per cent.[38] Harry
Roberts, a doctor in the East End of London who was very much in
favour of the NHI scheme, commented that 'insured persons nowa-
days see very much more of their doctors than they used to do.'[39] The

36 *Medical World*, 9 April 1914.
37 E. Balint, and J. S. Norell, *Six Minutes for the Patient, Interactions in General Practice Consultations* (Tavistock Mind and Medicine Monograph 23, 1973).
38 *Medical World*, 9 April 1914.
39 PRO Pin 4/202, Evidence to Royal Commission on National Health Insurance.

Government Actuary had estimated that under the 1911 act, each insured working-class person would see their doctor between one and two times a year (1.7 times on average), an under-estimate influenced by previously low rates of contact.[40] Some practitioners, who were more critical of the NHI scheme, thought that it had led to greatly increased malingering.[41] Since the doctor now stood in a 'gatekeeping' role in relation to unemployment benefits, there may have been an element of imposture in such 'malingering'. Arguably, a sounder explanation for much of this patient consultation was that, for the first time, working-class people were able to take relatively minor ailments to the doctor – as their betters had long been accustomed to do. These figures for later practitioner–patient contact suggest a large amount of untreated sickness for working-class men before 1911, since they were the main beneficiaries of the legislation. Corroboration for this was the *Lancet's* earlier statement that the 'tendency of the working classes is to ignore disease in its earliest and most manageable stages.'[42] Working-class female dependants were left outside the 1911 act, so that many of their medical conditions remained untreated. Evidence of these was described in the sufferers' own words in *Maternity Letters*, published in 1915. These vividly suggested the large amount of untreated complaints among mothers – backache, neuralgia, varicose veins, headaches, and prolapsed wombs. Significantly, the women regarded their ailments – some of a painful and highly inconvenient kind – with fatalism. 'In my early motherhood I took for granted that women had to suffer. I dragged about in misery', commented one. Others wrote of being 'a martyr to suffering' or that 'my life was a perfect burden to me.'[43] Such everyday discomfort was what life had taught them that wives and mothers might expect as their lot; it was not an occasion for even contemplating a visit to the doctor. Attitudes to sickness within 'illness-behaviour', were thus culturally differentiated, varying over time, and between classes and amongst individuals.[44] What one saw as sickness another perceived as, if not an inevitable part of the human condition, nevertheless a predictable one, and as such a situation to be endured. Whether a sick-role was assumed and patient status adopted was variable, and whether a regular practitioner was summoned, depended to an important extent

---

[40] PRO MH 77/182 Evidence to Spens Committee by Bradford Hill and BMA.
[41] PRO Pin 4/202, Evidence to Royal Commission on National Health Insurance by National Medical Union.
[42] *Lancet*, ii, p. 654 (3 November 1877).
[43] M. Llewellyn Davies, *Maternity Letters from Working Women* (second edn, 1978), pp. 24, 29, 33, 104, 111.
[44] D. Mechanic, 'The Concept of Illness Behaviour', *Journal of Chronic Diseases*, 15 (1962).

on ability to pay. Other things being equal, cultural parameters moved in the doctor's favour with an increase in medical authority.

Did doctors prosper?

Although the domestic management of health inhibited the expansion of activities by doctors and thus implicitly challenged the practitioner's authority, a set of older beliefs on providential healing complemented it.[45] In the context of the overall themes of this book Benjamin Franklin's remark seems apposite, 'God heals and the doctor takes the fee.'[46] Certainly, the art of medicine was more highly developed than the science of medicine. Relying on symptomatology and a critical evaluation of the testimony of patients meant that communicating with the client, making sense of what was said (or not said), and thus of psychological insight into personality, was vital to the practitioner's ability to make a diagnosis. So too, in a holistic interpretation of the body's afflictions, was a knowledge of hereditary predispositions through familiarity with family history, together with awareness of the environment in which the patient lived. Such professional encounters were likely to be more effective in dealing with chronic afflictions and therefore with those arising from the patient's lifestyle. Management of the affluent patient was thus among the more successful medical encounters; it might achieve alleviation of pain, easing of discomfort, and the provision of psychological or physical strategies for living with long-term ailments. This caring, rather than curing, role was the stuff of everyday doctoring. We have seen that such consultations needed to be leisurely if they were to be effective, and were mainly the preserve of the propertied classes. Customarily, poorer sufferers did without such expensive advice or psychological reassurance; retaining control of their conditions and providing what solace they could through home remedies, the cheaper medicines of the chemist or druggist, or the affordable option of the sixpenny doctor's advice at the end of the period. For acute conditions there was less class differentiation, since a good range of provision was available under the poor law, through medical charities and the voluntary hospital system. Indeed, where surgery was concerned the poor patient was to some extent advantaged in that major scientific advances occurred in hospital operating facilities that had been

---

45 See, for example, M. Macdonald, 'Religion, Social Change and Psychological healing in England, 1600–1800', in W. J. Shiels, ed., *The Church and Healing* (Oxford, 1982).
46 B. Franklin, *Poor Richard's Almanac* (1744), quoted in R. and D. Porter, *In Sickness and in Health*, p. 54.

designed for the impoverished sector of the population. Women and children also benefited through the provision of specialist hospital facilities. In physic, by contrast, there was an epistemological revolution in the way that disease was understood, although within our period the therapeutic consequences of germ theory in disease-specific interventions were very limited.[47]

Given restricted advances in the medical profession's healing powers, patients displayed a robust scepticism about the disinterestedness of doctors' intentions. This can be seen in Georgian and early-Victorian cartoons and poems which also provided a graphic depiction of the crudity of medical methods. Doctors' shortcomings were not readily concealed as was indicated by popular contemporary epithets for practitioners – Sawbones, Fillgrave or Slasher – which continued into the Victorian period. Another accusation made against the Georgian medical profession was its allegedly mercenary nature:

> For in ten words the whole art is comprised
> For some of the ten are always advised
> Piss, spew or spit
> Perspiration and sweat
> Purge, bleed and blister
> Issues and clyster
>
> Most other specifics
> Have no visible effects
> But the getting of fees
> For a promise of ease.[48]

Where money was concerned, there was not a world of difference between contemporary perceptions of the regular practitioner and of the quack. Of the latter, Crabbe wrote nearly a century later, in 1810:

> But now our quacks are gamesters, and they play
> With craft and skill to ruin and betray;
> With monstrous promise they delude the mind,
> And thrive on all that tortures human-kind.
> Void of all honour, avaricious, rash,
> The darling tribe compound their boasted trash –
> Tincture or syrup, lotion, drop or pill;
> All tempt the sick to trust the lying bill.[49]

This tradition continued, if less stridently, during the Victorian period. The feminist, Frances Power Cobbe, alleged that 'the pecuniary interests of the [medical] profession continually over-ride the

---

[47] Kunitz, 'Personal Physician ', pp. 251–3.
[48] Baynard, *Health, A Poem, Shewing How to Procure, Preserve and Restore It* (first edition, 1719). This poem was very popular and went through numerous editions.
[49] *The Borough*, Letter vii, lines 71–8.

312   *Making a medical living*

interests of patients' and concluded that 'the individual doctor's profits are in one scale and the patient's in another.'[50] Victorian novels showed great cynicism about the therapeutic effectiveness of doctors.[51] M. J. Peterson has suggested that this lack of therapeutic power was linked to low social status.[52] Socially, the medical man was seen as occupying an ambiguous position, and there is a well-known example of this in George Eliot's *Middlemarch*, set in the 1830s. Dr Lydgate was from a well-connected military family, yet he became a country practitioner, and the ladies of the county did not know how to place him. Was he a gentleman or not? Lady Chettam mused about Lydgate's birth, 'One does not expect it in a practitioner of that kind. For my own part, I like a medical man more on a footing with the servants, they are oftener all the cleverer.' In contrast, the eponymous hero of Anthony Trollope's *Dr Thorne*, set in a period some twenty years later, was criticised not so much by the social élite as by his colleagues. They disliked his 'tradesmanlike' dispensing of his own medicines, the publication of his charges (7s 6d within a circuit of seven miles, and more for longer distances), and his failure to make the monetary relationships with the patient unobtrusive.

A physician should take his fee without letting his left hand know what his right hand was doing; it should be taken without a thought, without a look, without a move of the facial muscles ... the true physician should hardly be aware that the last friendly grasp of the hand had been made more precious by the touch of gold. Whereas, that fellow Thorne would lug out half a crown from his breeches pocket and give it in change for a ten-shilling piece.[53]

The practitioner's perception was increasingly that medicine was not a branch of commerce but a reputable profession dedicated to healing. Luke Fildes' 'The Doctor', painted in 1891 exemplified this ideal. Fildes apparently obtained his inspiration for the painting from a historical event: the illness and death of his own little son Philip in 1877, and the attendance by a devoted family doctor, Dr Murray. (See Plate 16) The painting was popular with the public (for whom childhood was a favourite subject) and phenomenally so with medical practitioners. Indeed, doctors amongst Fildes' acquaintance had competed amongst themselves to sit for the subject of the painting. In Britain today it often adorns medical schools, and in the USA it was

50 Cobbe, 'Medicine and Morality', pp. 225, 316.
51 M. F. Brightfield, 'The Medical Profession in Early Victorian England, as Depicted in the Novels of the Period', *BHM*, 35 (1961).
52 M. J. Peterson, 'Gentlemen and Medical Men: the Role of Professional Recruitment', *BHM*, 58 (1984), p. 470.
53 A. Trollope, *Dr Thorne* (World's Classics edition, Oxford, 1980), pp. 32–3.

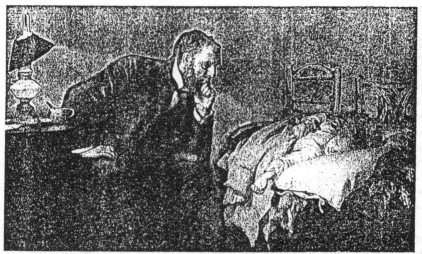

Plate 16   Detail from L. V. Fildes, 'The Doctor' (1891)

chosen for the postage stamp commemorating the centenary of the oldest medical society.[54] In its respectful treatment the painting contrasts with the visual lampoons of an earlier age: the doctor had become an honourable professional rather than a tradesman of dubious integrity. The painting shows a thoughtful male doctor, head propped against his hand, sitting looking in a concerned fashion at a child patient, lying prone across two chairs in the cottage of a Devon fisherman's family. What aspects of the painting might appeal to the medical profession? The doctor is depicted as dedicated and disinterested; prepared to spend time with the patient, even if the material reward from this poor family was likely to be negligible. Equally, there was acknowledgement of the doctor's inability to save the child's life, despite his best efforts, and the anguish that this caused him. The portrait was thus a brilliant synthesis: sufficiently realistic – in depicting a common predicament – to gain recognition as an honest portrayal, yet sufficiently idealised to appeal to medical practitioners' self-image of what they wished professional life was like. In art, but not in practice, the doctor could afford to give ample time even to his poorer patients.

   Why had doctors as an occupational group not achieved the prosperity that would have made this feasible? Urbanisation had led to an increasingly diverse range of practices within the medical market – rural, suburban, inner-city, family or élite – enabling practitioners to operate in an increasingly segmented market for their patients. Reinforcing this increasing variety had come a growing range of appointments – voluntary, charitable, public – which in their prestigious or mundane character further assisted practitioners in attracting particular sorts of patients. At the same time there was a long-term trend towards larger practices in which the economically more successful sustained a larger volume of work through taking on partners and employing assistants. Although this would have enhanced the chances of achieving prosperity, it was offset by a failure to control the numbers entering medicine. An over-supply of doctors had severe repercussions on practitioners' standards of living, particularly in the period after the Napoleonic Wars, and again during late-Victorian and Edwardian times, when hidden underemployment and practice failures were conspicuous. The experience of doctors contrasted with the slower expansion and greater financial success of those practising law.[55] Alternative practitioners also undercut the regular practitioner in the medical market. And of importance for the sense of well-being of doctors, from élite physicians or surgeons to GPs, was the challenge posed to medical authority by lay control of medical institutions, clubs and insurance schemes. The more financially precarious was the practice, the greater seemed to have been the resentment, since each gnawed away at the doctor's struggling self-esteem.

At the end of our period a rare address to doctors on medicine as business – revealingly one that had been requested by practitioners – remarked that 'As a rule, we do not care to discuss the proper reward of our services, for it is said to savour of commercialism but … scientific ability and business capacity are not incompatible.'[56] Insecure in their professional role, and in their aspirations to gentility, doctors were reluctant to adopt these business methods, even though they might have gained them a better living and thus helped them attain the higher social status for which they yearned. Deprived of a comfortable bank balance, most took comfort in high-sounding rationales of their function in society. Eminent members of the profession delivered *Addresses* at the start of each year in medical schools, which were a skilful juggling act in warning of the hard economic road to be

---

[55] Between 1881 and 1911 numbers of medical practitioners increased by 63% compared with legal practitioners who increased by only 23% (Perkin, 'Middle-class Education', p. 129).

[56] Sir John Collie, 'Address on the Business Side of Medical Practice', *BMJ*, 21 March 1914.

travelled, but in which flights of rhetoric on the respectable state of their putative occupation provided compensation for this. For example, 'The hope that it may one day yield you an honourable subsistence ... may also enable you to cultivate those qualities which serve to distinguish a Christian gentleman.'[57] Or again, 'Your know-ledge, your skill, your good character, will constitute your fortune.'[58] Famous doctors inspired their humbler colleagues with the disinter-ested ideals that had informed their work. Thus, Percival Pott is said to have expired with the words 'My lamp is nearly extinguished. I hope that it has burned for the benefit of others.'[59] Indeed, altruism in medicine was an important element in practice as discussion in Chapter 8 indicated. Even a stern feminist critic of the medical pro-fessions' morality and economic motivation recognised that 'The ordi-nary English country practitioner, with his small pay, his rough work in all weathers, and his general kindliness and honesty, is one of the most respectable members of the community.'[60] Counteracting the tradesmanlike image that the low income of many practitioners would otherwise have engendered was a hard-won public respect for what were perceived to be the doctor's high ideals.

Respect for the individual doctor was indivisible from a more general rise in medical authority. Within this period a general improvement in health and in life expectancy owed more to rising living standards and to environmental improvements in public health, yet in public perception may have been credited to the medical pro-fession alone. Credence in the doctor's powers was a seductive option in an age when faith in progress was strong, but where advancing secularism had undercut alternative religious belief. To some extent this growth in medical influence was connected with the rise of professionalism; enhanced pretensions, improved social presentation, and an increased command of specialist skills in the market.[61] This social phenomenon was underpinned by some notable developments in surgical practice, and by theoretical advances in scientific under-standing. These important – yet still restricted advances – lent a mantle of scientific competence to all members of the medical pro-fession. That many of the scientific discoveries did not immediately lead to a greater therapeutic effectiveness was not widely understood,

---

[57] H. W. Fuller, *Advice to Medical Students* (St. George's Hospital, 1857), p. 5.
[58] Brodie, *An Introductory Discourse on the Duties and Conduct of Medical Students and Practitioners* (1843). This was delivered at St George's Hospital.
[59] Quoted in Brodie, *Discourse*, p. 27. [60] Cobbe, 'Medical Profession', p. 306.
[61] See Perkins, *Professional Society*; Friedson, *Profession of Medicine*; Illich, *Disabling Professions*.

except by doctors themselves. In order to offset their limited therapeutic competence and partial success in achieving economic prosperity, practitioners maintained self-esteem by reference to their honourable intentions to patients, and their disinterested contribution to humanity. John Haygarth expressed this clearly:

Their thoughts, in the daily exercise of their profession, are so constantly and so anxiously exerted to save life and to relieve misery, that they enjoy perhaps a higher satisfaction than others from the gratification of these humane sentiments.[62]

[62] J. Haygarth, *An Inquiry into How to Prevent Smallpox* (Chester, 1784), p. 220.

Select bibliography

Manuscript sources

Barnes Medical Library, University of Birmingham

MS 1, Notes on John Hunter's Lectures on Surgery
MS 49, Cases in Surgery of J. Badley, 1802–3
MS 51, Notes on Abernethy's Lectures on the Theory and Practice of Surgery
MS 44, Birmingham School of Medicine Minute Book, 1831–8

Bath City Reference Library

MS 1495, Directions to Sir Alexander Fraser, 1675

Brotherton Library, University of Leeds

MS 551, Notes on Abernethy's Lectures, 1796
MS 566, Mr J.Tatham's Notes on William Cullen's Lectures, 1772–3
MS 560, Notes of Richard Hey, 1785–6

Buckinghamshire RO

Box 5, Diary of A. W. Blyth

Carlisle Public Library

E 104, Case Book of W. Brownrigg , 1737–42

Chester RO

H1/5, Chester Royal Infirmary Minutes

Devon RO

MS 64/8/8/1–9, Diaries of John Haddy James, 1788–1851
MS 73/12/1/1–9, Letters of John Haddy James, 1812–6

HR 1–3, Patients Journal, Devon and Exeter Hospital, 1753–61
HS 1, Statutes and Rules of the Devon and Exeter Hospital, 1743

Dorset RO

BG/SH A1/12–16, Sherborne Union Minutes, 1854–63
D/48/18/25, Legal papers of White and Harston
PE/POY/OV/1, Contract of Mr Fussell with Poyntington Parish, 1834
PE/SPV/OV/5, Agreements of Stour Provost Parish , 1787, 1804
PE/WM OV 18/3, Register of Medical Relief in the Wimborne District, Wimborne Union, 1861–3

E. Suffolk RO

ADA 9/AH5/1/1, Agreement for Building a Pest House at Shipmeadow, 1767
HD 365/1–3, Diaries of W. Goodwin of Earl Soham, 1785–1809
HA 93/9/419, Letters of Dr E. Beck, 1858
HA 61, 436/26, Accounts of Dr Beck, 1858

Gloucestershire RO

D 637 II/3/C6, Correspondence on Irregular Medical Practice, 1863–64
D 2071 B6, Pest House Erection in Chipping Sodbury Parish, 1757
P 31/OV 2/3, Overseers Accounts of Badgeworth Parish, 1732
P 81/OV 7/2, Agreements with Surgeons in Chipping Camden Parish,
P 317/VE 2/1, Vestry Book of Stow on the Wold Parish,
P 336/VE 2/1, Select Vestry Book of Toddenham Parish, 1819–34
Pc 1159 'Quack' advertisement

Leeds Archives

Uncatalogued, Newby Hall Papers

Leicestershire RO

DE 513/500, Testimonials of Thomas Macauley, 1866
DE 2934/44, Surgeon's Agreement for Watton in the Wolds Parish, 1817
DG 24/859/3, Payment for Royal Attendance on George IV to Henry Halford
DG 24/941–943, Diaries of Henry Halford, 1832–4
DG 24/812/25–31, Halford MSS, Doctors' Disagreement over Death Certificate, 1806
Leicester Infirmary, MS 3/D/9, Reports of House Visitors, 1826–52

Library of the Society of Friends, London

Microfilms 178–182, Hodgkin MSS (Originals in the Bodleian Library, Oxford)

Lincolnshire RO

Flinders MS 1–3, Diary and Accounts of Matthew Flinders
Miscellaneous Don 477, Ledger of Lincolnshire Surgeon, 1875–85

Manchester RO

M134/1/1/1–16, Miscellaneous Papers of Dr E. Lyon, 1790–1862
M134/1/2/8, Papers of E. Lyon

Norfolk RO

MS 49/5, House Surgeon Notes of M. Beverley, 1865–71
MS 470, Letters and Diaries of J. G. Crosse
MS 471, Letter Book of J. G. Crosse
MS 476, Memoirs of J. G. Crosse, 1819–47
MS 564, Rules and Orders for the Norfolk and Norwich Hospital, 1804
MS 20789, J. G. Crosse's Surgery Cases, 1826–7
MS 20795, J. G. Crosse's Correspondence, 1829–46
MS 5249, Descriptions and Plates of Bayly's Surgical Cases, 1806–10 by J. G. Crosse
NNH 49/1–2, Case Book of B. Norgate, 1828–57
PD 50/49, Overseers' Accounts for Gissing Parish,
Uncatalogued, Le Strange Collection, Account Book of Charities to the Sick and Poor
Uncatalogued, Forehoe Incorporation Minutes
Uncatalogued, Smallburgh Incorporation Minutes

Public Record Office

MH 32/101, Report of H. Jenner Fust, 1896,
MH 32/102, Reports of H. G. Kennedy, 1896, 1900
MH 62/130, Interdepartmental Committee, 1920
MH 77/182, Evidence to Spens Committee, 1945
PIN 4/202, Evidence to Royal Commission on National Health Insurance, 1926

Royal College of Physicians, London

MSS 597–602, Ledgers of Dr J. S. Taylor
MS 629, Minutes of the Governors of the Westminster General Dispensary, vol. 1
MS 2437, Medical Diary of Dr S. T. Taylor, 1882–8
MS 2468, Minutes of Carey Street Dispensary
MS 2508, Accounts of Carey Street Dispensary 1782–93
MS 2509/1, Plan and Reports of the Carey Street Dispensary, 1783

Royal College of Physicians, Edinburgh

James Gregory, MS 4, Clinical Cases at the Royal Infirmary, Edinburgh, 1780–1
James Gregory, MS 7, Lectures in Medicine, c. 1805
James Hamilton, MS 5, Heads of Lectures on the Diseases of Infancy and Childhood, 1815
James Hamilton the Younger, MS 14, Miscellaneous correspondence
Cullen MS 30/1–21, Letters from Cullen, 1755–90
Cullen MS 31/1–17, Letters to Cullen, 1774–90

Miscellaneous MS, Edinburgh Royal Maternity Hospital Indoor Case Book, 1844–71

Royal College of Surgeons of London

Uncatalogued, MS of Alexander Marcet on Hospital Practice, 1804–17
Uncatalogued, Edward Jenner Correspondence
Uncatalogued, William Hunter Correspondence
Uncatalogued, William Thomson Correspondence

Royal Society of Medicine, London

MS 165, Hodgkin's Notes of Post-Mortem Examinations, 1845–52

Scottish RO

CS 96/1301–2, Account Books of David Wishart
CS 236/Miscellaneous 9/1 nos. 90–1, Bankruptcy Papers of G. Scrimzeour
CS 237/F9/13 nos. 4347–8, Bankruptcy Papers of W. C. Johnstone
GD 18/2131–43, Clerk of Penicuick Papers
GD 35/236/13, Diary of Dr D. Dundas
GD 80/932, Letters of J. Clark, 1793–1804
GD 110/976/1–2, Letters of A. Walker, 1745–56
GD 136/1085/1–2, Medical Bills of Dr Sinclair
GD 253/143/2–3, Medical Papers of Dr J. Hope

Sheffield City Archives

Em 888, Medical Ledger of W. Elmhirst, 1768–73
TC 166, Appointment of Surgeons to Sheffield Workhouse, 1756

Somerset RO

DD/8AS/TN 54, Correspondence of H. Norris, 1812
DD/SAS/TN 28, Accounts of James Billett
DD/TB 13/7–8, Medical Bills of Carew Family
DD/TB 15/30, Medical Bills of Carew Family
DD/WY box 1, Medical Diary of J. Wyndham, 1674–1750
D/P/Can 13/2/2, Poor Book of Cannington Parish, 1752–1832
DD/FS/48, Ledger of B. Pulsford, 1757–60
D/P/Bra 13/2/2, Overseers' Account Book of Bradford on Tone Parish, 1762–88
D/P/Back 13/2/6, Overseers' Vouchers of Backwell Parish, 1756–1850
D/P Badg P3/2/4–5, Bills of Badgworth Parish, 1768–1810
D/P/Broo 13/2/3, Bills of Broomfield Parish
D/P/bh/13/10/3, Reports of the Taunton and Somerset Hospital, 1828
DD/SAS TN 54, Reports of the Taunton and Somerset Hospital, 1832

Wellcome Institute for the History of Medicine, London

AL 67582, Correspondence of Dr Baillie, 1807
AL 67615, Correspondence of J. Anderson

MS 1094, Rules and Orders of the Bath Casualty Hospital, 1788–1817
MS 1145, Notes on Patients at St Bartholomew's Hospital by S. Berry, 1829–36
MS 1856, Diary of Assistant Physician at the Westminster Hospital, 1786
MS 2596, Notes on Clinical Cases in the Edinburgh Infirmary by James Gregory, 1783–4
MS 2598, Notes on Lectures on the Practice of Physic by James Gregory, 1795
MS 2966, Notes on Lectures on Obstetrics by W. Hunter, 1775–83
MS 3218, Diary of Robert Lee, 1793–1872
MS 3245, Autobiographical Fragment by J. C. Lettsom
MS 3246–8, Fugitive Pieces by J. C. Lettsom
MS 3820 Case book of Richard Paxton
MS 3958, Notes of Lectures on the Practice of Surgery by Percival Pott, 1782
MS 4337, Notes of House Surgeon at St Bartholomew's Hospital, 1778–81
MS 5005, Case Book of R. Wilkes, 1737–51
MS 5006, Diary of R.Wilkes, 1739–51
MS 5103, Notes on Thomas Young's Lectures on Midwifery
MS 91800, Correspondence of Sir G. Baker, 1806

Wiltshire RO

J6/196/3, Consultations at Savernake Cottage Hospital, 1873–9
1269/7–8, Ledgers of Dr G. Salter, 1858–1911
J8/110/1, Auditors Reports on Salisbury Infirmary, 1766–1814
Uncatalogued Ailesbury papers

York District Hospital Medical Library

York Hospital Court of Governors Minute Books

Parliamentary papers

Report of Royal Commission of Enquiry into Scottish Universities, 1830 XII
SC on Medical Education, 1834, XIII
SC on Medical Poor Relief, 1844, IX
SC on Medical Relief, 1854, XII
Report on Candidates for the Medical Department, 1878–9, XLIV
Report of Royal Commission into Medical Acts, 1882, XXIX
Report of Royal Commission on Medical Acts, 1882, XXIX
Board of Trade Returns of Expenditures by Working Men, 1889, LXXXIV
SC on Metropolitan Hospitals, 1890, XVI
Report of the Registrar General, 1900, XV
Report to the Board of Trade on British and Foreign Trade and Industrial Conditions, 1903, XVIII
Interdepartmental Committee on the Inspection and Feeding of Children, 1906, XLVII
RC on the Poor Laws and Relief of Distress, 1909, XL, XLI, XXXVII, LIII
Report of the Chief Medical Officer of the Board of Education, 1910, XXIII
Report as to the Practice of Medicine and Surgery by Unqualified Persons, 1910, XXXXVII
41st Report of Local Government Board, 1912–13, XXXV
Report of Sir William Plender in Respect of Medical Attendance and Remuneration in Certain Towns, 1912–13, LXXVIII

Some Notes on Medical Education by G. Newman, 1918, xix
An Outline of the Practice of Preventive Medicine by G. Newman, 1919, xxix
Returns from Universities in Receipt of Treasury Grant, 1921, viii

Periodicals and newspapers

British Medical Journal
Contemporary Review
Cornhill Magazine
Edinburgh Medical Journal
English Woman's Journal
Fortnightly Review
Gentleman's Magazine
Lancet
Medical Women's Federation Newsletter
Medical Women's Journal
Medical World
Modern Review
Nineteenth Century
Provincial Medical and Surgical Journal
Punch
The Times
Westminster Review
Women's Medical Journal

Pre 1910 printed books and articles

A Narrative of the Efficacy of the Bath Waters in Paralytic Disorders (Bath, 1787)
A Tariff of Medical Fees Recommended by the Shropshire Ethical Branch of the BMA
     (Shrewsbury, 1870, 1874, 1889)
Aitken, G. A., *The Life and Works of John Arbuthnot* (second edn, New York, 1892)
Alcock, T., *Essay on the Education and Duties of the General Practitioner in Medicine
     and Surgery* (1823)
Alford, H., 'The Bristol Infirmary in My Student Days, 1822–1828', *Bristol
     Medical and Chirurgical Journal* (September 1890)
Allen, J. M., 'On the Differences in the Minds of Men and Women,' *Journal of
     the Anthropological Society of London*, 7 (1869)
Arbuthnot, A., *An Essay Concerning the Nature of Aliments* (1731)
Armstrong, G., *A General Account of the Dispensary for the Relief of the Infant Poor*
     (1769)
Armstrong, G., *An Essay on the Diseases Most Fatal To Infants* (second edn, 1771)
Autobiography of the Late Benjamin C. Brodie, (1865)
Baxter, R. D., *National Income* (1868)
Bell, J. *Letters on Professional Character and Manners* (Edinburgh, 1810)
Birkbeck Hill, G., ed., *Letters of Samuel Johnson* (2 vols. 1892)
Brodie, B., *An Introductory Discourse on the Duties and Conduct of Medical
     Students and Practitioners* (1843)
Buchan, W., *Domestic Medicine* (second edn, 1772)
Bull, T., *Hints to Mothers* (1837)
Cadogan, W., *An Essay upon the Management of Children* (tenth edn, 1777)

Campbell, R., *The London Tradesman* (1747)

Carlisle, A., *Practical Observations on the Preservation of Health* (1838)

Cases of Persons Admitted into the Infirmary at Bath under the Care of Doctor Oliver (Bath, 1760)

Castle, T., ed. *The Principles and Practice of Obstetricy by James Blundell* (1834)

Cheyne, G., *An Essay on Regimen* (second edn, 1740)

Clarke, J., *Commentaries On Some Of The Most Important Diseases Of Children* (1815)

Clarke, J. F., *Autobiographical Recollections* (1874)

Colquhoun, P., *A Treatise on Indigence* (1806)

Colquhoun, P., *A Treatise on the Wealth, Power and Resources of the British Empire* (second edn, 1815)

Copeman, E., ed., *John Green Crosse. Cases in Midwifery* (1851)

Crompton, S., *Memoir of Edmund Lyon, MD* (Manchester, 1881)

Cullen, W., *First Lines of the Practice of Physic* (Edinburgh, 1829)

Dale, W., *The State of the Medical Profession in Great Britain and Ireland* (Dublin, 1875)

Darwin, F., ed. *The Life and Letters of Charles Darwin* (1888)

Davenant, F., *What shall my son be* (1870)

Davies, D., *Elements of Obstetric Medicine* (second edn, 1841)

Davis, J. B., *A Cursory Inquiry Into Some Of The Principal Cause Of Mortality Among Children* (1817)

Day, W. H., *Essays on the Diseases of Children* (1873)

de Styrap, J., *The Young Practitioner* (1890)

Denman, T., *Aphorisms on the Application and Use of Forceps* (fourth edn, 1793)

Denman, T., *Introduction to the Practice of Midwifery* (2 vols., second edn, 1794)

Duffey, E. B., *What Should Women Know* (1873)

Eden, F. M., *The State of the Poor* (3 vols., 1797)

Falconer, R. W., *The Bath Mineral Waters* (1861)

Fuller, H. W., *Advice to Medical Students* (St George's Hospital, 1857)

Gooch, R., *An Account of some of the Most Important Diseases Peculiar to Women* (1829)

Good, J. M., *The History of Medicine, so far as it relates to the Profession of the Apothecary* (1795)

Goodhart, J. F., *The Diseases of Children* (third edn, 1888)

Granville, A. B., *The Spas of England and Principal Sea-Bathing Places* (3 vols., 1841)

Granville, P. B., ed., *The Autobiography of A. B. Granville* (two vols., second edn, 1874)

Gregory, J., *On the Duties and Qualifications of a Physician* (second edn, 1820)

Gregory, S., *Female Physicians* (1864)

Hamilton, A., *Elements of the Practice of Midwifery* (1775)

Hamilton, A., *A Treatise on the Management of Female Complaints* (seventh edn, Edinburgh, 1813)

Haygarth, J., *A Letter to Dr Percival on the Prevention of Infectious Fevers* (1801)

Haygarth, J., *An Inquiry on How to Prevent Smallpox* (Chester, 1784)

Heberden, W., *Commentaries on the History and Cure of Diseases* (reprint, New York, 1962)

Hill, J., *Cases in Surgery* (Edinburgh 1772)

Hodgkin, T., *An Essay on Medical Education* (1828)

Hodgkin, T., *Lectures on the Morbid Anatomy of the Serous and Mucous Membranes* (2 vols., London, 1836, 1840)

Hodgkin, T., *Medical Reform. An Address Read to the Harveian Society* (1847)

The Household Encyclopaedia or Family Dictionary (1858)

Hunter, A., *A Treatise on the Mineral Waters of Harrogate* (1830)

Keeteley, C. B, *The Student and Junior Practitioner's Guide to the Medical Profession* (second edn, 1885)

King, G, *National and Political Observations and Conclusions upon the State and Condition of England* (1696)

Langslow, R., *The Case of Master Day of Yoxford* (Bungay, 1800)

Leake, J., *A Lecture Introductory to the Theory and Practice of Midwifery* (1782)

Lee, R., *Lectures on the Theory and Practice of Midwifery* (1844)

Lettsom, J. C., *Medical Memoirs of the General Dispensary in London for part of the Years 1773 and 1774* (1774)

Macpherson, J., *The Baths and Wells of Europe* (1869, 1873, and 1888 edns).

Manley, M., *On the Nature and Treatment of the Most Frequent Diseases of Children* (1830)

Mason, S., *The Philosophy of Female Health* (1845)

Mathews, J. M., *How to Succeed in the Practice of Medicine* (Louisville, 1902)

McClintock, A. H., ed., *Smellie's Treatise on the Theory and Practice of Midwifery* (3 vols., New Sydenham Society, 1876)

Mears, M., *The Pupil of Nature* (1797)

The Medical Works of Richard Mead (Dublin, 1767)

Men-Midwives and Female Physicians (1864)

Munk, W., *The Life of Henry Halford* (1895)

Munk, W., *Roll of the Fellows of the Royal College of Physicians of London* (3 vols., 1861 and 1878)

Newdigate-Newdegate, Lady, *The Cheverels of Cheverel Manor* (1898)

Nightingale, F., *Introductory Notes on Lying-In Institutions* (1871)

Norford, W, *A Letter to Dr Sharpin in Answer* (Bury, 1764)

Paget, J., 'What becomes of Medical Students?', *St Bartholomew's Hospital Reports*, 5 (1869)

Paget, S., ed., *Memoirs and Letters of Sir James Paget* (1901)

Percival, T., *Medical Ethics* (Manchester, 1803)

Percival, T., *Philosophical, Medical and Experimental Essays* (1776)

Percival, T., *Works* (4 vols., 1807)

Playfair, W. S., *A Treatise on the Science and Practice of Midwifery* (1876)

Ramsbotham, F. H., *Principles and Practice of Obstetric Medicine and Surgery* (1841)

Rivington, W., *The Medical Profession* (Dublin, 1879)

Rogers, J., *Reminiscences of a Workhouse Medical Officer* (1889)

Rules and Regulations Agreed and Entered into by Medical Gentlemen of Blackburn (Blackburn,1819)

Russell, J., *The Character and Claims of the Medical Profession* (Birmingham, 1853)

Scott, W., *The Surgeon's Daughter* (Waverley Novels, vol. xlviii, Edinburgh, 1833)

Sharpin, Dr, and Steward, M, *An Appeal to the Public etc* (Bury, 1764)

Simpson, W., *Hydrologia Chymica* (1669)

Smellie, W., *A Treatise on the Theory and Practice of Midwifery* (3 vols., 1752–64)

Smollett, *An Essay on the External Use of Water* (1752)

Stevens, J., *Man-Midwifery Exposed* (1862)
Stevenson, W. E., *The Medical Act (1858) Amendment Bill and Medical Reform: A paper read before the Abernethian Society at St Bartholomew's Hospital* (1880)
Stone, S., *A Complete Practice of Midwivery* (1737)
Storer, W. O., ed., *J. Y. Simpson's Obstetric Memoirs and Contributions* (2 vols., Edinburgh, 1855)
Surtees, R. S., *Ask Mamma. The Richest Commoner in England* (1874)
Talley, W., *He or Man-Midwifery* (1863)
Taylor, J. M., *The Physician as Businessman* (Philadelphia, 1891)
Thackeray, W., *The History of Pendennis* (1848–50)
Thomson, H. B., *The Choice of a Profession* (1857)
Thomson, J., *An Account of the Life, Lectures and Writings of William Cullen, MD* (2 vols., Edinburgh, 1859)
Thoughts on Brightelmston Concerning Sea-Bathing and Drinking Sea-Water with some Directions for their Use (1768).
Tilt, E. J., *On the Preservation of the Health of Women* (1851)
Wakefield, E. G., *England and America: a Comparison of the Social and Political State of Both Nations* (1833)
Walsh, J. H., *A Manual of Domestic Economy* (1857, 1890)
Walsh, J. H., *A Manual of Domestic Economy* (1890)
Ward, E., *A Step to the Bath* (1700)
Warne's Household Manual (1879)
Warren, S., *Passages from the Diary of a Late Physician* (2 vols., Paris, 1839)
Wesley, J., *Primitive Physic* (second edn, 1791)
West, C., *On Hospital Organisation with Special Reference to the Organisation of Hospitals for Children* (1877)
West, C., *Lectures on the Diseases of Infancy and Childhood* (1848)
West, C., *The Profession of Medicine* (1896)
White, C., *The Management of Pregnant and Lying-In Women* (1773)
Wilde, J., *The Hospital, a Poem in Three Books, Written in the Devon and Exeter Hospital, 1809* (Norwich, 1809)
Willan, R., *Miscellaneous Works* (1821)
Withers, T., *A Treatise on the Errors and Defects of Medical Education* (York, 1794)
The Works of Alexander Monro, MD, Published by His Son Alexander Monro (Edinburgh, 1781)

Post 1910 printed books and articles

Abel Smith, B., *The Hospitals* (1964)
Abel Smith, B., 'The Rise and Decline of Early Health Maintenance Organisations: Their International Experiences', *Social History of Medicine*, 2 (1989)
Abraham, J. J., *Lettsom, His Life and Times, Friends and Descendants* (1933)
Ackernecht, E. W., *Medicine at the Paris Hospital, 1794–1848* (Baltimore, 1967)
Agnew, L. R. C., 'Quackery' in A. G. Debus, ed., *Medicine in Seventeenth-Century England* (Berkeley, 1974)
Alexander, W., *First Ladies of Medicine. The Origins, Education and Destination of Early Women Medical Graduates of Glasgow University* (Wellcome Unit for the History of Medicine, Glasgow, 1987)

Altier, G., and Riley, J. C., 'Frailty, Sickness and Death: Models of Morbidity and Mortality in Historical Populations', *Population Studies*, 43 (1989)

Anderson, O., *Suicide in Victorian and Edwardian England* (Oxford, 1987)

Andrews, C. B., ed., *The Torrington Diaries* (4 vols., 1935)

Anning S. T., and Wallis, W. K. J., *A History of Leeds School of Medicine* (Leeds, 1982)

Armstrong, B. N., *The Health Insurance Doctor. His Role in Britain, Denmark and France* (Princeton, 1939)

Askwith, B., *Piety and Wit* (1982)

Aveling, J. H., *English Midwives, their History and Prospects* (second edn, 1967)

Balint, E., and Norell, J. S., *Six Minutes for the Patient, Interactions in General Practice Consultations* (Tavistock Mind and Medicine Monograph 23, 1973)

Balint, M., *The Doctor, His Patient and the Illness* (1964)

Bartrip, P. W. J., *Mirror of Medicine. A History of the British Medical Journal* (Oxford, 1990)

Batty Shaw, A., 'Benjamin Gooch, Eighteenth-Century Surgeon' *Medical History*, XVI (1972)

Batty Shaw, A., 'The Norwich School of Lithotomy' *Medical History*, XIV (1970)

Berridge, E., ed., *The Barretts at Hope End. The Early Diary of Elizabeth Barrett Browning* (1974)

Blundell, M., ed., *Blundell's Diary and Letter Book, 1702–1728* (Liverpool, 1952)

Bonner, T. N., 'Abraham Flexner as Critic of British and Continental Medical Education' *Medical History*, 33 (1989)

Borsay, P., *The English Urban Renaissance in the Provincial Town, 1660–1770* (Oxford, 1991)

Bradford Hill, A., 'The Doctor's Pay and Day', *Journal of the Royal Statistical Society*, CIV (1951)

Brewer, J., and Porter, R., eds., *Consumption and the World of Goods* (1993)

Brightfield, M. F., 'The Medical Profession in Early Victorian England, as Depicted in the Novels of the Period', *Bulletin of the History of Medicine*, 35 (1961)

Brock, R. C., *The Life and Work of Astley Cooper* (1952)

Brockbank, W., *Portrait of a Hospital, 1752–1948* (1952)

Brockbank, W., 'Country Practice in Days Gone By', *Medical History*, 6 (1962)

Brockbank W. and Kenworthy, F., eds., *The Diary of Richard Kay, 1716–1751* (Chetham Society, vol. CVI, third series, Manchester,1968)

Bryne, P. S., and Long, B. E., *Doctors Talking to Patients* (DHSS, 1976)

Burdett's Hospitals and Charities (1919)

Burkhardt, F. and Smith, S., eds., *The Correspondence of Charles Darwin* (6 vols., Cambridge, 1985)

Burnby, J. G. L., *A Study of the English Apothecary from 1660 to 1760* (Medical History Supplement Number 3, Wellcome Institute, London, 1983)

Butler, S. V. F., 'A Transformation in Training: the Formation of University Medical Faculties in Manchester, Leeds and Liverpool, 1820–1884', *Medical History*, 30 (1986)

Bynum, W. F., 'Medicine and the English Court, 1688–1837', in V. Nutton, ed., *Medicine at the Courts of Europe, 1500–1837* (1990)

Bynum, W. F., 'Physicians, hospitals and career structures in eighteenth-century London' in W. F. Bynum and R. Porter, eds., *William Hunter and the Eighteenth Century Medical World* (Cambridge, 1985)

Leake, C. D., ed., *Percival's Medical Ethics* (Baltimore, 1927)

Carr Saunders A. M., and Wilson, P. A., *The Professions* (second edn, 1964)

Cassell, E. J., *Talking with Patients* (2 vols., MIT, 1985)

Chamberlain, M., *Old Wives Tales* (1981)

Chambers, P., *A Doctor Alone: a Biography of Elizabeth Blackwell* (1956)

Cherry, S., 'The Hospitals and Population Growth', *Population Studies*, XXIV (1980)

Coleman, W., 'Health and Hygiene in the *Encyclopédie*. A Medical Doctrine for the Bourgeoise', *Journal of the History of Medicine*, 29 (1974)

Coley, N. G., '"Cures without care". "Chymical physicians", and mineral waters in seventeenth-century English medicine', *Medical History*, 23 (1979)

Coley, N. G.,'Physicians and the Chemical Analysis of Mineral Waters in Eighteenth-Century England', *Medical History*, 26 (1982)

Colp, R., *To Be An Invalid. The Illness of Charles Darwin* (Chicago, 1977)

Comrie, J. D., *History of Scottish Medicine* (1927)

Cooter, R., ed., *Studies in the History of Alternative Medicine* (1988)

Cope, Z., *The Versatile Victorian, Being the Life of Sir Henry Thompson, Bt, 1820–1904* (1951)

Cope, Z., *William Cheselden, 1688–1752* (1953)

Cope, Z., 'The Private Medical Schools of London (1746–1914)', in F. N. L. Poynter, ed., *The Evolution of Medical Education in Britain* (1966)

Cope, Z., 'The Influence of the Free Dispensaries upon Medical Education in Britain', *Medical History*, XII (1969)

Cox, A., *Among the Doctors* (1950)

Crafts, N., *British Economic Growth during the Industrial Revolution* (1985)

Crellin, J. K., and Scott, J. R., 'Pharmaceutical History and its Sources in the Wellcome Collections, II, Fluid Medicines', *Medical History*, 14 (1970)

Crosse, V. M., *A Surgeon in the Early Nineteenth Century. The Life and Times of J. G. Crosse, 1790–1850* (1968)

Crowther, M. A., *The Workhouse System* (1981)

Crowther, M. A.,'Paupers or Patients? Obstacles to Professionalization in the Poor Law Medical Service before 1914', *Journal of the History of Medicine*, 39 (1984)

D. King-Hele, *Letters of Erasmus Darwin* (Cambridge, 1981)

Daniels, A. K., 'How Free Should Professions Be', in E. Friedson, ed., *The Professions and their Prospects* (1971)

de Moulin, D., *A Short History of Breast Cancer* (Boston, 1983)

Defoe, D., *A Tour Through the Whole Island of Great Britain* (2 vols., 1974)

Dewhurst, K., *John Locke, Physician and Philosopher* (1963)

Digby, A., *Madness, Morality and Medicine. A Study of the York Retreat, 1796–1914* (Cambridge, 1985)

Digby, A., *Pauper Palaces* (1978)

Digby, A., 'Women's Biological Straitjacket' in S. Mendus and J. Rendall, eds., *Sexuality and Subordination* (1989)

Digby, A., and Bosanquet, N., 'Doctors and Patients in an Era of National Health Insurance and Private Practice', *Economic History Review*, second series, XLI, (1989)

Dobson, M., 'Mortality Gradients and Disease Exchanges: Comparisons from Old England and Colonial America', *Social History of Medicine*, 2 (1989)

Donnison, J., *Midwives and Medical Men. A History of Inter-Professional Rivalries and Women's Rights* (New York, 1977)

Dupree, M. W., and Crowther, M. A., 'A Profile of the Medical Profession in Scotland in the Early Twentieth Century: the Medical Directory as a Historical Source', *Bulletin of the History of Medicine*, 65 (1991)

Earle, P., *The Making of the English Middle Class. Business, Society and Family Life in London, 1660–1730* (1989)

Eccles, A., *Obstetrics and Gynaecology in Tudor and Stuart England* (1982)

Edel, L., *The Diary of Alice James* (New York, 1964)

Ehrenreich, B., and English, D., *For Her Own Good. 150 Years of the Experts' Advice to Women* (1979)

Eland, G., ed., *Purefoy Letters* (2 vols., 1935)

Elwin, M., *The Noels and the Millbankes. Their Letters for 25 Years* (1967)

English, B. H., *Five Generations of a Whitby Medical Family* (Whitby, 1977)

Eyler, J. M., *Victorian Social Medicine* (Baltimore, 1979)

Feinstein, C. H., 'A new look at the cost of living, 1870–1914' in J. Foreman Peck, ed., *New Perspectives on the Late Victorian Economy* (Cambridge, 1991)

Feinstein, C. H., 'The Rise and Fall of the Williamson Curve', *Journal of Economic History*, XLVIII (1988)

Fildes, V., *Breasts, Bottles and Babies* (Edinburgh, 1986)

Fildes, V., *Wet Nursing. A History from Antiquity to the Present* (Oxford, 1988)

Fildes, L. V., *Luke Fildes, R. A., A Victorian Painter* (London, 1968)

Fissell, M. E., *Patients, Power, and the Poor in Eighteenth Century Bristol* (Cambridge, 1991)

Fissell, M., '"The Sick and Drooping Poor" in Eighteenth Century Bristol and its Regions', *Social History of Medicine*, 2 (1989)

Fletcher, R., *The Parkers at Saltram* (1970)

Flinn, M. W., 'Medical Services under the New Poor Law' in D. Fraser, ed., *The New Poor Law in the Nineteenth Century* (1976)

Floud, R., 'Standards of Living and Industrialisation' in A. Digby and C. H. Feinstein, eds., *New Directions in Economic and Social History* (1989)

Floud, R., Wachter, K., and Gregory, A., *Height, Health and History. Nutritional Status in the United Kingdom* (Cambridge, 1990)

Foster, W. D., 'The Finances of a Victorian General Practitioner', *Proceedings of the Royal Society of Medicine*, 66 (1973)

Foucault, M., *The Birth of the Clinic. An Archaeology of Medical Perception* (New York, 1973)

Foxon, G. E., 'Thomas Hodgkin, 1798–1866. A Biographical Note', *Guy's Hospital Reports*, 115 (1966)

Franklin, A. W., 'Children's Hospitals' in F. N. L. Poynter, ed., *The Evolution of Hospitals in Britain* (1964)

French, R., and Wear, A., eds., *British Medicine in an Age of Reform* (1992)

Friedson, E., *Professional Powers. A Study of the Institutionalisation of Formal Knowledge* (Chicago, 1986)

Friedson, E., *Profession of Medicine* (New York, 1975)

Friedson, E., 'The Theory of the Professions: State of the Art', in R. Dingwall, and P. Lewis, eds., *The Sociology of the Professions* (1983)

Garlick, K. and Macintyre, A. eds., *The Diary of Joseph Farington* (8 vols., 1978)

Gelfand, T., *Professionalizing Modern Medicine. Paris Surgeons and Medical Science and Institutions in the 18th Century* (Westport, Connecticut, 1980)

Gillespie, J., *The Price of Health: Governments and Medical Politics, 1910–1960* (Cambridge, 1991)

Gittins, D., *Fair Sex. Family Size and Structure, 1900–1939* (1982)

Glynn, A., *Elinor Glynn – A Biography* (1955)

Granshaw, L., ' "Fame and Fortune by Means of Bricks and Mortar": the Medical Profession and Specialist Hospitals in Britain', in L. Granshaw and R. Porter, eds., *The Hospital in History* (1989)

Gray, E., *Papers and Diaries of a York Family, 1764–1839* (1927)

The Great Diurnall of Nicholas Blundell (Record Society of Lancashire and Cheshire, 1968)

Greer, A. W., *Tubbs. A Nineteenth Century GP* (King's Lynn, 1988)

Hamilton, B., 'The Medical Professions in the Eighteenth Century', *Economic History Review*, IV (1951)

Hannah, L. *Inventing Retirement. The Development of Occupational Pensions in Britain* (Cambridge, 1986)

Hemlow, J., ed., *Journals and Letters of Fanny Burney* (5 vols., Oxford, 1975)

Hobhouse, E., *The Diary of a West Country Physician* (1934)

Holloway, S. W. F., *Royal Pharmaceutical Society of Great Britain, 1841–1991. A Political and Social History* (1991)

Holloway, S. W. F., 'The Apothecaries Act', *Medical History*, 10 (1966)

Holmes, G., *Augustan England, Professions, State and Society, 1680–1730* (1982)

Holroyd, M., *Bernard Shaw. Vol. II, 1898–1918. The Pursuit of Power* (London, 1989)

Honigsbaum, F., *The Division in British Medicine. A History of the Separation of General Practice from Hospital Care, 1911–1968* (1979)

Howie, W. B., 'Complaints and Complaints Procedures in the Eighteenth Century and Early Nineteenth Century Provincial Hospitals in England', *Medical History*, 25 (1981)

Hunt, T., *The Medical Society of London, 1773–1973* (1972)

Illich, I., *Disabling Professions* (1977)

Inkster, I, 'Marginal Men. Aspects of the Social Role of the Medical Community in Sheffield, 1790–1850', in J. Woodward and D. Richards, eds., *Health Care and Popular Medicine in Nineteenth-Century England* (1977)

Jackson, R. V., 'The Structure of Pay in Nineteenth-Century Britain', *Economic History Review*, second series, XL, (1987)

Jacyna, L. S. ed., *A Tale of Three Cities. The Correspondence of W. Sharpey and A. Thomson* (Medical History Supplement 9, 1989)

Jalland, P., and J. Hooper eds., *Women from Birth to Death* (1986)

Jenkinson, J., 'The Role of Medical Societies in the Rise of the Scottish Medical Profession, 1730–1939', *Social History of Medicine*, 4 (1991)

Jewkes, J. and S., *The Genesis of the British NHS* (Oxford, 1962)

Jewson, N. D., 'Medical Knowledge and the Patronage System in 18th Century England', *Sociology* 8 (1974)

Johnson,P., *Saving and Spending. The Working Class Economy in Britain, 1870–1939* (Oxford, 1988)

Jolly, H., *Diseases of Children* (third edn, 1976)

Jordanova, L., 'The social sciences and the history of science and medicine' in P. Corsi and P. Weindling, eds., *Information Sources in the History of Science and Medicine* (1983)

Kerr, J. M. ed., *Historical Review of British Obstetrics and Gynaecology, 1800–1950* (Edinburgh, 1954)

Kett, J. F., 'Provincial Medical Practice in England, 1730–1815', *Journal of the History of Medicine*, XIX (1964)

King, L. S., *The Growth of Medical Thought* (Chicago, 1963)

King, L. S., *The Medical World of the Eighteenth Century* (Chicago, 1958)

King, L. S.,'The Development of Scientific Medicine' in L. S. King, ed., *Mainstreams of Medicine. Essays on the Social and Intellectual Context of Medical Practice* (San Antonio, 1971)

King, L. S., 'George Cheyne, Mirror of Eighteenth Century Medicine', *Bulletin of the History of Medicine*, 48 (1974)

King Hele, D., *Letters of Erasmus Darwin* (Cambridge, 1981)

Kunitz, S. J., 'The Personal Physician and the Decline of Mortality in the Late Nineteenth and Early Twentieth Centuries', in R. Schofield, D. Rehur, and A. Bideau eds., *The Decline of Mortality in Europe* (Oxford, 1991)

Laidler, P. W., and Gelfand, M., *South Africa. Its Medical History, 1652–1898* (Cape Town, 1971)

Landers, J., 'Mortality and Metropolis: the case of London, 1625–1825', *Population Studies*, 41 (1987)

Lane, J., 'Eighteenth-Century Medical Practice: a Case Study of Bradford Wilmer, Surgeon of Coventry, 1737–1813', *Social History of Medicine*, 3 (1990)

Lane, J. 'The Medical Practitioners of Provincial England in 1783', *Medical History*, 28 (1984)

Lane, J., 'The Provincial Practitioner and His Services to the Poor, 1750–1800', *Bulletin of the Society for the Social History of Medicine*, 28 (1981)

Lane, J., 'The Role of Apprenticeship in Eighteenth-Century Medical Education' in W. F. Bynum and R. Porter, *William Hunter and the Eighteenth Century Medical World* (Cambridge, 1985)

Lane, J. E., 'Robert Willan', *Archives of Dermatology and Syphilology*, 13 (1926)

Langdon-Davies, J., *Westminster Hospital* (1952)

Langford, P., *A Polite and Commercial People: England, 1727–1783* (Oxford, 1992)

Larson, M. S., *The Rise of Professionalism. A Sociological Analysis* (Berkeley, 1978)

Lawrence, S. C., '"Desirous of Improvements in Medicine": Practitioners in the Medical Societies at Guy's and St Bartholomew's Hospitals, 1795–1815', *Bulletin of the History of Medicine*, 59 (1985)

le Fanu, W. R., 'The lost half century in English Medicine, 1700–1750', *Bulletin of the History of Medicine*, 46 (1972)

Leake, C. D., *Percival's Medical Ethics* (Baltimore, 1927)

Lee, E., *The Watering Places of England Considered with Reference to their Medical Topography* (third edn, 1914)

Lewis, J., *The Politics of Motherhood* (1980)

Lewis, R., and Maude, A., *Professional People* (1952)

Lindert, P., and Williamson, J. G., 'Revising England's Social Tables, 1688–1812', *Explorations in Economic History*, (1982)

Llewellyn Davies, M., *Maternity Letters from Working Women* (second edn, 1978)

Loudon, I., *Medical Care and the General Practitioner, 1750–1850* (Oxford, 1986)

Loudon, I., 'The Concept of the Family Doctor', *Bulletin of the History of Medicine*, 58 (1984)

Loudon, I., 'A Doctor's Cash Book. The Economy of General Practice in the 1830s', *Medical History*, 27 (1983)

Loudon, I., 'The Nature of Provincial Medical Practice in Eighteenth Century England', *Medical History*, 20 (1985)

Loudon, I., 'On Maternal and Infant Mortality 1900–1960', *Social History of Medicine*, 4 (1991)

Loudon, I., 'The Origins and Growth of the Dispensary Movement in England', *Bulletin of the History of Medicine*, 55 (1981)

Loudon, I., 'Two Thousand Medical Men in 1847', *Bulletin of the Society for the Social History of Medicine*, 33 (1983)

MacAlpine, I., and Hunter, R., *George III and the Mad-Business* (1969)

Macdonald, M., 'Anthropological Perspectives on the History of Science and Medicine', in Corsi and Weindling, eds., *Information Sources in the History of Science and Medicine* (1983)

Macdonald, M., 'Religion, Social Change and Psychological Healing in England, 1600–1800', in W. J. Shiels, ed., *The Church and Healing* (Oxford, 1982)

MacKenzie, N. and J., eds., *The Diary of Beatrice Webb, 1873–92* (4 vols., 1982)

Manton, J., *Elizabeth Garrett Anderson* (1965)

Manton, J., *Sister Dora* (1971)

Marland, H., *Medicine and Society in Wakefield and Huddersfield, 1780–1870* (Cambridge, 1987)

Marland, H., 'The Medical Actitivities of Chemists and Druggists in Wakefield and Huddersfield', *Medical History*, 31 (1987)

Marshall, J. D., *The Autobiography of William Stout of Lancaster 1665–1752* (Chetham Society, third series XIV, Manchester, 1967)

Massey, P., '1360 British Middle-Class Households in 1938–9', *Journal of the Royal Statistical Society*, (1942)

Maulitz, R., 'Metropolitan Medicine and the Man-Midwife: the Early Life and Letters of Charles Locock', *Medical History*, 26 (1982)

Maulitz, R. C., *Morbid Appearances* (Cambridge, 1987)

McDonald, M., *Mystical Bedlam. Madness, Anxiety and Healing in Seventeenth Century England* (Cambridge, 1981)

McInnes, A., 'The Emergence of a Leisure Town: Shrewsbury 1660–1760', *Past and Present*, 120 (1988)

McKendrick, N., Brewer, J., Plumb, J. H., eds., *The Birth of a Consumer Society. The Commercialization of Eighteenth century England* (1983)

McKeown, T., *The Modern Rise in Population* (New York, 1976)

McKeown, T., 'A Historical Appraisal of the Medical Task' in G. McLachlan and T. McKeown, eds., *Medical History and Medical Care: A Symposium of Perspectives* (Oxford, 1971)

Mechanic, D., 'The Concept of Illness Behaviour', *Journal of Chronic Diseases*, 15 (1962)

Miller, G., *The Adoption of Inoculation for Smallpox in England and France* (Oxford, 1957)

Mitchell, B. R., *Abstract of British Historical Statistics* (Cambridge, 1962 and 1988)

Mitchison, R., *British Population Since 1860* (1977)

Moberley Bell, E., *Storming the Citadel* (1953)

More Secret Remedies (BMA, 1912)

Moscucci, O., *The Science of Women. British Gynaecology 1849–1890* (Cambridge 1990)

Mossner, E. C. and Rose, I. S., eds., *The Correspondence of Adam Smith* (Oxford, 1977)

Mui, H. C., and L. H., *Shops and Shopkeeping in Eighteenth Century England* (Kingston, Canada, 1989)

Mullett, C., *Public Baths and Health in England from the Sixteenth to the Eighteenth Century* (Baltimore, 1946)

Mullett, C. F., ed., *The Letters of Dr George Cheyne to the Countess of Huntingdon* (San Marino, 1940)

Mullett, C. F., ed., *The Letters of Dr George Cheyne to Samuel Richardson* (University of Missouri Studies, Columbia, 1943)

Mumford, E. M., *Chester Royal Infirmary, 1756–1956* (1956)

Neve, M., 'Orthodoxy and Fringe: Medicine in Late Georgian Bristol', in W. F. Bynum and R. Porter, eds., *Medical Fringe and Medical Orthodoxy, 1750–1850* (1987)

Newman, C. 'Diagnostic Investigation before Laennec', *Medical History*, 4 (1960)

Newman, C., 'Physical Signs in London Hospitals' *Medical History*, 2 (1958)

Newsholme, A., *The Ministry of Health* (1925)

Nicholson, J. L., 'Variations in Working Class Expenditure', *Journal of the Royal Statistical Society*, (1949)

Oakley, A., *Women Confined. Towards a Sociology of Childbirth* (New York, 1980)

Oakley, A., *The Captured Womb* (Oxford, 1984)

Oppenheim, J., *'Shattered Nerves'. Doctors, Patients and Depression in Victorian England* (Oxford, 1991)

Parfitt, J., *The Health of a City: Oxford, 1770–1974* (1987)

Parsons, T., *The Structure of Social Action* (New York, 1949)

Parsons, T., 'Illness and the Role of the Physician: a Sociological Perspective', *American Journal of Orthopsychiatry*, 21, (1951)

Pelling, M., 'Healing the Sick Poor: Social Policy and Disability in Norwich 1550–1640', *Medical History*, 29 (1985)

Pelling, M., 'Medical Practice in Early Modern England: Trade or Profession', in W. Prest, ed., *The Professions in Early Modern England* (1987)

Pelling, M., 'Occupational Diversity and the Trades of Norwich, 1550–1640', *Bulletin of the History of Medicine*, 56 (1982)

Pelling M., and Webster, C., 'Medical Practitioners' in C. Webster, ed., *Health, Medicine and Mortality in the Sixteenth Century* (Cambridge, 1979)

Pemberton, J., *Will Pickles of Wensleydale* (1970)

Pensabene, T. A., *The Rise of the Medical Profession in Victoria* (1980)

PEP, *Report on the British Health Services* (1937)

Perkin, H. J., *Origins of Modern English Society* (1969)

Perkin, H. J., *The Rise of Professional Society. England Since 1880* (1989)

Perkin, H. J., 'Middle-Class Education and Employment in the 19th Century: A Critical Note', *Economic History Review*, 14 (1961–2)

Peterson, M. J., *The Medical Profession in Mid-Victorian London* (Berkeley, 1978)

Peterson, M. J., 'Dr Acton's Enemy: Medicine, Sex and Society in Victorian England', *Victorian Studies*, 29 (1986)

Peterson, M. J., 'Gentlemen and Medical Men: the Role of Professional Recruitment,' *Bulletin of the History of Medicine*, 58 (1984)

Pickstone, J. V., *Medicine and the Industrial Society* (Manchester, 1985)

Pinner, M., and Miller, B. F., eds., *When Doctors are Patients* (New York, 1952)

Plarr, *Lives of the Royal College of Surgeons of England*, (2 vols., 1930)

Ponsonby, A, *English Diaries* (1923)

Pooler, H. W., *My Life in General Practice* (1948)

Porter, R., 'Medicine and the Enlightenment in Eighteenth Century England', *Bulletin of the Society for the Social History of Medicine*, 25 (1979)

Porter, R., *Doctor of Society. Thomas Beddoes and the Sick Trade in Late-Enlightenment England* (1992)

Porter, R. *English Society in the Eighteenth Century* (1982)

Porter, R., *Health for Sale. Quackery in England, 1660–1850* (1989)

Porter, R., ed., *The Medical History of Waters and Spas* (1990)

Porter, R., ed., *Patients and Practitioners. Lay Perceptions of Medicine in Pre-industrial Society* (Cambridge, 1985)

Porter, R., ed., *The Popularisation of Medicine* (1992)

Porter, R, 'The Gift Relation: Philanthropy and Provincial Hospitals in Eighteenth-Century England', in L. Granshaw and R. Porter, eds., *The Hospital in History* (1989)

Porter, R., 'I think ye Both Quacks', in W. F. Bynum and R. Porter, eds., *Medical Fringe and Medical Orthodoxy* (1987)

Porter, R., 'The Language of Quackery', *Bulletin of the Society for the Social History of Medicine*, 33 (1983)

Porter, R., 'Lay Medical Knowledge in the Eighteenth Century: the Evidence of the Gentleman's Magazine', *Medical History*, 29 (1985)

Porter, R., 'William Hunter: a Surgeon and a Gentleman', in W. F. Bynum and R. Porter, eds., *William Hunter and the Eighteenth Century World* (Cambridge, 1985)

Porter, R., and D., *Patient's Progress. Doctors and Doctoring in Eighteeenth-Century England* (1989)

Poynter, F. N. L. ed., *The Evolution of Medical Education in Britain* (1966)

Poynter, F. N. L., 'A Unique Copy of George Armstrong's Printed Proposals for Establishing the Dispensary for Sick Children, 1769', *Medical History* (1957)

Prest, W. R., 'Why the History of the Professions is not Written', in G. R. Rubin and D. Sugarman, eds., *Law, Economy and Society. Essays in the History of English Law, 1750–1914* (1984)

Prest, W., ed., *The Professions in Early Modern England* (1987)

Price, R., 'Hydropathy in England 1840–1870', *Medical History*, 25 (1981)

Radbill, S. X., 'Paediatrics', in A. G. Debus, ed., *Medicine in the Seventeenth Century* (Berkeley, 1971)

Radcliffe, W., *Milestones in Midwifery* (Bristol, 1967)

Ramsey, M., *Professional and Popular Medicine in France, 1770–1830. The Social World of Medical Practice* (Cambridge, 1988)

Rather, L. J., *Mind and Body in Eighteenth Century Medicine* (1965)

Rather, L. J., 'The "Six Things Non-Natural": A Note on the Origins and Fate of a Doctrine and a Phrase', *Clio Medica*, 3 (1968)

Razzell, P. E., *The Conquest of Smallpox* (Firle, Sussex, 1975)

Razzell, P. E., 'Population Change in Eighteenth Century England: A Re-interpretation', *Economic History Review*, second series, xviii (1965)

Reader, W. J., *Professional Men. The Rise of the Professional Classes in Nineteenth-Century England* (1966)
Reilly, T. F., *Building a Profitable Practice* (Philadelphia, 1912)
Reiser, S. J., *Medicine and the Reign of Technology* (Cambridge, 1990)
Rendall, J., 'The Influence of the Edinburgh Medical School on America in the Eighteenth Century', in R. G. W. Anderson and A. D. C. Simpson, eds., *The Early Years of the Edinburgh Medical School* (Edinburgh, 1976)
Rendle-Short, J., 'William Cadogan, Eighteenth Century Physician', *Medical History*, 4 (1960)
Richardson, R., *Death, Dissection and the Destitute* (1988)
Riley, J. C., *The Eighteenth Century Campaign to Avoid Disease* (1987)
Risse, G. B., *Hospital Life in Enlightenment Scotland. Care and Teaching at the Royal Infirmary of Edinburgh* (Cambridge, 1986)
Risse, G. B., '"Doctor William Cullen, Physician, Edinburgh": A Consultation Practice in the Eighteenth Century', *Bulletin of the History of Medicine*, 48 (1974)
Roberts, E., *A Woman's Place. An Oral History of Working-Class Women, 1890–1940* (1984)
Roberts, H., ed., *Women, Health and Reproduction* (1981)
Roberts, R. S., 'The Personnel and Practice of Medicine in Tudor and Stuart England. Part 1. The Provinces', *Medical History*, VI (1962)
Rolleston, H. D., *Sir Thomas Allbutt. A Memoir* (1929)
Rook, A., 'General Practice, 1793–1803. Transactions of a Huntingdonshire Medical Society', *Medical History*, 4 (1960)
Rosen, G., *The Structure of American Medical Practice, 1875–1941* (Philadelphia, 1983)
Rosen, G., 'Medicine as a Function of Society' in L. S. King, ed., *Mainstreams of Medicine. Essays on the Social and Intellectual Context of Medical Practice* (San Antonio, 1971)
Rosen, G. and Rosen, B. C., eds., *400 Years of a Doctor's Life* (New York, 1947)
Rosenberg, C., 'The Practice of Medicine in New York a Century Ago' in J. W. Leavitt and R. L. Numbers, eds., *Sickness and Health in America* (Madison, 1978)
Rosenberg, C., 'The Shape of Traditional Practice, 1800–1875' in G. Rosen, ed., *The Structure of American Medical Practice 1875–1941* (Philadelphia, 1983)
Rosner, L., *Medical Education in the Age of Improvement. Edinburgh Students and Apprentices, 1760–1826* (Edinburgh, 1990)
Routh, G., *Occupation and Pay in Great Britain, 1906–1979* (1980)
Rowntree, B. S. and Kendall, M., *How the Labourer Lives* (1913)
Ruhrah, J., ed., *William Cadogan. His Essay on Gout* (New York, 1925)
Russell, P. M. G., *A History of the Exeter Hospitals, 1170–1948* (Exeter, 1976)
Sadler, E., 'An Historical Survey of Children's Hospitals', in L. Granshaw and R. Porter, eds., *The Hospital in History* (1990)
Schofield, R., 'Did Mothers really Die?', in L. Bonfield, P. Laslett, and R. M. Smith, eds., *The World We Have Gained* (Cambridge, 1985)
Schumpeter, J. A., *Imperialism and Social Classes* (Oxford, 1951)
A Seventeenth-Century Doctor and His Patients, John Symcotts (Bedfordshire Record Society, XXXI, 1951)
Shaw, G. B., *Prefaces*, (1934)

Shorter, E., *Bedside Manners. The Troubled History of Doctors and Patients* (New York, 1985)

Shryock, R. H., *The Development of Modern Medicine* (second edn, 1947)

Sigsworth, E. 'A Provincial Hospital in the Eighteenth Century', College of General Practitioners' *Yorkshire Faculty Journal* (June 1966)

Sigsworth, E., and Brady V., *The Ledger of William Elmhirst* (Hull, ND)

Slack, P., 'Mirrors of Health and Treasures of Poor Men: the Uses of the Vernacular Medical Literature of Tudor England', in C. Webster, ed., *Health, Medicine, and Mortality in the Sixteenth Century* (Cambridge, 1979)

Smith, F. B., *The People's Health, 1830–1910* (1979)

Smith, J. R., *The Speckled Monster* (Essex Record Office, Chelmsford, 1987)

Smith, R., 'The Development of Guidance for Medical Practitioners by the General Medical Council', *Medical History*, 33 (1993)

Smith, W. D. A., 'A History of Nitrous Oxide and Oxygen Anaesthesia: Henry Hill Hickman in his Time', *British Journal of Anaesthesia*, 50 (1978)

Spencer, H. R., *The History of British Midwifery, 1650–1800* (1927)

Stamp, J. C., *British Incomes and Property* (1916)

Stamp, W., *'Doctor Himself'. An Unorthodox Biography of Harry Roberts, 1871–1946* (1949)

Starr, P., 'Medicine, Economy and Society in Nineteenth Century America,' *Journal of Social History*, 10 (1977)

Stevens, R., *Medical Practice in Modern England. The Impact of Specialization and State Medicine* (New Haven, 1966)

Stout, G.,'A Ledger initialled "G P"', *Cleveland and Teesdale Local History Society*, 48 (1985)

Sturdy, S., 'The Political Economy of Scientific Medicine and Science: Education and the Transformation of Medical Practice in Sheffield, 1890–1922', *Medical History*, 36 (1992)

Szasz, T. S. and Hollender, M. C., 'A Contribution to the Philosophy of Medicine. The Basic Models of Doctor-Patient Relationship', *AMA Archives of Internal Medicine*, 97 (1956)

Szasz, T. S., Knott, W. F. and Hollander, M. H, 'The Doctor-Patient Relationship in Historical Context', *American Journal of Psychiatry*, 115 (1958)

Szreter, S., 'The Importance of Social Intervention in Britain's Mortality Decline c. 1850–1914: a reinterpretation of the Role of Public Health', *Social History of Medicine*, 1 (1988)

Szreter, S., 'Mortality and Public Health, 1815–1914', *ReFRESH*, 14 (1992)

Taylor, S., *Good General Practice* (1954)

Temkin, O., *Galenism. The Rise and Decline of a Medical Philosophy* (Ithaca, 1973)

Temkin, O., 'The Role of Surgery in the Rise of Modern Medical Thought', *Bulletin of the History of Medicine*, 25 (1951)

Thirsk, J., *Economic Policy and Projects. The Development of a Consumer Society in Early Modern England* (Oxford, 1988)

Thomas, E. G., 'The Old Poor Law and Medicine', 5, *Medical History*, 24 (1980)

Thornton, E. M., *Marianne Thornton. A Domestic Biography* (1956)

Towler, J., and Bramall, J., *Midwives in History and Society* (1986)

Trollope, A., *Dr Thorne* (World's Classics edn, Oxford, 1980)

Verney, Lady Margaret Maria, *Verney Letters of the Eighteenth Century from the MSS at Claydon House* (1930)

Waddington, I., *The Medical Profession in the Industrial Revolution* (1984)
Waddington, I., 'The Development of Medical Ethics – a Sociological Analysis', *Medical History*, 19 (1975)
Wain, J., *Johnson on Johnson* (1976)
Wake, J., *The Brudenells of Deane* (second edn, 1954)
Wallis, P. J. and R. V., *Eighteenth Century Medics* (Newcastle on Tyne, 1988)
Walter, J., 'Famine, disease and crisis mortality in early modern society' in J. Walter and R. S. Schofield, eds., *Famine, Disease and the Social Order in Early Modern Society* (Cambridge, 1989)
Warner, J. H., 'Therapeutic Explanation and the Edinburgh Bloodletting Controversy', *Medical History*, 24 (1980)
Waterhouse, R., *Children in Hospital. A Hundred Years of Child Care in Birmingham* (1962)
Wear, A., 'Medical Practice in Late Seventeenth and Early Eighteenth Century England: Continuity and Union', in R. French and A. Wear, eds., *The Medical Revolution of the Seventeenth Century* (Cambridge, 1989)
Webb, S., and B., *The State and the Doctor* (1910)
Webster, C., *The Health Services Since the War* (1988)
Weindling, P., 'Linking Self Help and Medical Science and Medical Science: the Social History of Occupational Health' in P. Weindling, ed., *The Social History of Occupational Health* (1985)
Weindling, P., 'Medical Practice in Imperial Berlin: The Casebook of Alfred Grotjahn', *Bulletin of the History of Medicine*, 61 (1987)
Williams, M., ed., *The Letters of William Shenstone* (Oxford, 1931)
Williamson, J. G., 'The Structure of Pay in Britain, 1710–1911', *Research in Economic History*, 7 (1982)
Wilmott, E., ed., *Journal of Dr John Simpson* (Bradford, 1981)
Wilson, A., 'Participant or Patient? Seventeenth-Century Childbirth from the Mother's Point of View', in R. Porter, ed., *Patients and Practitioners. Lay Perceptions of Medicine in Pre-Industrial Society* (Cambridge, 1985)
Winter, A., 'Mesmerism and the Introduction of Inhalation Anaesthesia', *Social History of Medicine*, 4 (1991)
Winter, J. M., *The Great War and the British People* (1985)
Wiseman, A. L., 'The Surgeoness: the Female Practitioners of Surgery, 1400–1800', *Medical History*, 28 (1984)
Wood, C., *Paradise Lost*, (1990)
Wood, N., *Spa Treatment: Selection of Patients and the Choice of a Suitable Spa* (1910)
Wood, N. F., *Dollars to Doctors* (Chicago, 1912)
Woodford, L., 'A Medical Student's Career in the Early Nineteenth Century', *Medical History*, XIV (1970)
Woodham Smith, C., *Florence Nightingale, 1820–1910* (1950)
Woods, R., 'The Effects of Population Redistribution on the Level of Mortality in Nineteenth Century England and Wales', *Journal of Economic History*, XLV (1985)
Woods, R., 'Public Health and Public Hygiene: The Urban Environment in the Late Nineteenth and Early Twentieth Centuries', in R. Schofield, D. Rehur and A. Bideau eds., *The Decline of Mortality in Europe* (Oxford, 1991)
Woods, R. and Hinde, P. R., 'Mortality in Victorian England: Models and Patterns', *Journal of Interdisciplinary History*, XVIII (1987)

Woodward, J., *To Do The Sick No Harm. A Study of the British Voluntary Hospital System to 1875* (1974)

Wrigley, E. A., 'The Growth of Population in Eighteenth Century England: A Conundrum Resolved', *Past and Present*, 98 (1983)

Wrigley E. A. and Schofield, R. S., *The Population History of England 1541–1871: a Reconstruction* (1981)

Wyke, T. J.,'Hospital Facilities for, and Diagnosis and Treatment of, Venereal Disease in England, 1800–1870', *British Journal of Venereal Diseases*, 49 (1973)

Wyman, A. L., 'The Surgeoness: the Female Practitioner of Surgery, 1400–1800' *Medical History*, 28 (1984)

Young, J. H., 'James Hamilton (1767–1839) Obstetrician and Controversialist', *Medical History*, 7, (1963)

Youngson, A. J., *The Scientific Revolution in Victorian Medicine* (1979)

Index of medical names

338

General index

Aberdeen 12
abortionists 64
accoucheurs 173–4, 255–6, 269–61, 263–8
accounts, practitioners' 41, 49, 115, 117,
    161, 166–7, 227, 243
    ledgers 3, 4, 41, 45, 114, 141, 185, 231
    see also bills, debts, fees, expenses
Acts of Parliament 7, 28, 31, 51, 309
    Anatomy (1832) 92, 237
    Apothecaries (1815) 28, 53
    Medical (1858) 13, 19, 20, 28, 31, 36, 53,
        57, 131
    Medical Amendment (1886) 31, 267
    Midwives (1902) 258
    National Health Insurance (1911) 3, 51,
        121
    Pharmacy (1868) 68
    Poor Law Amendment (1834) 44, 244
    Sale of Food and Drugs (1875) 68
Ailesbury family 177
Albert, Prince 270
alternative medicine 32, 63, 68
    acupuncture 26
    balneology 221
    bonesetting 26, 41, 64, 225
    cataract couching 41
    faith healing 64
    herbalism 26, 64
    homeopathy 26
    hydropathy 26, 215, 221, 306
    medical galvanism xix, 26
    mesmerism 26
    old wives' practices 64, 231, 258–9
    osteopathy 26
    phrenology 26
    uroscopy 64, 68
alternative practitioners
    and medical competition 7, 21, 26, 35–6,
        42, 64, 68, 178, 305–6

and legislation 28, 68
    see also alternative medicine, quacks
America, see USA
anaesthesia 83, 95, 260, 270, 273, 274
anatomy 55–6, 91–3, 94
anatomy schools 13, 55, 126
antisepsis 95, 274
apothecaries
    entrepreneurialism by 41, 112
    numbers of 13, 217
    training of 28, 53
    types of work of 29, 107, 235, 241
    see also chemists, druggists,
        surgeon-apothecaries
apothecaries' shops 29, 31–2, 41, 53, 201,
    305
Apothecaries, Society of 28, 57
appointments, medical
    club appointments 38, 50, 122
    of medical women 293–5
    poor law 50, 109, 225–33, 244–9, 245
    role in expanding practice 6, 109, 120–5,
        137, 142, 171–3, 191, 289–90, 314
    salaried 161
    Scottish 166
    see also Medical Officers of Health,
        School Medical Officers
apprenticeship 12, 28, 32, 52–4, 126, 128,
    137, 172, 266
Armstrong, George 280, 282, 284
assistants 20, 54, 58, 108, 120, 125–33, 138,
    161, 171–2, 244, 257, 266, 295, 314
Association of Registered Medical
    Women of the UK 293
Atholl, Duke of 161
Australia 122, 161, 168

Baker, John 220
bankruptcies, medical 162, 166

Cambridge Studies in Population, Economy and Society in Past Time

Titles available in paperback are marked with an asterisk

Printed in the United States
By Bookmasters